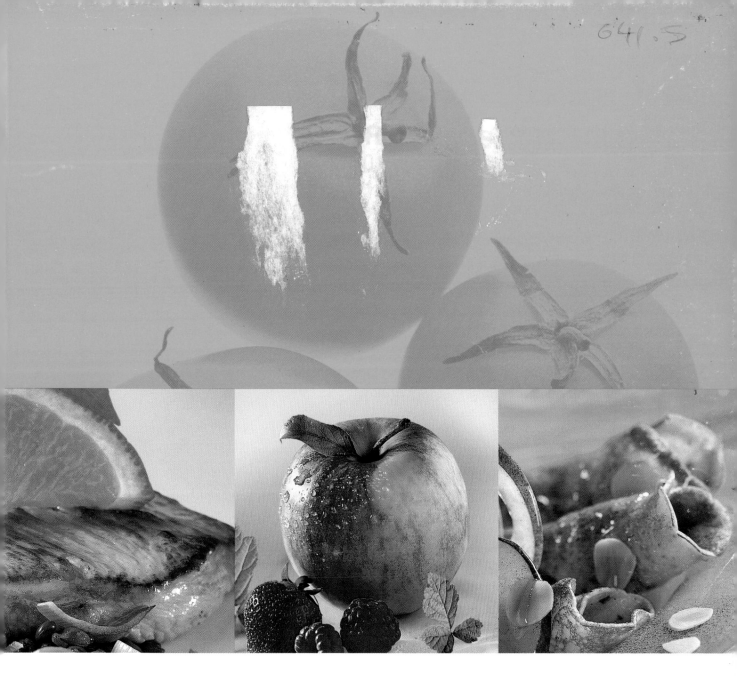

Healthy Diabetic Cooking

250 easy and delicious recipes for a nutritionally balanced diet

MEDICAL AND DIETARY INFORMATION: DR. HANS
HAUNER, ROSALIE LOHR AND AXEL BACHMANN
RECIPES: FRIEDRICH BOHLMANN, ERIKA
CASPAREK-TÜRKKAN AND BETTINA KÖHLER
RECIPE PHOTOGRAPHS: MICHAEL BRAUNER

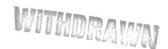

APPLE

Published in the UK in 2003 by
Apple Press
Sheridan House
112-116a Western Road
Hove BN3 1DD

www.apple-press.com

ISBN 1-84092-401-2

Design: Peter Maher
Electronic formatting: Jean Peters

Printed and bound in Spain

03 04 05 06 07 5 4 3 2 1

Contents

Living Well with Diabetes   4
Foreword by Dr. Hans Hauner
What You Need to Know About Diabetes   6
Regulating Blood Glucose   6
So You Have Diabetes. Now What?   6
Types of Diabetes   7
Metabolic Syndrome   8
A Lifelong Diet?   8
Hypoglycemia   8
Proper Nutrition for People with Diabetes   9
Healthful Eating—What Does That Mean?   9
The Right Combination Makes All the Difference   9
How Many Meals a Day?   9
The Nutrition Pyramid   10
Carbohydrates   11
Fiber   11
The Glycemic Index   11
What Sweetener to Use?   11
Protein   12
Fat   13
Vitamins and Minerals   14
Beverages   14
Diabetes and Excess Weight   16
How Much Energy Do I Need?   16
Tips on Losing Weight   16
The Body Mass Index (Chart)   17
Physical Activity   18
Daily Activity   18
Recreational Activity   18
Sports and Strenuous Physical Activity   19

Practical Tips   20
Low Fat   20
Fiber   20
Sugar and Spice   20
Baking   20
Diabetic Products   21
Supplements   21
Additional Tips   21
Hypoglycemia   21
Breakfasts and Snacks   22
Eat breakfast like a king...
Salads and Soups   52
Cold and crunchy or hot and drinkable?
Vegetables   72
A meal with plenty of crunchy fresh vegetables leaves you feeling fit and full of energy
Fish and Seafood   94
Eating fish means filling up on energy!
Meat and Poultry   112
Less is more...
Pasta, Rice and Company   138
Potatoes and pasta, rice, whole grains and legumes—anywhere, anytime!
Sweets and Desserts   158
Not always, but more often
Savory Baked Goods, Breads, Rolls, Cakes and Pies   174
Delicious baked goods for guests and fests
Index   228

Living Well with Diabetes

Type 2 diabetes mellitus is now one of the major diseases in the general population. Over the past few decades, the number of people afflicted has risen to epidemic proportions and continues to increase. The main reasons are poor diet and lack of exercise. We now know that excess weight combined with a poor diet is by far the leading cause of this disease—the majority of those who suffer from type 2 diabetes are overweight, even obese.

It is clear that the first and most important treatment for type 2 diabetes lies in modifying a person's diet, if only to control his or her weight. Those who succeed in this will experience a surprisingly rapid improvement in their blood glucose level, not to mention the reduction of other risk factors such as blood pressure and metabolism of fat. In fact, weight loss and a change in diet usually lead to lower blood glucose more rapidly than any medication designed for the purpose. But a healthier, more diabetic-friendly diet is seldom pursued, mainly because many people with diabetes would rather swallow their medication than change their eating habits.

Our attitudes about the ideal diet for those with diabetes have changed radically over the last 20 years. The days when diabetics had to restrict alcohol and sugar intake, not to mention traveling with a kitchen scale, have long since passed. Today, it's easier to maintain a healthful and interesting diet than many believe and a healthful diet can offer a variety of foods, as well as scope for personal preferences. And this type of diet can also reduce the likelihood of heart disease, stroke and some kinds of cancer.

So what exactly is a diabetic diet? The most important elements can be summarized in a few sentences. First, greatly reduce fat intake, especially the type found in animal fats such as butter, meats and cheeses. Second, avoid foods high in sugar and starch in favor of fiber-rich foods that help to lower blood glucose levels gradually. Third, eat plenty of fruit and vegetables to provide your body with valuable nutrients and leave you feeling satisfied.

This book also covers other important factors for an optimal diabetic diet and ways you can incorporate them into daily life. You'll quickly discover how diverse and delicious the modern diabetic diet is, and you'll find that you won't have to give up all sweet treats. It's primarily a question of approaching serving sizes and food combinations in an intelligent and balanced way. If you're interested in controlling your diabetes through healthful, pleasurable eating, you'll relish this book.

Dr. Hans Hauner
Düsseldorf, Germany

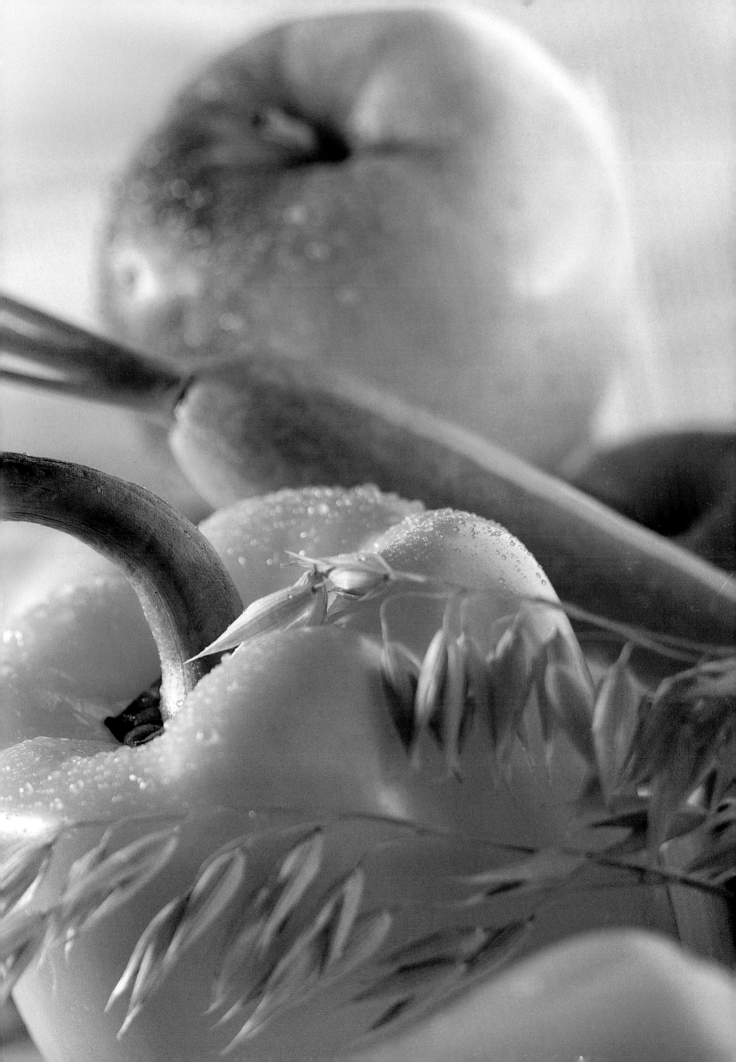

What You Need to Know About Diabetes

You may still remember your reaction when your doctor first diagnosed type 2 diabetes mellitus. Many people are shocked. All they know about this disease is that it is a chronic metabolic disorder they will have to live with for the rest of their lives. But today the future isn't so bleak. Current treatment is so sophisticated that it can be designed to meet individual needs and circumstances.

The term "diabetes mellitus" is derived from Greek and literally means "flow sweet as honey"—an appropriate concept, as the main symptom of those who suffer from irregular insulin production is the glucose eliminated in urine.

What causes this?

Regulating Blood Glucose

The most important hormone in the regulation of blood glucose is insulin, which is produced in the pancreas and released according to need. The higher the intake of carbohydrates (sugars and starches) is during a meal, the more insulin is released.

All high-carbohydrate foods—such as potatoes, rice, pasta, fruit, bread and other grain products—are broken down in the pancreas into their individual building blocks, or glucose molecules (a simple sugar).

The body's cells need this simple sugar to produce energy. Glucose is circulated to the body's cells by the blood. Red blood cells, particularly those going to the brain, need a steady supply of glucose.

Insulin is released to regulate rising blood glucose levels. It helps transfer the sugar to the body's cells by "unlocking" them like the key to a castle door. Your blood glucose then sinks to a normal level, between 3.5 and 6.0 millimoles per liter, or mmol/L (between 65 and 110 milligrams per deciliter, or mg/dL). Following a meal, the level ranges from 6.0 to 10.0 mmol/L (110 to 180 mg/dL).

In type 2 diabetes, the pancreas usually produces enough insulin. The main problem is that the body's cells barely react to it. Muscle, fat and liver cells develop a sensitivity, or resistance, to insulin—they no longer open up when the insulin links up with their receptors, and the glucose can't enter the cell.

To reduce a chronically high blood glucose level, the pancreas produces even more insulin. The cells that produce insulin aren't designed to react in this piecemeal way over the long term, however, and blood glucose remains chronically high because

of the insulin lack. Since such a high level no longer falls within the tolerance levels of a healthy organism, the body takes additional measures to regulate the problem by eliminating excess sugar by way of the kidneys.

The presence of sugar in urine indicates that the regulation of blood glucose is malfunctioning. At what point this so-called kidney threshold is crossed depends on the individual and his or her age.

The first symptoms of an increase in blood glucose include
- increased thirst
- frequent urination
- fatigue, listlessness
- weakness, lack of drive
- impaired vision
- itchiness
- skin inflammations
- poor healing
- urinary tract infections
- genital infections
- impotence

The appearance and extent of these symptoms vary according to the individual.

So You Have Diabetes. Now What?

When diabetes is diagnosed, it is essential to learn more about it. Once you do, you'll quickly realize that your daily life won't be seriously restricted. Much of your therapy can be worked out with your family physician and his or her colleagues.

An essential element of therapy is changing your diet. By optimizing your metabolism in this way, you can delay or completely avoid other problems, such as those that relate to the kidneys, nerves, eyes and blood vessels.

Control is important: regular testing of blood glucose and physical checkups help determine an optimal blood glucose level. This is key to your well-being and your quality of life. Your local diabetes association can provide helpful information about this disease and its control.

Types of Diabetes

The goal of every type of diabetic therapy is to avoid unpleasant symptoms and complications in everyday life.

The nutritional recommendations for managing diabetes mellitus are clearly defined, yet they take individual circumstances into account. If you are elderly, pregnant or very active physically, you should discuss your special needs with your physician.

Type 1 Diabetes

In North America, only 5% to 10% of those with diabetes have type 1. Also known to as juvenile-onset diabetes, it often begins in

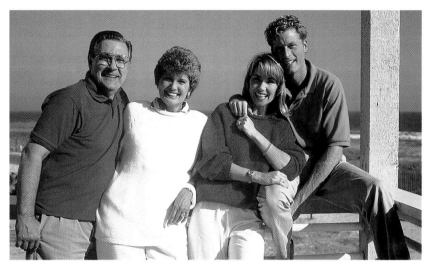

childhood, although it can also occur in adults up to about age 40.

Type 1 diabetes mellitus is caused by a combination of viral infections, hereditary factors and the so-called autoimmune disorders. In type 1 diabetes, insulin-producing cells have been destroyed and do not release insulin, so blood glucose is no longer transferred to the cells.

Since the body no longer produces it, insulin is the most important component of therapy

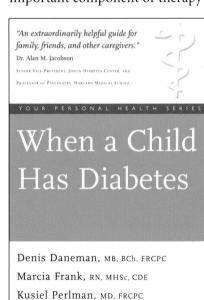

"An extraordinarily helpful guide for family, friends, and other caregivers."
Dr. Alan M. Jacobson
Senior Vice-President, Joslin Diabetes Center, and
Professor of Psychiatry, Harvard Medical School

YOUR PERSONAL HEALTH SERIES

When a Child Has Diabetes

Denis Daneman, MB, BCh, FRCPC
Marcia Frank, RN, MHSc, CDE
Kusiel Perlman, MD, FRCPC

for type 1 diabetes. Generally, people with type 1 diabetes need to take medication, as their pancreas is unable to produce enough insulin, and it is essential that people with type 1 diabetes balance the amount of insulin they take with the amount of carbohydrates they eat. Otherwise, there are no specific dietary recommendations other than eating healthful, well-balanced meals.

Type 2 Diabetes

Because it occurs largely in adults, type 2 has been commonly referred to as adult-onset diabetes, and 90% to 95% of all diabetics in North America are of this type.

The probability of inheriting a predisposition to diabetes mellitus is 40%, but lifestyle factors that result in the body's inability to regulate blood glucose also come into play. These factors tend to be characteristic of western industrialized nations, where the number of people who have type 2 diabetes mellitus is rising rapidly and younger people are increasingly affected.

Such factors include
- excess weight
- high consumption of animal fats and white-flour products
- insufficient amounts of vitamins, minerals and other essential nutrients
- too little fiber
- lack of exercise
- high stress

Few type 2 diabetics are slim or even normal in weight.

Metabolic Syndrome

Excess weight, high blood glucose, high blood pressure and type 2 diabetes often go hand in hand. An array of risk factors like these is sometimes called "metabolic syndrome." The sooner diabetes is diagnosed, the better the chances of preventing associated disorders.

A Lifelong Diet?

All the above is why changing to a nutritious low-fat diet and becoming more active are important measures in controlling type 2 diabetes. For those who are overweight, losing some pounds can be decisive in normalizing blood glucose levels. Losing weight always leads to an improved response to insulin by the body's cells.

It's important to note that we no longer talk about special foods or a restricted diet for people with diabetes mellitus. On the contrary, the recommended foods are only slightly different from the guidelines for people who do not have diabetes. Meals can and should be low-fat, nutritious and varied—as well as appetizing and delicious.

Hypoglycemia

When blood glucose drops below 4.0 mmol/L (70 mg/dL), it is called hypoglycemia. In less serious cases, hypoglycemia can result in paleness, sweating, tremors, pounding heart, headache, nervousness, a vora-

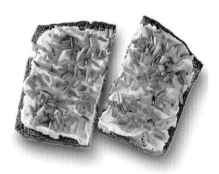

cious appetite and a furry feeling in the mouth. It can also lead to substantial problems in concentration, vision and speech, as well as lightheadedness, which can ultimately lead to hypoglycemic shock. Always have glucose or fruit juice on hand to control a sudden drop in glucose due to medications used to lower blood glucose.

Hypoglycemia can also result from too much insulin or, rather, too few carbohydrates. The most common causes of hypoglycemia are alcohol consumption and too much physical stress.

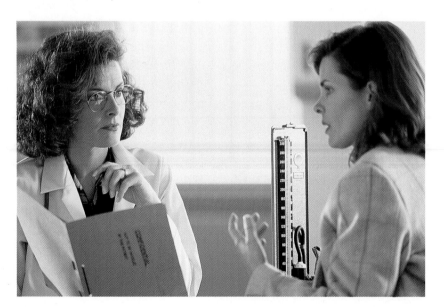

Proper Nutrition for People with Diabetes

Healthful Eating— What Does That Mean?

The secret behind a nutritious meal is simply eating the right amount of foods in the right combinations—this applies to everyone! Enjoy a variety of foods, and choose only the best. This overall approach will enhance your quality of life and allow you to live a long, healthy life.

Beyond that, an appropriate eating strategy for those with diabetes is fundamental to therapy. The risk of cardiac and circulatory problems, blood-vessel damage, kidney disease and nervous disorders can be reduced, while a sense of well-being and a high quality of life can be maintained and even enhanced.

The big advantage of a diabetic diet is that you are eating healthily and paying attention to your weight. By following the advice of qualified professionals, dietitians and your physician, you'll be able to develop a personalized meal plan that meets your particular needs while keeping in mind that your dietary requirements may change over time.

The Right Combination Makes All the Difference

Healthful eating emphasizes the need to derive energy from a balanced variety of foods. These provide the body with the carbohydrates, protein, fat, vitamins, minerals, trace elements and protective vegetable matter it needs. Carbohydrate- and fiber-rich vegetables, legumes, grains and specific types of fruit have an especially positive effect on blood glucose levels and also leave you feeling satisfied.

How Many Meals a Day?

There is no general rule about the number of meals you should eat daily. Consult your physician to find out if three meals a day are enough or if more are necessary to counteract the effect of pills or insulin.

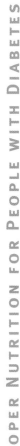

The Nutrition Pyramid

Eat sparingly: Spreads such as butter or margarine. Vegetable oils are clearly more healthful for cooking and baking. Beware of hidden fats in sweets and prepared foods as well.

In moderation: Dairy products also contain carbohydrates. High-fat cheeses and products made from whole milk or cream are also high in fat. Select low-fat products instead.

2 to 3 times a week: Meat and poultry should be eaten only 2 to 3 times a week as a main course.
In moderation: Cold cuts for sandwiches should be replaced as often as possible by low-fat cheese, vegetable spreads, herbs and vegetables.
At least 6 times a month: Consume plenty of fish because of its healthful fatty acids and iodine content.

Not always, but more often: Fresh fruit contains fructose. Eat up to 3 servings (about 4 oz/125 g per serving) a day as a snack.

Help yourself: Fresh vegetables can be eaten any time you're hungry. Vegetables should be the largest portion on your plate at mealtimes.

Selecting grain products: Choose whole-grain foods.
High carb content, but they're good for you: Potatoes and legumes.

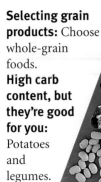
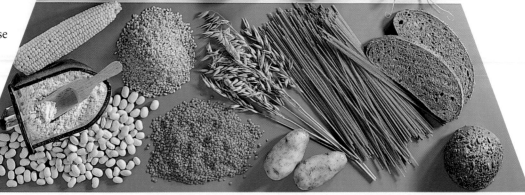

Select foods from every level of the nutrition pyramid. The sizes of the different levels indicate the food groups you can eat plenty of and those you should eat sparingly. Eat more of the foods in the lower levels than the ones in the upper levels.

Carbohydrates

There's no reason to avoid carbohydrates if you have diabetes. On the contrary, since carbs produce energy and raise blood glucose levels, the body needs carbs as quick fuel. Your first choice for foods that deliver carbohydrates are whole grains and whole-grain products, followed by potatoes, brown rice and legumes. Fresh fruit is also a good source of carbs (fructose, for example) and is also rich in fiber, minerals, vitamins and secondary vegetable matter. Choose unprocessed or lightly processed foods because processing removes many of the nutrients.

How Much Is Best?

The amount of carbohydrates you need depends on how much it takes to maintain the greatest feeling of well-being and increase your physical activity. The proportion of carbohydrates to daily energy requirements should be 50% or more, the same as for people with a normal metabolism. For example, if you consume 1,800 calories per day, you will need between 8 and 9 oz (225 to 270 g) a day. This content can come from various sources (cereals and grains, fruits and vegetables, milk, sugar), and if you are counting carbs, it will be between 15 and 18 carbohydrate choices of 15 g each.

Fiber

Fiber slows the rate at which carbohydrates are broken down into simple sugar, so the more fiber you eat, the slower the rate at which your blood glucose will rise. What's more, fiber and vegetable matter from legumes, oats, pasta, brown rice and fruit not only protect your health but can also substantially reduce blood glucose levels. The recommended amount of fiber—about 1 oz (30 to 35 g) a day—prevents digestive problems and helps eliminate toxins.

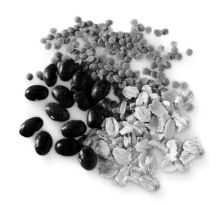

The Glycemic Index

A helpful tool for everyday use. The effect of carbohydrate-rich food on blood glucose does not depend entirely on the amount of carbohydrates consumed. The amount of fat, protein and fiber in your food also play a major role. The different components of foods mean that each type has a different effect on blood glucose. The rate at which carbohydrates enter the bloodstream after a meal depends on how your meals are organized. This is expressed in terms of the glycemic index (GI), where the number assigned shows which foods raise and which foods lower blood glucose levels. The higher the GI of a food, the faster and higher blood glucose will rise after eating it.

Foods that have a high GI—such as glucose, lemonade, honey, sugar, jujubes and jelly beans, gummi bears and jellied fruit—are suitable for raising blood glucose levels quickly to prevent hypoglycemia. These should only be eaten in small quantities, if at all. Foods that have a low GI rating (see page 12) are much better. They allow blood glucose to rise gradually and leave you feeling satisfied longer.

- Competitive athletes, especially those in endurance sports, are familiar with the glycemic index and take it into account when choosing carbohydrates that increase energy levels.
- Those who perform mental tasks can concentrate longer if they eat carbohydrate-rich foods with a low glycemic index.
- Many weight-conscious people pay careful attention to the glycemic index when choosing their foods, since those with a low glycemic index can prevent a craving for sweets and reduce a big appetite.

Sugar should represent no more than 10% of the total number of calories consumed (1 to 2 oz/30 to 50 g a day). It's easy to reach this amount, since sugar is added to many prepared foods.

What Sweetener to Use?

Although diabetics can add small amounts of sugar to sweeten their food, they should generally use sugar-free (and therefore calorie-free) sweeteners. For example, you can sweeten drinks with additives such as saccharin, cyclamate, aspartame, sucralose (Splenda) or acesulfame K. All sweeteners available in Canada, the U.S. and Great Britain go through rigorous testing. Once approved, they are deemed suitable for use by all who reside in those countries, including those with diabetes, if used in moderation. Used in small amounts, they should pose no risk to your health. Check with your dietitian if you have any questions.

Other sugar substitutes, such as fructose, sorbitol, xylitol, mannitol, isomalt, lactitol, maltitol and polydextrose, depend partly on

insulin to be metabolized. Baked goods containing sugar substitutes are often high in fat, so they should be eaten only in very small quantities or not at all.

Protein

Since protein has little bearing on blood glucose, a higher percentage of protein has long been recommended in the overall diabetic diet. Too much protein, however, can lead to negative health effects in diabetics already suffering from kidney damage.

Protein must be consumed daily because it is essential in building body cells, but in some countries, protein consumption is generally higher than the daily recommended maximum of 10% to 20% of total calories. Even

athletes and diabetics do not need more protein than this.

Protein is largely available through animal sources such as dairy products, fish, meat and eggs. If the kidneys are already damaged, increasing protein intake can lead to further damage or kidney failure, so the amount of protein should be controlled.

Foods rich in vegetable protein include grains, legumes and nuts. Protein obtained by combining legumes and corn, potatoes and eggs, potatoes and quark, potatoes and legumes, whole grains and dairy products or legumes and dairy products is even better for the body.

Please note that milk, yogurt and other dairy products also contain carbohydrates that affect blood glucose levels.

Protein Consumption — Less Is More

Make vegetable dishes the mainstay of your meal plan, and eat fish at least twice a week. Lean fish in particular deliver large amounts of protein and low amounts of healthful fat. Omega-3 fatty acids contained in fatty fish have a healthful effect on cholesterol levels and blood vessels, and saltwater fish contain iodine.

This glycemic index table refers to the carbohydrate content of various foods. By combining foods rich in fat, protein and fiber, you can lower their glycemic index and reduce their effect on blood glucose.

Foods with a high glycemic index	Foods with a low glycemic index
Glucose, maltose, fried potatoes, very light white-flour products, mashed potatoes, honey **> 90**	Whole-grain bread, bran bread, brown rice, peas, granola with no sugar added **> 40**
Carrots, cornflakes, popcorn **> 90**	Oatmeal, kidney beans, unsweetened fruit juices, whole wheat noodles, pumpernickel bread, peas, dairy products, ice cream **> 30**
Pumpkin, watermelon, sugar (sucrose), baguettes, granola with sugar added, chocolate bars, boiled potatoes (skin off), cookies, corn, white rice **> 70**	Legumes, fresh fruit, jams (total sugar content 40 g), dark chocolate (cocoa content > 70%), fructose **> 20**
Dried fruit, multigrain bread, boiled potatoes (skin on), bananas, melons, jams **> 60**	Peanuts, soy products **> 15**
Noodles (semolina) **approx. 55**	Fresh vegetables, mushrooms **< 15**

Fat

The body needs some fat to function, but eating too much fat is one cause of excess weight. The type of fat you eat is also important. Fat serves as a fuel for the heart and muscles, carries fat-soluble vitamins A, D, E and K, keeps the skin looking smooth and supports many other bodily functions. The problem is that many people consume more fat than they need. And what's worse, the fats they consume come primarily from animal products, which leads to excess weight and metabolic disorders. In general, reduce your fat consumption and eat mainly vegetable fats.

How Much Fat Should You Eat?

Fat should represent no more than 30% of your daily caloric intake, roughly 2 to 3 oz (60 to 80 g) a day. Per person, this translates to 1 tablespoon (15 mL) of oil for cooking and frying and 1 tablespoon (15 mL) as a topping. You can also add 1 teaspoon (5 mL) per serving of salad.

Choose lower-fat cheeses, no more than 20% of total weight (part-skim mozzarella has 17% fat, and some other cheeses are lower), and reduce your meat consumption.

Which Fat Is Best?

Each type of fat is made up of different fatty acids. For example, there are saturated, monounsaturated and polyunsaturated fats. Vegetable oils are rich in the latter two types and are also cholesterol-free. Animal products, on the other hand, contain mostly saturated fats. The exception is

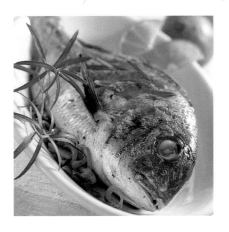

fish. Fish contain primarily unsaturated fats, including omega-3 fatty acids, which are good for the heart and circulatory system. To improve your health and increase your energy level, your diet should be rich in monounsaturated fats. For cooking and frying or for dressing salads, choose good-quality vegetable oils, but use them sparingly. The best sources are olive oil and canola oil.

When selecting animal products, choose the lowest-fat types: dairy products with 1%, 2% or no fat, cheese with no more than 20% of total weight (30% to 40% by dry weight). Lean sausage and sliced meats include corned beef, turkey and chicken sausage, smoked ham and smoked beef. Stay away from obviously fatty foods such as bacon, and if you can't avoid margarine or butter, use them sparingly.

Rich in saturated fats	Rich in unsaturated fats	Rich in polyunsaturated fats
butter	olive oil	wheat germ oil
palm oil	canola oil	corn oil
coconut oil	peanut oil	thistle oil
	margarine	flaxseed oil
	sesame oil	sunflower seed oil
	soybean oil	pumpkin seed oil
		diet margarine(but beware of trans fats)
		walnut oil

Vitamins and Minerals

Nutritional guidelines recommend eating fresh fruit and vegetables 5 times a day. The more you enjoy these on a daily basis, the more likely you are to get enough vitamins, fiber and other healthful and protective vegetable matter.

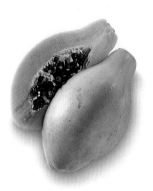

It isn't difficult to eat 5 servings of vegetables, salad and fruit every day—1 serving of salad at each main meal, at least 1 vegetable serving with one of your main meals, and peppers, kohlrabi or other vegetable sticks for between-meal snacks. What matters most is that they taste good. Only peas, broad beans and corn need to be monitored for carb content. You can also eat a juicy fruit up to twice a day. Choose fruit of a modest size and avoid overripe fruit, which can make blood glucose levels rise too quickly.

Enjoy fruit and vegetables raw or only slightly cooked so the valuable vitamins and protective vegetable matter are not destroyed.

Beverages

The body needs at least 6 cups (1.5 L) of fluids a day to balance its water needs. The beverage pyramid illustrated here shows clearly that mineral water and herbal and fruit teas are ideal thirst-quenchers, and they're calorie-free.

Diet soft drinks containing sweeteners don't have to be included when calculating the amount of carbohydrates, but such drinks should be enjoyed in moderation because of the fructose and sugar substitutes they contain, which can raise blood glucose levels.

After playing sports, a juice spritzer made from pure fruit juice and mineral water in a ratio of 1:4 is ideal since it replaces lost minerals and carbohydrates.

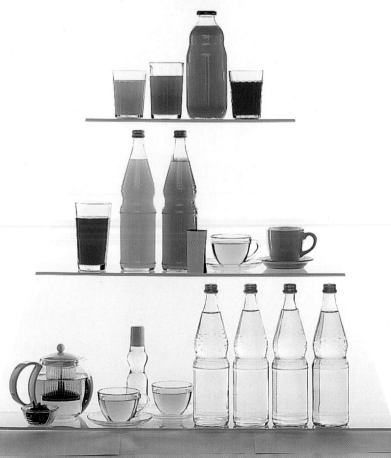

The best thirst-quenchers are calorie-free drinks such as mineral water and herbal and fruit teas.

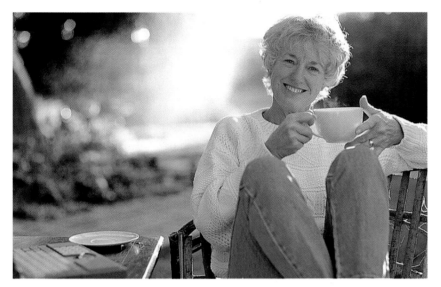

Alcohol

Women should not drink more than ½ oz (15 mL) of pure alcohol daily, and men should not consume more than 1 oz (30 mL). If you have high blood glucose and high triglyceride levels, avoid alcohol altogether. Alcohol's ability to reduce blood glucose can seriously affect those with diabetes. Under alcohol-free conditions, the liver mobilizes sugar reserves to maintain blood glucose at normal levels, but energy reserves stored in the body as glycogen and fat can't be released in the presence of alcohol. The oxidization of alcohol reduces the oxidization of energy-producing substances in the body and can thus lead to serious and lengthy hypoglycemia and unconsciousness (hypoglycemic coma or hypoglycemic shock). Consuming alcohol after a strenuous workout is particularly dangerous, especially if the carbohydrates used up during strenuous activity are not replaced by eating.

- Enjoy alcohol only in small amounts.
- Never drink on an empty stomach. Try to eat before and while drinking.
- Alcohol's ability to lower blood glucose levels will continue as long as it remains in the bloodstream, and it takes 1 hour to break down one unit of alcohol—the amount typically found in 12 oz (375 mL) of American (3.5% alc./vol) beer; 4 oz (50 mL) of wine; or 1 oz (30 mL) of 50 proof liquor.
- Don't count the carbohydrate content of alcoholic beverages as part of your daily carbohydrate requirement.
- When drinking alcohol, reduce the dosage of any medication taken to lower blood glucose, if necessary. Always consult your physician first.
- If you've consumed a lot of alcohol, measure your blood glucose before bed and eat extra carbohydrates as needed before going to sleep. Talk to your physician about the safest blood glucose level for you.

Average Alcohol Content in Beverages:

Amount	Beverage	Alcohol content
1 pint (500 mL)	alcohol-free beer	2 g
1 pint (500 mL)	diet pilsener	24 g
1 pint (500 mL)	3.5% alc./vol. beer	17.5 g
1 pint (500 mL)	5.5% alc./vol. beer	27.5 g
1 pint (500 mL)	wheat beer	20 g
¾ cup (175 mL)	cider	10 g
½ cup (125 mL)	red or white wine	12 g
½ cup (125 mL)	sparkling wine, champagne	10 g
¼ cup (50 mL)	sherry	9 g
3 tbsp (45 mL)	Irish whiskey, 45% alc./vol.	20 g
4 tsp (20 mL)	kirsch, 40% alc./vol.	8 g

Diabetes and Excess Weight

One of the fundamental elements of treating diabetes is weight control. Most people suffering from type 2 diabetes mellitus are also overweight. Losing only a few pounds can make a difference to blood glucose and related complications.

Whether you should lose weight, and how much, is best determined by your physician. In the case of a little excess weight (BMI 25 to 29.9), you should lose at least 7 to 11 pounds (3 to 5 kg). If you're severely overweight (BMI 30 or more), then you need to lose more. To find your BMI, see opposite.

How Much Energy Do I Need?

The days of painstakingly counting calories and carbs are definitely done. Dropping pounds by starving only meant they came rapidly back once the diet was over. In fact, people often became heavier than they were before dieting.

The new motto is: eat a variety of low-fat foods. Energy requirements vary according to each individual, but a rough guide might follow this formula: 30 calories per kilogram of body weight (about 13.6 calories per pound) per day. To calculate the number of calories to eat if you want to lose weight, multiply your weight in kilograms by 30 (or your weight in pounds by 13.6) and subtract 500. You should never consume less than 1,200 calories a day. And remember these goals: balance your energy intake with energy expenditure, and keep your BMI under 25.

The Way to Your Desired Weight

The most effective measures for reaching your desired weight involve reducing your intake of fat and increasing physical activity. Crash diets are harmful to the heart and circulatory system and have no long-term effect. Ideally, you should try to lose 2 to 4 pounds (1 to 2 kg) a month over a period of 3 to 6 months—12 months at the most.

Lose weight in consultation with your physician. In the case of obesity (BMI over 35), eating therapy in a specialized center may be beneficial.

Diabetes Diet: That Was Then, This Is Now!

When you say the words "weight loss," most people automatically think of deprivation. Now is the time to turn this thinking around. Everything is allowed, but in the right amounts! You do *not* have to maintain a boring diet, and you can continue to eat your favorite foods. Some changes to your diet will allow you to eat a variety of healthful and satisfying foods without completely depriving yourself of the treats you love.

To change your lifestyle and eating habits, the same rules apply as for people who do not have a metabolic disorder:

- Reduce your weight slowly but permanently. To do this, you need to control the amount of fat, fiber and carbohydrates in every meal.
- Physical activity helps you lose weight and raise your spirits. And there is another plus— your cells will react better to insulin.

Tips on Losing Weight

- Set small, realistic goals that you can achieve—to lose 2 pounds (1 kg) a month, for example.
- Avoid distractions such as watching television or reading while eating. This can lead you to unconsciously eat more than you actually need.
- Drink a glass of water or eat raw vegetables or a salad before each meal to help fill your stomach.
- Prepare attractive, appetizing meals, even if you're eating alone. Set your table nicely and enjoy your meal.
- Try to determine whether you're actually hungry or you just feel like eating.
- Chew your food thoroughly.
- Quench your thirst with-calorie-free drinks: mineral water, herbal or fruit teas

flavored with lemon juice or diet soft drinks with sweetener.

- Never go grocery shopping when you're hungry, and stick to your shopping list.
- "Light" on a food label does not always mean low fat or low sugar. Read the list of ingredients carefully. If fat is listed as the first ingredient, then it's a high-calorie product. If sugar appears as the last ingredient, then it's probably insignificant.

To find out if your weight is normal, use the Body Mass Index (BMI), which measures body weight in relation to height.

$$BMI = \frac{body\ weight\ (kg)}{[body\ height\ (m^2)]}$$

In the chart below, you can find your BMI at a glance without having to do any complicated calculations. Find your height along the vertical axis, and your weight along the horizontal axis. If your BMI falls within the obese zone, then you must lose weight. Your physician can help you.

Note: These numbers are not to be used for children, teenagers or the elderly.

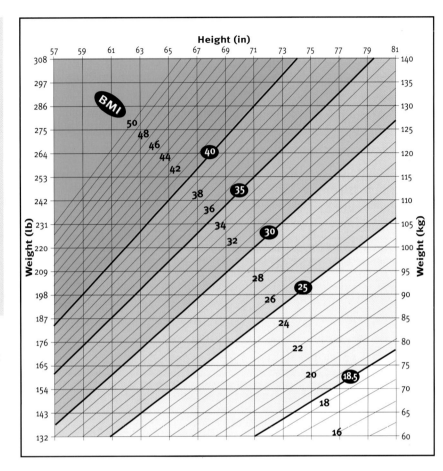

To estimate BMI, locate the point on the chart where height and weight intersect. Read the number on the dashed line closest to this point. For example, if you weigh 69 kg and are 173 cm tall, you have a BMI of approximately 23, which is in Normal Weight.

You can also calculate your BMI using this formula:

$$BMI = weight(kg)/height(m^2)$$

Health Risk Classification According to Body Mass Index (BMI)

Classification	BMI Category (kg/m2)	Risk of developing health problems
Underweight	<--- 18.5	Increased
Normal Weight	18.5–24.9	Least
Overweight	25.0–29.9	Increased
Obese class I	30.0–34.9	High
Obese class II	35.0–39.9	Very high
Obese class III	--->= 40.0	Extremely high

Source: Health Canada. Canadian Guidelines for Body Weight Classification in Adults. Ottawa: Minister of Public Works and Government Services Canada; 2003.

Note: For persons 65 years and older the "normal" range may begin slightly above BMI 18.5 and extend into the "overweight" range.

To clarify risk for each individual, other factors such as lifestyle habits, fitness level, and presence or absence of other health risk conditions also need to be considered.

Physical Activity

Physical activity is another important element in the treatment of diabetes. What's more, regular exercise is fun, it increases your sense of well-being, and it helps control weight. In short, exercise has a positive effect on weight, cholesterol, blood pressure and blood glucose. And you don't need to become a competitive athlete to improve your sense of well-being. Even small changes to your daily routine can have a positive effect on your blood glucose and consequently on your health.

You can do very simple things to increase your physical activity, although, depending on your health, not every activity is advisable. Start with a mild to moderate exercise program, then gradually increase the level of activity. If you haven't exercised for some time, consult your physician before starting a program. And give your body enough time to get used to strenuous activity.

Regardless of the activity you choose, do yourself an extra favor—endurance exercise. This trains the heart and circulatory system, makes the muscle cells more sensitive to the effects of insulin and leads to the secretion of the body's own "feel-good" hormones. Endurance activities are also ideal for burning off fat. The longer you maintain the activity, the more fat is taken from the body's reserves. Steady exercise for more than 20 to 30 minutes at a time is best for burning fat—but you should still be able to talk without puffing, and your pulse rate should not exceed 130 beats per minute.

The most appropriate exercises are easy on the joints. They include such activities as
- walking
- speed walking
- cycling
- swimming
- dancing

Activities that require quick changes in direction, pressure or weight stress the joints. If you are overweight or have back or knee problems, avoid
- jogging
- tennis
- soccer

Strength training builds muscles. Because muscle burns more calories than fat, the need for energy remains high. Strength training won't help you lose weight, but your body will become slimmer and you'll have better muscle tone.

Combining endurance exercise and strength training is ideal. For example, you could walk at a brisk pace for 30 minutes 3 to 4 times a week and do strengthening exercises once a week.

Daily Activity

Take advantage of the many opportunities for exercising on a daily basis:
- Walk or bicycle short distances.
- If you use your car or public transit frequently, park your vehicle or get off the bus several blocks from your final destination and continue on foot.
- Use stairs instead of elevators or escalators as often as possible.
- If you spend much of your day sitting, take a break and do small leg exercises. These give you additional activity and also help maintain flexibility.

Recreational Activity

Fit in more opportunities to increase your physical activity in your free time and on weekends. Whether you exercise alone, with a partner or friend, or in an organized setting, team or club is up to you.
- Instead of watching television in the evening, take a short walk.
- Take care of small errands near home on foot or by bicycle.
- Go swimming once a week.
- Instead of buying a lot of food at once, shop more often on foot.
- Visit a fitness center with friends or on your own. These centers offer a variety of activities—weight training,

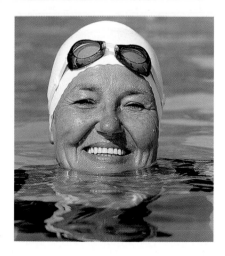

stretching and strength classes, aerobics and dancing are typical.

- Join a club that does something you like: racquet sports, rowing, hiking, bicycling, Tai Chi, recreational team sports.

Sports and Strenuous Physical Activity

Increasing your physical activity means more work for your muscles. This is a big advantage, because using your muscles

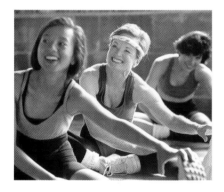

increases the amount of insulin absorbed by your body's cells.

Muscles that are forced to work harder also need more energy. More carbohydrates are burned and blood glucose sinks, so athletes who have diabetes must carefully coordinate their carbohydrate intake with their insulin dosage to prevent hypoglycemia.

You can avoid hypoglycemia by making sure you have a supply of carbohydrates available when you're making greater physical demands of your body than usual. If you take medication to lower blood glucose, consult your

physician about how much to take before, during and after any strenuous physical activity.

In the case of unplanned activities, be sure that you have some small snacks, including energy drinks and other carbonated beverages, to provide your body with additional carbohydrates. If you're planning any endurance activities, or if you do them on a regular basis, you can plan a reduction in medication ahead of time.

Any glucose-reducing medication needs to correspond to the positive effect physical activity has on blood glucose. Otherwise, hypoglycemia may result, as greater use of your muscles during physical activity leads to more glucose flowing from the blood to muscle cells. If the medication isn't adjusted accordingly, blood glucose levels could drop too low.

Measure your blood glucose before and after exercising (if you are doing an activity over an

extended period, measure partway through as well). Eat a banana or drink a glass of apple juice or orange juice, for example, depending on the results.

Symptoms of hypoglycemia:
- sweating
- shaking
- voracious appetite
- weakness
- weak knees
- rapid heartbeat
- impaired vision

Guideline: Eat an additional carbohydrate choice (15 g)— for example, 1 cup of low-fat unsweetened yogurt, a small fruit, ½ cup of fruit juice, 1 slice of bread or ½ a small bagel or English muffin—for every 30 minutes of physical activity or reduce the dose of your medication after consulting your physician.

Always carry some glucose so that you can act quickly at the first signs of hypoglycemia.

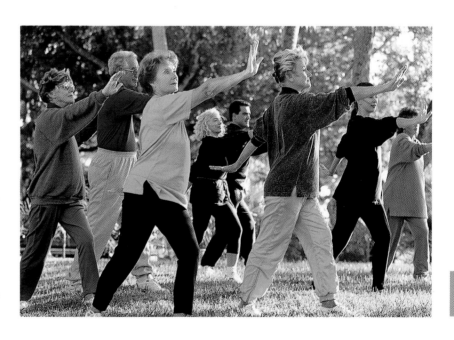

Practical Tips

Low Fat

- Use a variety of oils and vinegars with distinctive flavors. Cold-pressed oils have a stronger taste.
- Avoid prepared dressings and choose vinegar and oil or yogurt dressings instead of creamy dressings.
- 1 tsp (5 mL) of oil is sufficient for a serving of salad.
- If you prefer a creamier dressing, add buttermilk, kefir, low-fat yogurt or low-fat sour cream instead of cream, crème fraîche or other high-fat dairy products.
- To prepare a good sauce base, simmer a variety of fresh vegetables together. Dark sauces are more aromatic if you add finely chopped carrots, tomatoes, onions, a piece of celery and some chopped leek. For lighter sauces, use the white leek parts, onions, celery or carrots.

- Instead of thickening a sauce with cream, purée the cooked vegetables and combine. A dash of low-fat condensed milk is also a good alternative.
- As with sauces, soups can be made creamier by adding a vegetable purée.
- Buttermilk, kefir, low-fat yogurt or low-fat sour cream can round off the gravy for a roast. Spoon some into a small dish, stir in a few tablespoons of the hot stock and return the mixture to the pot. No further cooking is necessary. It will taste just as good as gravy made with higher-fat sour cream.

- Stir-frying, braising and browning in nonstick pans and woks are low-fat ways to cook and retain vitamins.
- The smaller the food to be cooked, the shorter the cooking time. Julienne or dice your vegetables. If using a wok, cut meat into fine strips.
- No need for whipping cream! Low-fat quark becomes light and creamy if you whisk in a few dashes of carbonated mineral water.
- Low-fat quark (or puréed cottage cheese) and low-fat yogurt combined in a 1:1 ratio make a light base for salad dressings, sauces and desserts.

Fiber

- Eat whole-grain products to increase your fiber intake. They don't have to contain the whole seed. Try products made of finely ground whole-grain flour such as whole-grain bread, rolls and crispbreads.
- Brown rice has a nutty flavor you'll enjoy.
- For an egg-free whole-grain pasta, try spelt noodles, which have a mild flavor.

Sugar and Spice

- Spices and fresh herbs enliven any meal and help eliminate the need for salt. Fresh herbs should be added to a warm meal just before serving; otherwise, they lose their flavor.
- Fiber-rich foods, protein and fat delay the transfer of sugar to the bloodstream. In combination with these nutrients, sugar won't raise blood glucose as much. Whole-grain cookies or whole-grain bread with marmalade and a little low-fat quark or puréed cottage cheese are ideal.
- Purée about half the quantity of fruit called for in a recipe when you're preparing a fruit dish. Fructose is quite sweet, so you can easily avoid other sweeteners.
- Sugar substitutes don't offer any advantages over everyday sugar. Use sweeteners in drinks and normal table sugar for cakes—but always in moderation. Reduce the amount of sugar you eat gradually so you don't crave it.
- Aspartame is not approved for cooking or baking.
- Choose vegetable thickeners such as carob flour or guar flour (available in health-food stores) over wheat and potato starches. They're based on indigestible fiber and not on starch. **Tip:** Use a pinch of thickener for each serving of sauce or soup, and give it a good 10 minutes to cook.

Baking

- Use coarsely ground whole-grain flour or half the amount of finely ground flour. You'll probably need to add a little extra to the amount of liquid called for in the recipe.
- When following regular recipes, reduce the amount of sugar called for by $\frac{1}{3}$ or $\frac{1}{4}$. No flavor will be lost.

Diabetic Products

- Enjoy a small sweet treat once in a while! The need for people with diabetes to avoid sugar has long since passed.
- Products containing sugar substitutes are usually not necessary. Such products are often more expensive, and the fat and calorie content is just as high, so they don't offer any advantages.
- Not all products bearing the label "diet" apply to those with diabetes.
- Instead of eating diet chocolate, you can snack on a piece of semisweet chocolate, which contains significantly less sugar than milk chocolate. Remember, however, that both are high in fat.
- If you want to treat yourself to something sweet once or twice a week, go ahead.

Supplements

- A multitude of vitamin, mineral and trace-element supplements are available for people with diabetes. Their effectiveness hasn't been proven, and they are only necessary in rare instances. If you need to take supplements, your physician will recommend them.

- The nutrients in fresh, natural foods are best for your body. A rich and varied diet that includes 3 servings of vegetables and 2 small servings of fresh fruit a day is your best source.
- Unprocessed or lightly processed foods retain their original fiber and many nutrients. Fresh fruit is better than juice, brown rice is better than white, boiled potatoes are better than French fries, and whole-grain bread is better than a baguette.

Additional Tips

- Eggs should be eaten no more than once or twice a week. Be aware that most noodles, cakes and cookies contain eggs.
- The processing and transformation of fats can lead to the so-called trans-fatty acids. These are indicated as "partially hydrogenated vegetable fats" and can have a detrimental effect on blood cholesterol.
- Use prepared foods only when there's no other choice and they won't produce negative effects when combined with other foods. Some prepared foods contain a lot of fat, sugar and salt.
- If you usually drink mineral water or tea to quench your

thirst, then a glass of wine with dinner is no problem.
- If you're eating a multi-course meal, you'll likely get more than the usual amount of carbohydrates, so pass on dessert altogether or ask for a cup of coffee or tea.
- To compensate for the excess calories and fat consumed on a day out, eat less—especially calorie-rich fatty foods—the next day.

Hypoglycemia

- A bedtime snack of whole-grain bread topped with low-fat quark, puréed cottage cheese or low-fat yogurt, or half a granola bar, can help prevent hypoglycemia during the night. Snacks like these, which have a low glycemic index, slowly raise blood glucose and are useful as a nighttime treat for people who need to inject insulin.
- Always carry glucose or fruit juice with you to raise blood glucose quickly in an emergency.
- Your blood glucose can still drop sharply hours after you've consumed alcohol or exercised heavily if you haven't eaten enough carbohydrates.

Breakfasts and Snacks

Eat breakfast like a king...

Both night owls and early birds can start their day full of energy after a colorful, nutritious breakfast. Combine a small serving of fruit, a grain such as bread and a dairy product to create an ideal morning meal—breakfast should be light and relaxed.

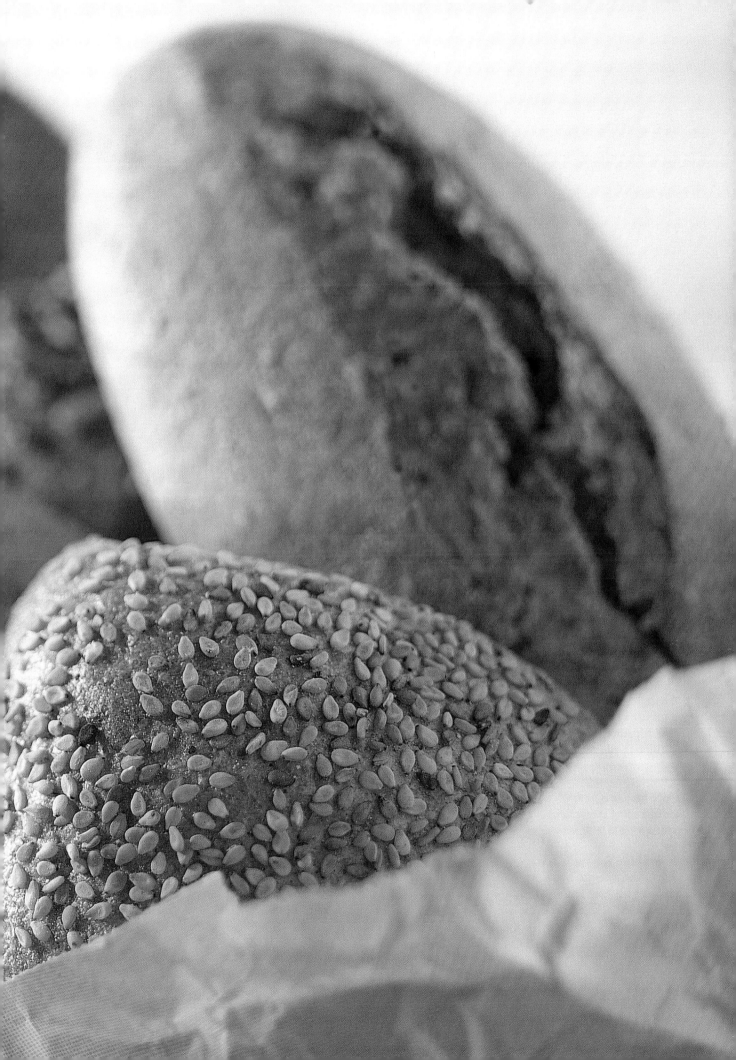

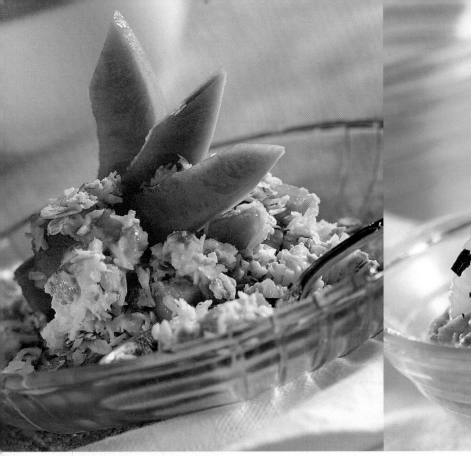
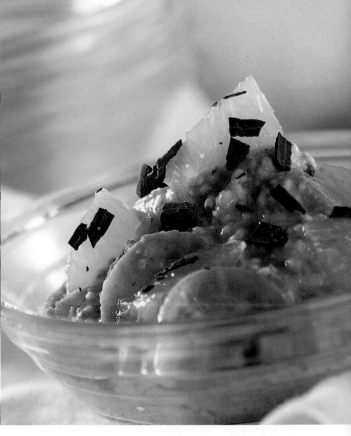

Coconut Muesli with Papaya

Carbohydrates	●●◖	20 min.
Fat	●●	
Fiber	●●	

Per serving: approx. 220 calories
7 g protein · 7 g fat · 29 g carbohydrates

FOR 2 SERVINGS:
1 small ripe papaya
2 tbsp (30 mL) unsweet-
ened flaked or shredded
coconut
1½ cups (375 mL/50 g)
multigrain flakes
¾ cup (175 mL/200 g) kefir
(health-food stores) or
low-fat yogurt
Pinch ground ginger
Pinch ground cinnamon
1 tbsp (15 mL) pear nectar

1 Peel the papaya, cut in half and remove the pit. Cut half the fruit into thin slices and dice the remainder.

2 Brown coconut in a dry nonstick skillet (frying pan). Combine with multigrain flakes and papaya in two small bowls.

3 Combine kefir, ginger, cinnamon and pear nectar. Pour over muesli and garnish with papaya slices.

!! TIP: Muesli ensures a good start to your day. If you buy prepared muesli, read the list of ingredients carefully. Avoid muesli that contains added sugar of any type.

Whole-Grain Muesli with Apricots and Yogurt

Carbohydrates	●●	15 min.
Fat	—	
Fiber	●	

Per serving: approx. 119 calories
4 g protein · 1 g fat · 23 g carbohydrates

FOR 2 SERVINGS:
3 tbsp (45 mL/30 g) wheat
berries
2 tbsp (30 mL) water
⅓ cup (75 mL/100 g) low-fat
yogurt
1 tsp (5 mL/15 g) liquid
honey
1 tsp (5 mL) unsweetened
sea buckthorn or cran-
berry juice (health-food
stores)
2 dashes liquid sweetener
¼ cup (50 mL/20 g) dried
apricots
½ orange
1 tsp (5 mL) chopped bittersweet chocolate

1 Coarsely grind the wheat berries, stir in the water and soak overnight, covered, in the refrigerator.

2 In the morning, stir in yogurt, honey, sea buckthorn juice and sweetener until smooth.

3 Cut apricots into fine strips. Combine with wheat–yogurt mixture.

4 Peel the orange, removing the white pith, and cut into bite-size pieces. Combine with muesli.

5 Spoon muesli into two small bowls. Garnish with chocolate and serve.

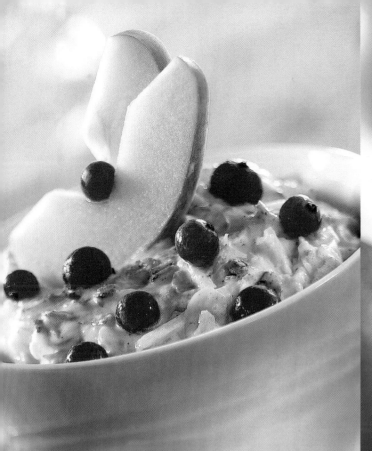

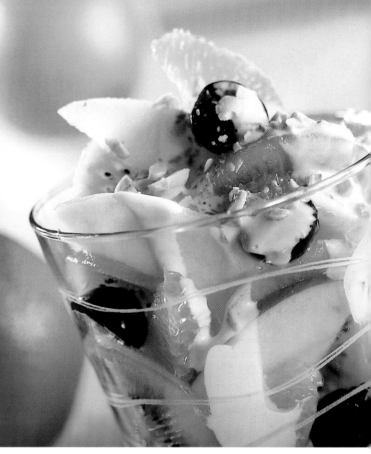

Crunchy Muesli with Apples and Bananas

Carbohydrates	●●●◖	15 min.
Fat	●●	
Fiber	●●	

Per serving: approx. 249 calories
4 g protein · 9 g fat · 38 g carbohydrates

FOR 2 SERVINGS:
1 banana
2 apples
5 tbsp (75 mL/75 g) low-fat
   yogurt
1 tbsp (15 mL/15 g) butter
½ tsp (2 mL) vanilla
1 tbsp (15 mL) sliced
   almonds or buckwheat
   groats
4 tbsp (60 mL) rolled oats
A few red currants

1 Peel the banana and mash with a fork. Core the apples, cut a few small wedges and set aside. Finely grate the remaining apple, skin on or off, and stir into the yogurt with the banana and vanilla.

2 In a small ovenproof pan or skillet (frying pan), heat butter and stir in sliced almonds and oats. Toast on top of the stove on medium heat, in a moderate (375°F/190°C) oven or under the broiler (grill) until golden, being careful not to burn them. Let the mixture cool slightly, then combine with the fruit–yogurt mixture.

3 Garnish with currants and remaining apple wedges.

Fruit Salad with Cashew Sauce

Carbohydrates	●●◖	25 min.
Fat	●	
Fiber	●	

Per serving: approx. 162 calories
4 g protein · 5 g fat · 25 g carbohydrates

FOR 2 SERVINGS:
1 small orange
⅔ cup (150 mL/100 g) red
   grapes
1 small kiwi fruit
1 small red apple
2 tbsp (30 mL) lemon juice
2 tbsp (30 mL) unsweet-
   ened cashew butter
   (health-food stores)
5 tbsp (75 mL/75 g) low-fat
   yogurt
2 tbsp (30 mL) cashews

1 Peel the orange, remove white pith and divide into sections, being careful to reserve any juice. Halve grapes and remove seeds. Peel kiwi, halve and slice.

2 Cut the apple into quarters and core it, then slice into wedges. Immediately immerse these in the lemon juice, stir and remove. Combine the fruit and arrange in small bowls.

3 Combine lemon juice and reserved orange juice with the cashew butter and stir into the yogurt.

4 Toast chopped cashews in a nonstick skillet (frying pan) on medium heat. Pour the cashew sauce over the salad. Garnish with additional nuts, coarsely chopped.

Cream Cheese and Fruit Sandwich

Carbohydrates	●●	15 min.
Fat	–	
Fiber	●	

Per serving: approx. 134 calories
4 g protein · 2 g fat · 24 g carbohydrates

FOR 2 SERVINGS:
4 slices whole-grain bread
½ cup (125 mL/50 g) raspberries
2 tbsp (30 mL) low-fat cream cheese
1 peach

1 Toast the bread. Wash and crush the raspberries and combine with the cream cheese. Add a little water as needed and stir until creamy. Spread on two slices of toast.

2 Halve and pit the peach, then cut into thin wedges. Arrange on top of the cream cheese mixture. Top with the remaining slices of toast and serve.

 TIP: You can use red currants or strawberries instead of raspberries.

Rolls with Ricotta Cream

Carbohydrates	●●●	15 min.
Fat	●●●	
Fiber	●●	

Per serving: approx. 288 calories
11 g protein · 12 g fat · 34 g carbohydrates

FOR 2 SERVINGS:
⅓ cup (75 mL/80 g) ricotta
1 to 2 tbsp (15 to 30 mL) skim milk
A few drops liquid sweetener
1 small apple
1 tbsp (15 mL) lemon juice
2 whole-grain rolls
2 tbsp (30 mL) pine nuts

1 Combine ricotta, milk and sweetener.

2 Peel and coarsely grate the apple, sprinkle with lemon juice and stir into the ricotta mixture.

3 Slice rolls in half and spread with ricotta cream. Coarsely chop the pine nuts and toast in a dry nonstick skillet (frying pan) on medium heat until golden, being careful not to scorch them, and sprinkle over the ricotta.

TIP: A mild fresh Italian cheese with a soft texture, ricotta is available in whole-milk, part-skim and skim-milk versions that have as much as 16% MF or as little as 5% MF.

Quark with Pear on Pumpernickel

Carbohydrates	●	15 min.
Fat	–	
Fiber	●	

Per serving: approx. 92 calories
8 g protein · 1 g fat · 14 g carbohydrates

FOR 2 SERVINGS:
½ cup (125 mL/100 g) low-fat quark
   or puréed cottage cheese
1 firm pear
Large pinch ground cinnamon
Salt
2 tbsp (30 mL/24 g) cranberry
   sauce, not sweetened with sugar
2 slices pumpernickel bread

1 Stir the quark until smooth. Halve and core the pear and grate into the quark. Mix lightly.

2 Season with a large pinch of cinnamon, or to taste, and a pinch of salt. Lightly stir in the cranberry sauce.

3 Spread on the pumpernickel.

TIP: Pumpernickel is ideal for your blood glucose. It contains far fewer carbohydrates than other types of bread, yet it is made from valuable whole grains. Although it contains more water and less salt, it delivers important vitamins and minerals. The small pumpernickel rounds are a nice alternative. You can also snack on these between meals when you feel those small hunger pangs.

Cream Cheese and Fruit
Sandwich, top
Rolls with Ricotta Cream,
bottom left
Quark with Pear on Pumpernickel,
bottom right

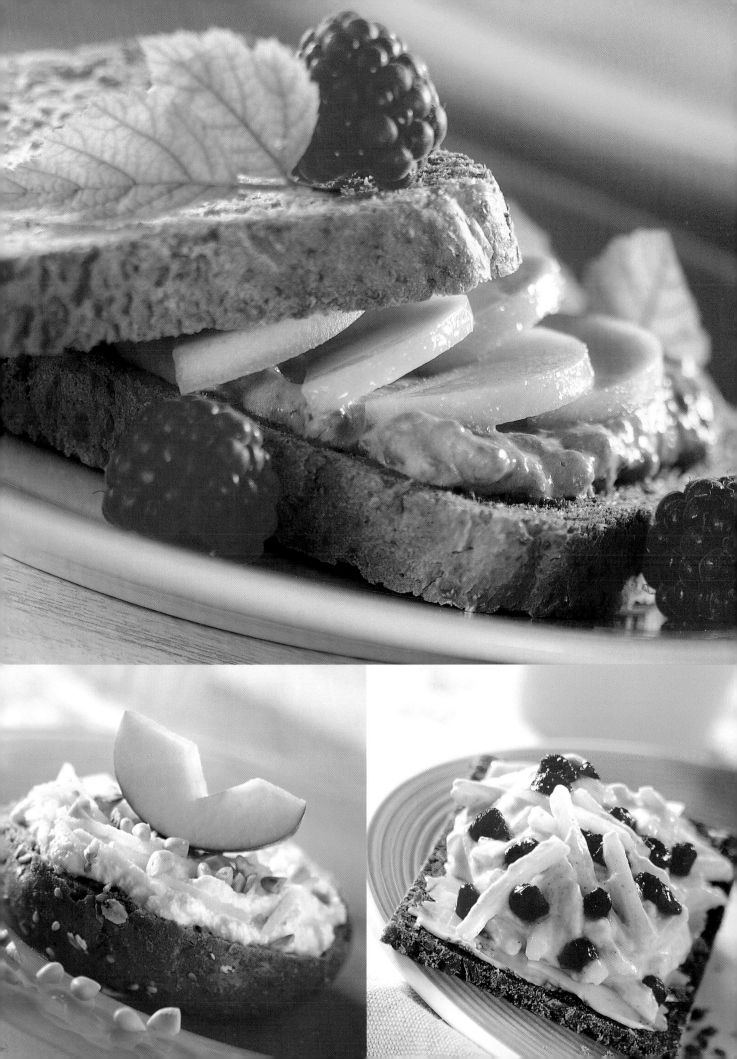

Pumpkin Rolls with Blue Cheese

Carbohydrates	●●◑	40 min.
Fat	–	(+ 1 hr. rising + 20 min. resting)
Fiber	●	(+20 min. baking)

Per serving: approx. 166 calories
9 g protein · 3 g fat · 26 g carbohydrates

FOR 8 ROLLS:
½ cup (125 mL/350 g) cooked or canned pure pumpkin
   purée
1 tsp salt, divided
2 cups (500 mL/250 g) coarsely ground whole wheat
   flour
1 (¼ oz/7 g/2¼ tsp) package dry yeast
Pinch sugar
1 tbsp (15 mL) chopped dried pumpkin seeds
4 tbsp (60 mL) lukewarm water
½ cup (125 mL/40 g) blue cheese (27% MF preferred)
1 shallot
2 tsp (10 mL) lemon juice
¾ cup (175 mL/160 g) low-fat quark or puréed cottage
   cheese
2 tbsp (30 mL) chopped Italian (flat-leaf) parsley
Freshly ground pepper

1 To make your own pumpkin purée, coarsely dice about 1 pound (450 g) of peeled pumpkin into a saucepan. Add a little water and 2 pinches of salt. Bring to a boil, turn down the heat and cook, covered, on low heat for 15 minutes, or until tender. Remove pumpkin, drain, and allow to cool. Squeeze in clean cheesecloth and measure out ½ cup (125 mL).

2 In a large bowl, combine flour, yeast, ½ tsp (2 mL) salt and a pinch of sugar. Using a handheld mixer, stir in the pumpkin purée and seeds and combine until smooth. Gradually mix in the water. Leave the dough to rise, covered, for 1 hour.

3 Preheat the oven to 350°F (180°C). Knead the dough on a lightly floured work surface. Divide and shape into 8 rolls and place on a baking sheet lined with parchment paper. Let rest for 20 minutes, then bake for 20 minutes.

4 Chop the shallot. In a bowl, cream the cheese with a fork. Stir in the shallot, lemon juice, quark and parsley. Mix in the pepper and serve with the pumpkin rolls.

 TIP: Fresh pumpkin rolls will keep for a day, and they are easy to freeze and reheat.

Supertoast with Cream Cheese

Carbohydrates	●	20 min.
Fat	–	
Fiber	●	

Per serving: approx. 78 calories
6 g protein · 1 g fat · 12 g carbohydrates

FOR 2 SERVINGS:
4 to 5 radishes
¼ cup (50 mL/50 g) low-fat cream cheese
Freshly ground pepper
2 slices whole-grain bread
¼ cup (50 mL/30 g) cucumber
1 tbsp (15 mL) watercress
1 medium tomato
Salt

1 Finely chop the rashes and combine with cream cheese. Season with a little pepper. Add a little water as needed and stir until creamy. Toast the bread slices, let cool slightly and spread with the cheese mixture.

2 Thinly slice the cucumber and arrange over the cream cheese. Place watercress on top of the cucumber slices.

3 Slice the tomato into thin wedges and arrange them on top of the watercress. Season with salt and pepper.

 TIP: To make this even tastier, stir ½ tsp (2 mL) Dijon mustard into the cream cheese. You can also thin the cream cheese with yogurt.

TIP: Toasted bread is generally more filling than plain. This applies to all types of bread, so try it!

Pumpkin Rolls with Blue Cheese, top
Supertoast with Cream Cheese, bottom

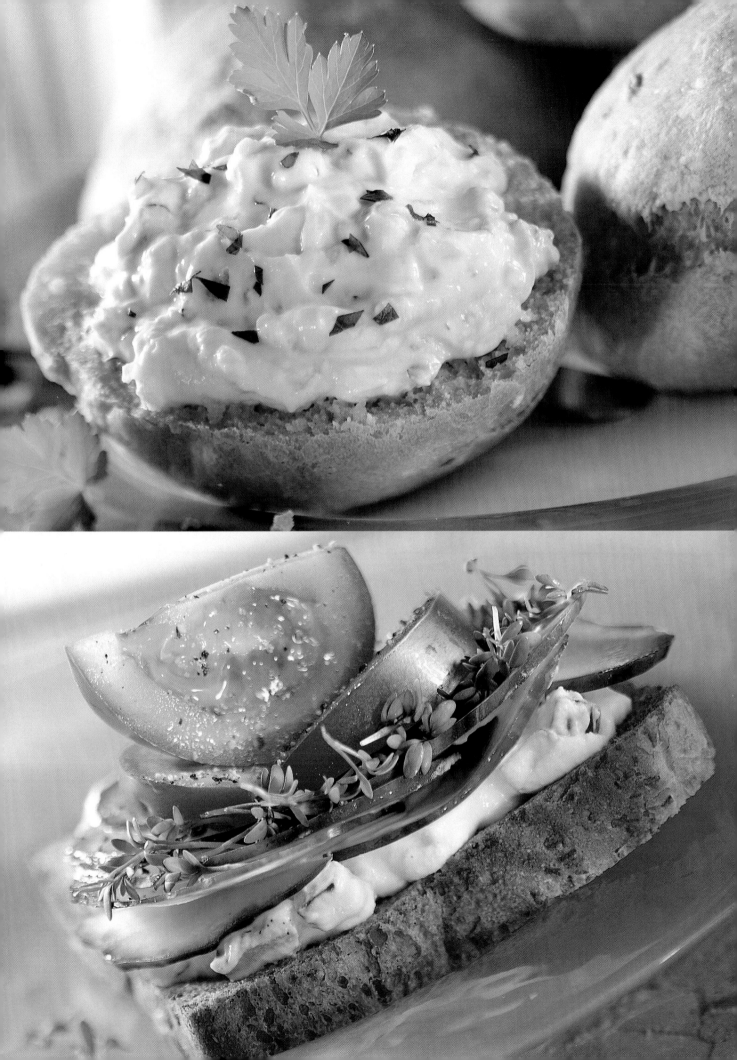

Open-Face Turkey Breast and Remoulade Sandwich

Carbohydrates	●◀	30 min.
Fat	●●	
Fiber	●	

Per serving: approx. 189 calories
9 g protein · 9 g fat · 18 g carbohydrates

FOR 2 SERVINGS:
1 hard-cooked egg
2 tbsp (30 mL/30 g) low-fat sour
 cream
3 tbsp (45 mL/20 g) finely chopped
 gherkins
1/2 tsp (2 mL) medium mustard
1 1/2 tsp (7 mL) finely chopped mixed
 fresh herbs, such as chives, parsley, dill, chervil
1 thick apple wedge
Worcestershire sauce
Salt
Liquid sweetener
2 slices (3 oz/85 g) whole-grain
 bread
2 tsp (10 mL/10 g) margarine
2 slices skinless boneless turkey
 breast
2 lettuce leaves

1 Peel and finely chop the hard-cooked egg. Mix about 1/2 with the sour cream, gherkins, mustard and herbs in a small bowl. Finely grate approximately 1 tsp (5 mL) of the apple and add to the remoulade. Slice the remaining apple, cut into small pieces and set aside. Season the remoulade with a dash of Worcestershire sauce, salt and sweetener.

2 Spread margarine on the bread. Place a lettuce leaf on each slice and cover with a slice of turkey.

3 Arrange remoulade on top and garnish with the remaining finely chopped hard-cooked egg and the apple pieces.

Creamed Ham on Rolls

Carbohydrates	●●	10 min.
Fat	●	
Fiber	●	

Per serving: approx. 212 calories
17 g protein · 6 g fat · 22 g carbohydrates

FOR 2 SERVINGS:
2 oz (60 g) lean cooked ham
1/2 cup (125 mL/100 g) low-fat quark
 or puréed cottage cheese
White pepper
Sweet paprika
2 whole-grain rolls
2 small gherkins
1 tbsp (15 mL) small capers
1 tbsp (15 mL) chopped chives

1 If necessary, remove any rind and then dice the ham.

2 Pulse the ham into the quark in a blender or food proces-sor, or mash and mix until smooth with a potato masher. Season with white pepper and paprika and mix well.

3 Slice rolls in half and spread with ham mixture. Slice the gherkins to use as a garnish and top with capers and chives.

!! **TIP:** Fresh herbs and homegrown sprouts will liven up any sandwich. They also provide energy, as well as valuable mineral and vitamin content.

Pesto and Sprouts on Rye Rolls

Carbohydrates	●●◀	15 min.
Fat	●●	
Fiber	●●	

Per serving: approx. 252 calories
16 g protein · 7 g fat · 31 g carbohydrates

FOR 2 SERVINGS:
1/2 cup (125 mL/100 g) low-fat cream
 cheese
1 tbsp (15 mL) flaxseeds
1 tbsp (15 mL) wheat germ
Salt and white pepper
2 whole-grain rye rolls
2 tsp (10 mL) pesto (prepared)
3/4 cup (175 mL/75 g) mixed sprouts:
 one or more of alfalfa, wheat,
 chickpeas, radish, flax
2 small tomatoes

1 In a small bowl, combine the cream cheese, flaxseeds and wheat germ. Season with salt and pepper. Add a little water as needed and stir until creamy.

2 Cut the rolls in half. Spread a thin layer of pesto on each half, then spread with the cream cheese.

3 Rinse and drain the sprouts and arrange on top of the rolls. Slice the tomatoes in wedges and serve on the side or on top.

**Open-Face Turkey Breast and Remoulade Sandwich, top
Creamed Ham on Rolls, bottom left
Pesto and Sprouts on Rye Rolls, bottom right**

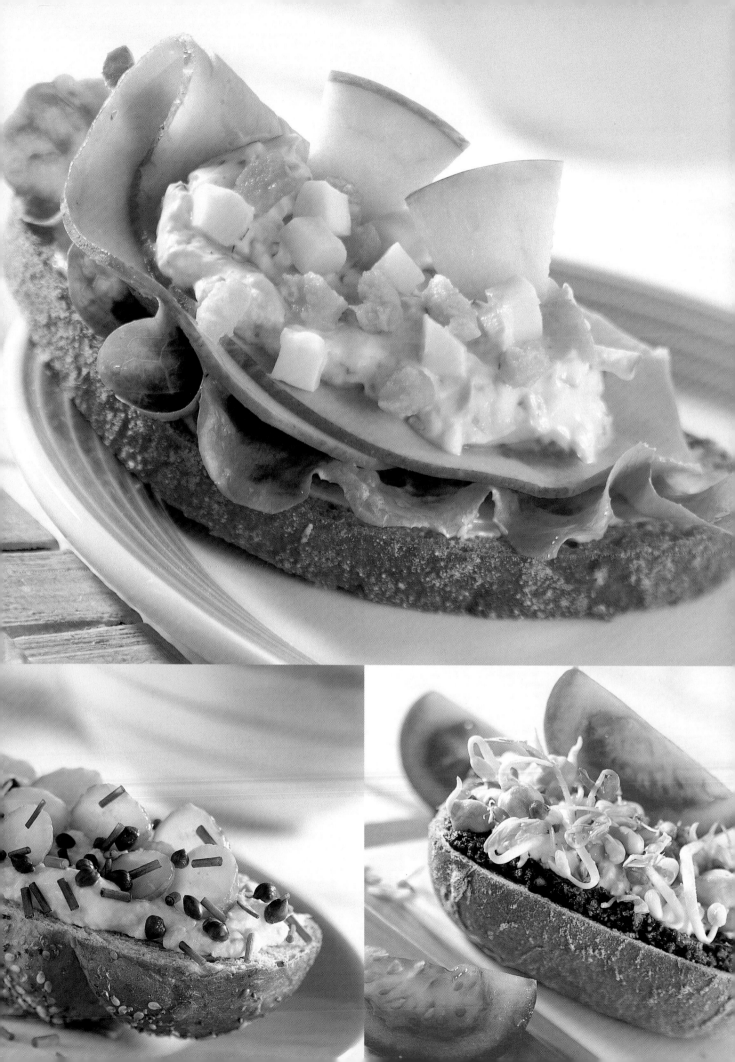

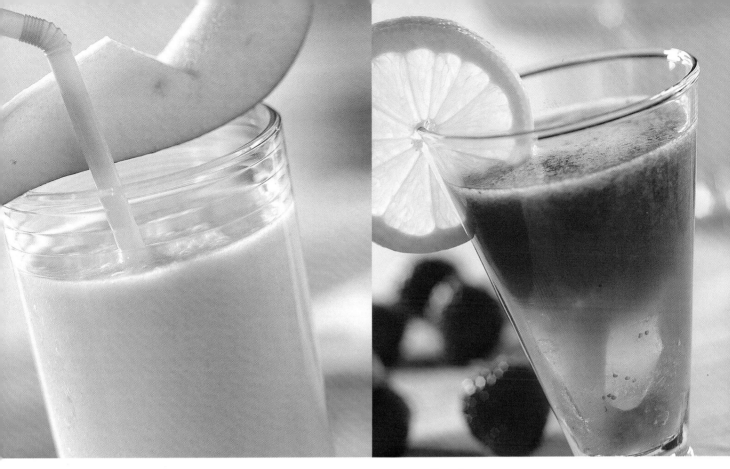

Pear–Buttermilk Flip

Carbohydrates	●◖	5 min.
Fat	—	
Fiber	●	

Per serving: approx. 82 calories
2 g protein · 0 g fat · 16 g carbohydrates

FOR 2 SERVINGS:
1 ripe pear
½ cup (125 mL/100 g) pear juice
¾ cup (175 mL/200 g) buttermilk
Pinch ground cinnamon

1 Halve and core the pear and chop finely.

2 Combine pear, pear juice and buttermilk in a blender or food processor, or mash and mix well with a potato masher.

3 Season with cinnamon, pour into two glasses and serve with thick straws.

Red Fitness Drink

Carbohydrates	◖	15 min.
Fat	—	
Fiber	—	

Per serving: approx. 37 calories
1 g protein · 0 g fat · 7 g carbohydrates

FOR 2 SERVINGS:
⅔ cup (150 mL/100 g) strawberries
⅔ cup (150 mL/100 g) watermelon
Mineral water
¼ tsp (1 mL) freshly grated ginger or ground cinnamon
½ lemon (organic preferred)
Liquid sweetener
4 ice cubes

1 Hull and wash strawberries and place in a blender or food processor.

2 Remove seeds, chop the watermelon and add it to the strawberries. Add the ginger and enough mineral water to reach 1⅔ cups (400 mL). Purée.

3 Cut 2 thin slices from the lemon and set aside. Grate a pinch of lemon zest from the remainder of the lemon and squeeze out 2 to 3 tsp (10 to 15 mL) juice.

4 Season the drink with the lemon zest, lemon juice and 3 to 4 dashes of liquid sweetener.

5 Place 2 ice cubes in a glass and pour in the drink. Cut reserved lemon slices to the center and garnish the rim of each glass.

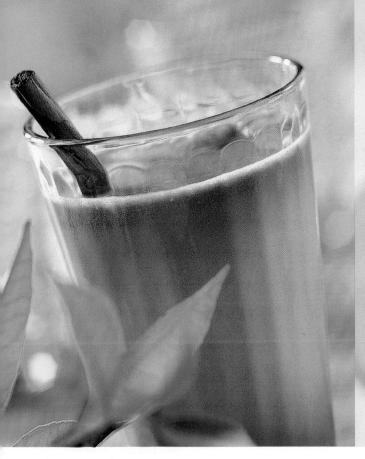

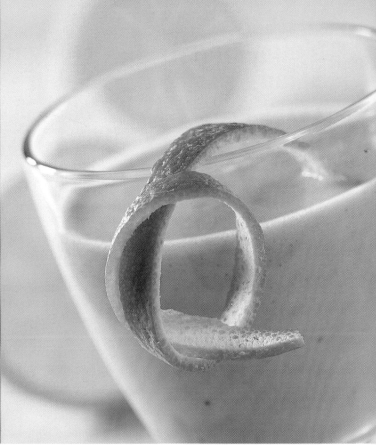

Cherry–Whey Cocktail

Carbohydrates	●◖	10 min.
Fat	–	
Fiber	–	

Per serving: approx. 81 calories
1 g protein · 0 g fat · 18 g carbohydrates

FOR 2 SERVINGS:
1 banana
½ cup (125 mL) cherry juice
1¼ cup (300 mL) whey
1 vanilla bean
2 cinnamon sticks

1 Peel banana, slice and place in blender or food processor. Pour in cherry juice and whey, and purée.

2 Slice the vanilla bean lengthwise. Using a pointed knife, scrape out the seeds, add to the drink and mix well. Pour the drink into two glasses, garnish each with a cinnamon stick and serve.

‼ TIP: Whey can be found in health-food stores, organic-food stores and in the refrigerated section of some grocery stores. Be sure to purchase pure, unflavored whey.

‼ TIP: When possible, buy only 100% pure fruit juice. If you can't find it in your grocery store, ask at your local natural- or health-food store.

Sea Buckthorn–Buttermilk Shake

Carbohydrates	●●	10 min.
Fat	–	
Fiber	–	

Per serving: approx. 112 calories
3 g protein · 1 g fat · 22 g carbohydrates

FOR 2 SERVINGS:
1 orange (organic preferred)
1 cup (250 mL) chilled buttermilk
¼ cup (50 mL) unsweetened sea buckthorn or cranberrry juice (health-food stores)
2 tbsp (30 mL) pear nectar
¼ tsp (1 mL) vanilla
Pinch ground ginger

1 Wash the orange in hot water and wipe dry. Cut two long spirals of the peel. Squeeze out the juice.

2 In a blender or food processor, combine buttermilk, sea buckthorn juice and pear nectar. Add the orange juice and blend until slightly frothy.

3 Season with vanilla and ginger and pour into two glasses. Garnish with orange spirals and serve chilled.

Melon–Berry Salad

Carbohydrates	●●◖	20 min.
Fat	–	
Fiber	●	

Per serving: approx. 157 calories
3 g protein · 2 g fat · 27 g carbohydrates

FOR 2 SERVINGS:
1¼ cups (300 mL/200 g) ripe
　honeydew or other melon
1⅓ cups (325 mL/200 g)
　strawberries
⅓ cup (75 mL/50 g) blackberries
¼ cup (50 mL) Marsala or sweet
　sherry
3 tbsp (45 mL/45 g) yogurt
2 tsp (10 mL) fresh lemon juice
1 tbsp (15 mL) maple syrup
Pinch ground cardamom
A few mint leaves

1 Cut the melon in half and remove the seeds. Use a melon baller to make small rounds of melon.

2 Rinse and drain the berries. Cut the strawberries in half and combine all the berries with the melon balls. Drizzle with the Marsala, mix gently and refrigerate, covered, for 15 minutes.

3 Meanwhile, combine yogurt, lemon juice and maple syrup in a small bowl and stir until smooth. Season with cardamom.

4 Arrange the fruit on plates, drizzle the yogurt sauce over and garnish with mint leaves.

TIP: This will have a slight flavor of the Middle East if you substitute 1 tsp (5 mL) rose water for the cardamom.

Fruity Rice Salad

Carbohydrates	●●●●	30 min.
Fat	●	
Fiber	●	

Per serving: approx. 268 calories
12 g protein · 5 g fat · 44 g carbohydrates

FOR 2 SERVINGS:
⅔ cup (150 mL) boiling salted water
⅓ cup (75 mL/60 g) long-grain con-
　verted (parboiled) rice
Salt
3½ oz (100 g) cooked frozen shrimp
½ small Galia or honeydew melon
1 small tart apple
1 tbsp (15 mL) vinegar
1 tbsp (15 mL) walnut oil
Freshly ground pepper
Mild curry powder

1 Add the rice to the water, cover, and cook on low heat for 20 minutes, stirring occasionally.

2 Thaw the shrimp. Seed the melon and form the flesh into balls with a melon baller. Core and finely dice the apple and toss with the vinegar.

3 Drain the rice well and combine with the shrimp, melon balls and apple. Drizzle in the walnut oil, season with salt, pepper and a little curry powder, and let stand for 15 minutes.

TIP: If you have time, use brown rice (which takes 35 to 45 minutes to cook) and substitute half a juicy papaya for the melon—a healthy combination.

Stuffed Grapefruit

Carbohydrates	●	15 min.
Fat	–	
Fiber	●	

Per serving: approx. 74 calories
2 g protein · 3 g fat · 11 g carbohydrates

FOR 2 SERVINGS:
1 large pink grapefruit
⅓ cup (75 mL/50 g) blueberries
2 tbsp (30 mL) old-fashioned rolled
　oats
1 tbsp (15 mL) unsweetened flaked
　or shredded coconut

1 Cut the grapefruit in half and loosen the flesh from the rind (a grapefruit knife is preferred, but a small sharp or serrated knife will suffice). Separate the fruit sections from the membranes and reserve the juice. Scrape the remaining membranes from the rind.

2 Wash and drain the blueberries. Combine with the oats, grapefruit sections and juice. Spoon mixture into grapefruit halves.

3 Toast the coconut in a dry nonstick skillet (frying pan) on medium heat until golden, being careful not to burn it. Sprinkle over the grapefruit halves.

TIP: Pink grapefruit is rich in carotenoids, which act as antioxidants, help prevent cancer, strengthen the immune system and help lower cholesterol.

TIP: If the mixture is too dry, stir in 2 to 3 tbsp (30 to 45 mL) low-fat yogurt or buttermilk.

Melon–Berry Salad, top
Fruity Rice Salad, bottom left
Stuffed Grapefruit, bottom right

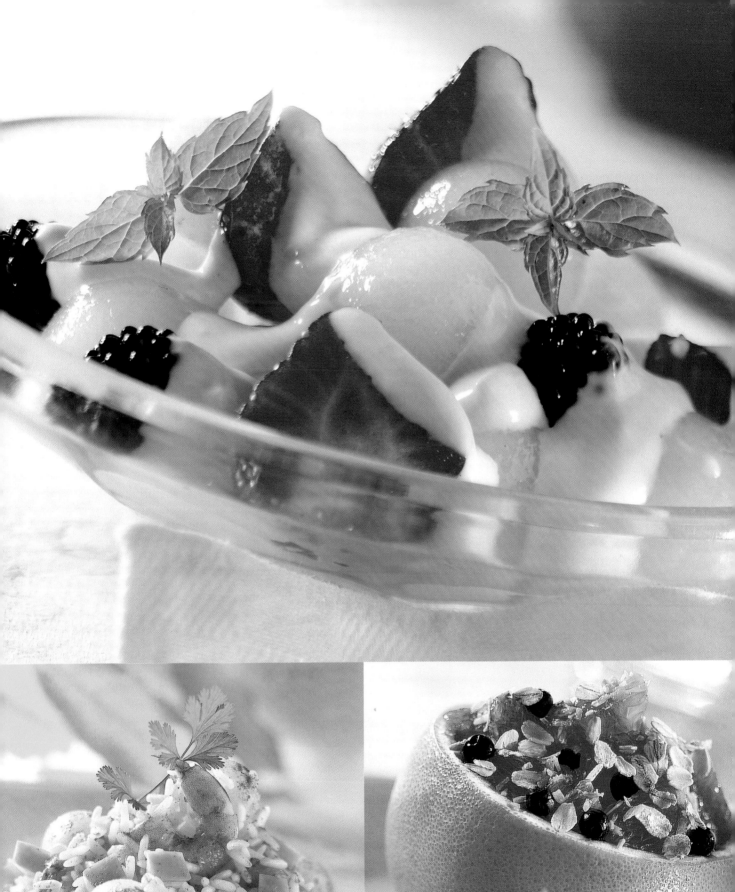

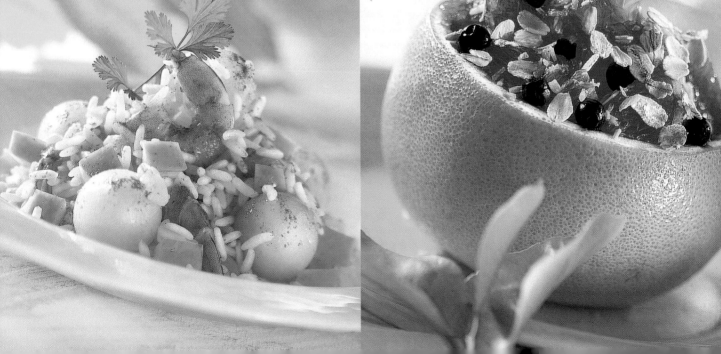

Carrot–Raisin Salad

Carbohydrates	●●	25 min.
Fat	–	
Fiber	●●	

Per serving: approx. 117 calories
2 g protein · 2 g fat · 20 g carbohydrates

FOR 2 SERVINGS:
¼ cup (50 mL) apple juice
1 tbsp (15 mL) raisins
3 medium carrots (about 1¾
   cups/425 mL/300 g)
1 apple
Juice of ½ small lemon
1 tsp (5 mL) walnut oil

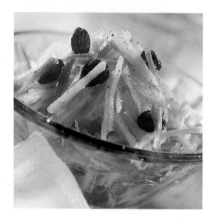

1 Heat the apple juice and soak the raisins in it for 15 minutes.

2 Peel carrots and grate finely. Peel, halve, core and finely grate the apple. Combine with the carrots.

3 Stir the lemon juice, walnut oil, raisins and apple juice into the carrot–apple mixture.

!! **TIP:** You can make this Carrot–Raisin Salad more exotic by using orange sections instead of grated apple. Soak the raisins in orange juice and season the salad with a mild curry powder.

Celery–Pear Salad

Carbohydrates	●●◗	30 min.
Fat	●●●	
Fiber	●●●	

Per serving: approx. 251 calories
5 g protein · 13 g fat · 27 g carbohydrates

FOR 2 SERVINGS:
½ cup (125 mL/250 g) pear juice
3 tbsp (45 mL) sherry vinegar
2 cups (500 mL/100 g) thinly sliced
   celery (about 4 ribs)
2 firm pears
1 oz (30 g) Roquefort cheese
2 tbsp (30 mL) walnut oil
Freshly ground pepper

1 Heat the pear juice and vinegar in a small saucepan. Add the celery and cook on low heat for 5 minutes.

2 Peel, halve, core and finely slice the pear. Remove celery from the cooking liquid and combine with the pear while still warm. Reserve cooking liquid.

3 Mash the Roquefort with a fork, stir in walnut oil and 4 tbsp (60 mL) of the vinegar–pear juice mixture. Pour over the salad. Leave to cool for 15 minutes before serving.

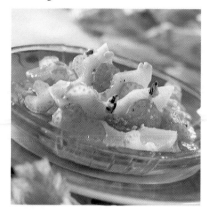

Turkey Snacks with Dip

Carbohydrates	◗	30 min.
Fat	●●	
Fiber	–	

Per serving: approx. 160 calories
17 g protein · 7 g fat · 7 g carbohydrates

FOR 2 SERVINGS:
4 oz (125 g) skinless boneless
   turkey breast
¼ tsp (1 mL) dried thyme
Salt
¼ tsp (1 mL) curry powder
¼ tsp (1 mL) sweet paprika
1 small onion
¼ apple, peeled
1 tbsp (15 mL) oil
1 tsp (5 mL) lemon juice
5 to 6 fresh basil leaves
⅔ cup (150 mL/150 g) yogurt
Sugar
¼ cucumber
6 cherry tomatoes

1 Dice the turkey into 12 medium cubes. Combine thyme, salt to taste, curry powder and paprika, and use this to season the meat.

2 Finely dice the onion and apple. Lightly sauté in hot oil on low heat for 5 minutes.

3 Add the turkey and brown on all sides. Cook, covered, on low heat for 5 minutes. Remove from pan and set aside to cool.

4 Cut or tear the basil into thin strips. Stir apple, onion, lemon juice and basil into the yogurt. Season with salt and a little sugar.

5 Peel the cucumber, slice lengthwise and cut into 12 pieces. Halve the tomatoes. Slide 1 piece of diced turkey, 1 piece of cucumber and 1 tomato half onto each of 12 small wooden skewers. Arrange on top of the yogurt sauce.

Turkey Snacks with Dip, right

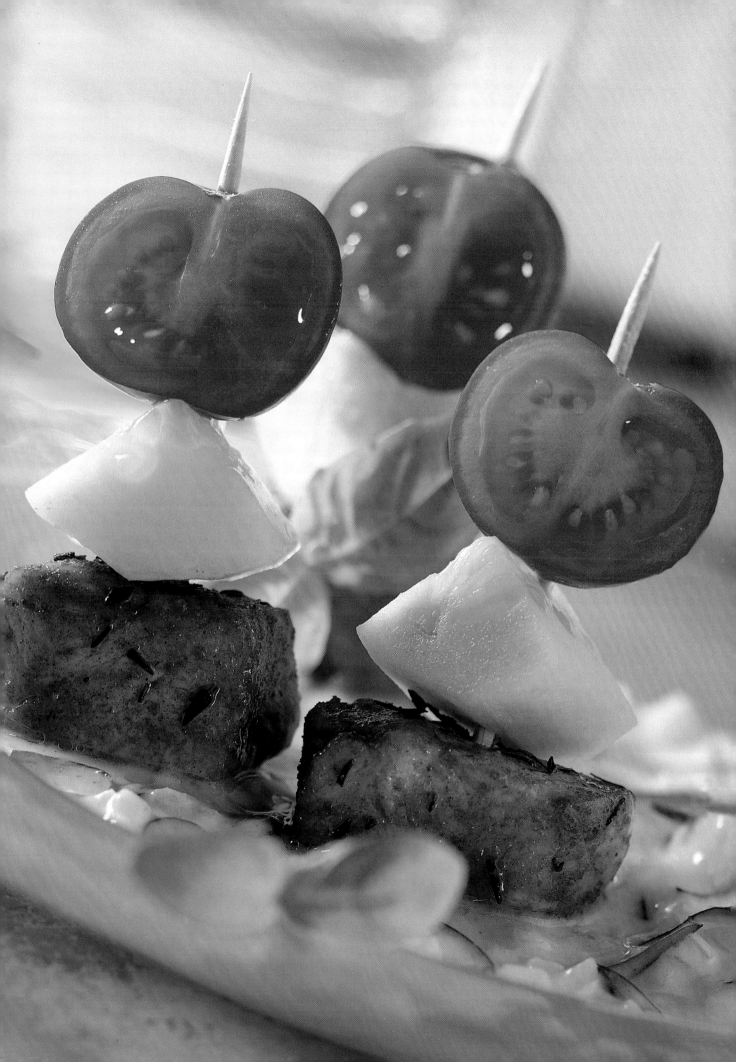

Open-Face Tomato Sandwich with Lovage

Carbohydrates	●●	20 min.
Fat	●	
Fiber	●	

Per serving: approx. 156 calories
5 g protein · 6 g fat · 20 g carbohydrates

FOR 2 SERVINGS:
5 lovage leaves
¼ cup (50 mL/50 g) sour cream
Salt
Freshly ground nutmeg
2 medium tomatoes
1 small red onion
1 tsp (5 mL) margarine
2 slices whole-grain bread
Freshly ground pepper
A few lovage leaves

1 Cut the 5 lovage leaves into fine strips. Stir into sour cream and season with a pinch of salt and a little nutmeg.

2 Slice the tomatoes. Halve and thinly slice the onion.

3 Spread margarine on the bread slices. Top with the tomato slices and season with pepper. Drizzle the sour cream over the tomatoes and garnish with half-moons of onion and additional lovage leaves.

!! TIP: The strong taste of lovage adds a certain "kick" to this snack, but you could use finely chopped celery or celery leaves instead.

Pumpernickel with Herbed Potato Cream

Carbohydrates	●●●	45 min.
Fat	–	
Fiber	●●●	

Per serving: approx. 177 calories
6 g protein · 1 g fat · 36 g carbohydrates

FOR 2 SERVINGS:
1 mealy (floury) potato
Salt
½ bunch mixed fresh herbs, such as chervil, chives, parsley, sorrel, borage
2 to 3 tsp (10 to 15 mL) low-fat quark or puréed cottage cheese
1 tsp (5 mL) mango chutney
½ tsp (2 mL) ground coriander seeds
Freshly ground pepper
12 pumpernickel rounds
½ bunch radishes

1 Peel the potato and cook, covered, for 20 minutes in salted water. Drain and press through a potato ricer or mash smooth while still hot.

2 Remove leaves from the herbs and set a few aside. Finely chop the remainder and combine with potato and quark. Stir in chutney and season with salt, ground coriander and pepper.

3 Spread the potato cream on the pumpernickel rounds. Garnish with decoratively cut radishes and reserved herb leaves.

Zucchini–Olive Crostini with Feta

Carbohydrates	●	30 min.
Fat	●●	
Fiber	●	

Per serving: approx. 170 calories
9 g protein · 9 g fat · 12 g carbohydrates

FOR 2 SERVINGS:
6 pitted black olives
2 oz (60 g) feta
1½ small zucchini (courgette)
1 small red onion
1 tsp (5 mL) olive oil
1 small clove garlic
Salt and freshly ground pepper
2 slices whole-grain bread

1 Preheat the oven to 475°F (250°C).

2 Depending on their size, halve or quarter the olives. Finely dice the cheese. Coarsely grate the zucchini. Finely dice the onion.

3 Heat the oil in a nonstick skillet (frying pan). Add onion and cook until translucent. Add zucchini. Peel and crush the garlic, and cook with the zucchini and onions on low heat for 5 minutes. Stir in olives, and season with salt and pepper.

4 Toast the bread. Spread the zucchini mixture on the toast. Sprinkle feta on top. Bake in the center of the oven for a few minutes, until the cheese has melted slightly.

Open-Face Tomato Sandwich with Lovage, top right
Pumpernickel with Herbed Potato Cream, bottom left
Zucchini–Olive Crostini with Feta, bottom right

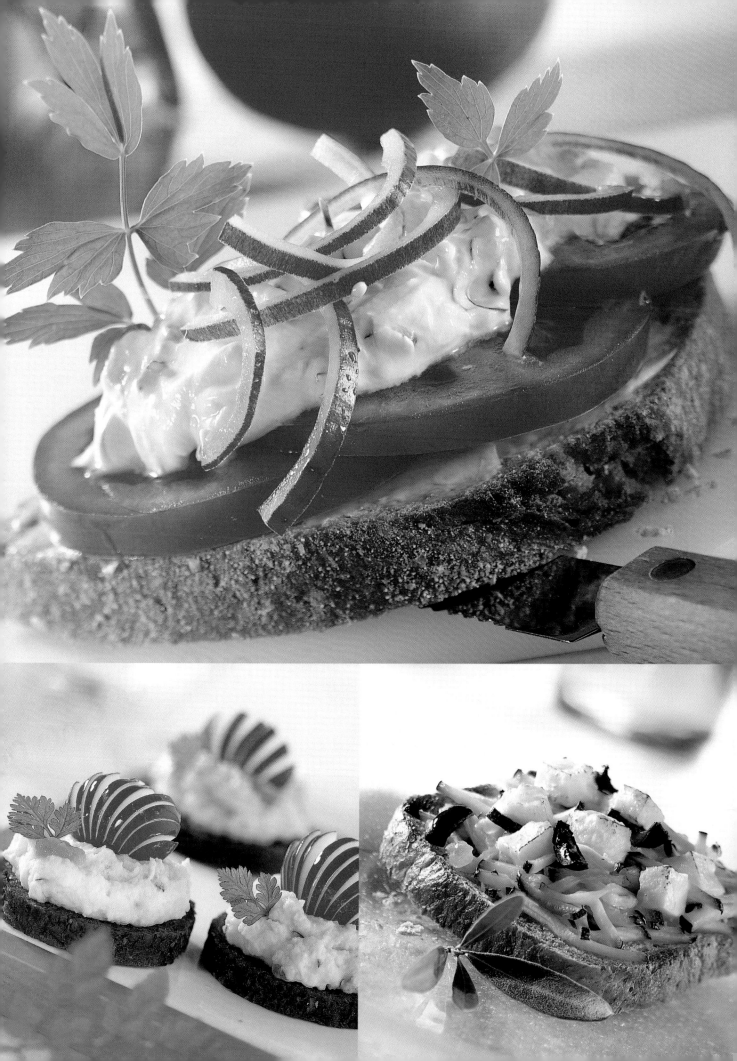

Red-Pepper Quark on Pumpernickel

Carbohydrates	●◖	20 min.
Fat	–	
Fiber	●	

Per serving: approx. 99 calories
6 g protein · 3 g fat · 13 g carbohydrates

FOR 2 SERVINGS:
¼ cup (50 mL/50 g) low-fat quark or
    puréed cottage cheese
4 tsp (20 mL/20 g) sour cream
¼ to ½ sweet red pepper
1 tsp (5 mL) capers
3 pinches dried herbes de Provence
Salt and freshly ground pepper
Freshly grated nutmeg
6 small pumpernickel rounds
Italian (flat-leaf) parsley leaves

1 Combine quark and sour cream in a small bowl.

2 Finely dice about ½ the red pepper and set some aside. Slice the rest into thin strips for garnish. Finely chop the capers. Stir the diced peppers and capers into the quark. Season with herbs, a pinch of salt and a little pepper and nutmeg.

3 Spoon the quark and red-pepper mixture onto the pumpernickel rounds. Garnish with the remaining red pepper and parsley.

Chickpea Pâté on Rye

Carbohydrates	●●●◖	1¼ hrs.
Fat	●	(+ 12 hrs.
Fiber	●●●	soaking)

Per serving: approx. 238 calories
10 g protein · 4 g fat · 40 g carbohydrates

FOR 2 SERVINGS:
½ cup (125 mL/75 g) dried
    chickpeas
1 tsp (5 mL) olive oil
1 large onion
¼ cup (50 mL) water
1 tsp (5 mL) salt
1 small clove garlic
1 tbsp (15 mL) chopped fresh
    parsley
1 tbsp (15 mL) lemon juice
2 slices rye bread

1 Cover the chickpeas with plenty of water and soak for 8 to 12 hours.

2 Drain and rinse the chickpeas. Cover with fresh cold water and bring to a boil. Cook, covered, on low heat for 1 hour. Leave to cool.

3 Coarsely chop the onion. Heat the oil in a skillet (frying pan). Add onion and cook on medium heat until translucent; season with a pinch of salt. Add the ¼ cup (50 mL) water, bring to a boil, cover, and cook on low heat for 5 minutes.

4 Drain chickpeas. Peel the garlic. Combine the chickpeas, garlic and onion with the cooking liquid in a blender or food processor, or mash and mix with a potato masher. Add a little more water if needed. Stir the parsley, salt and lemon juice into the chickpea mixture.

5 Toast the bread and spread thickly with the pâté while still warm.

Crostini with Tomato Ragout

Carbohydrates	●●◖	45 min.
Fat	●	
Fiber	●●	

Per serving: approx. 174 calories
6 g protein · 5 g fat · 25 g carbohydrates

FOR 2 SERVINGS:
1 small zucchini (courgette)
2 small tomatoes
2 shallots
1 small clove garlic
1 tsp (5 mL) olive oil
Salt and white pepper
Pinch dried, crushed chili pepper
4 to 6 slices whole-grain baguette
4 to 6 pitted black olives, sliced

1 Coarsely grate or julienne the zucchini. Finely dice the tomatoes. Peel shallots and garlic. Finely dice the shallots.

2 Using a pastry brush, coat a small nonstick skillet (frying pan) with olive oil, then heat on medium. Cook the shallots on low heat until translucent. Crush the garlic and add to the shallots. Turn up the heat, quickly wilt the zucchini, then stir in the tomatoes. Season with salt, pepper and chili pepper, and bring to a boil.

3 Lightly toast the baguette slices. Spread the zucchini–tomato mixture on each slice and garnish with olives.

Red-Pepper Quark on Pumpernickel,
right
Chickpea Pâté on Rye, bottom left
Crostini with Tomato Ragout,
bottom right

BREAKFASTS AND SNACKS

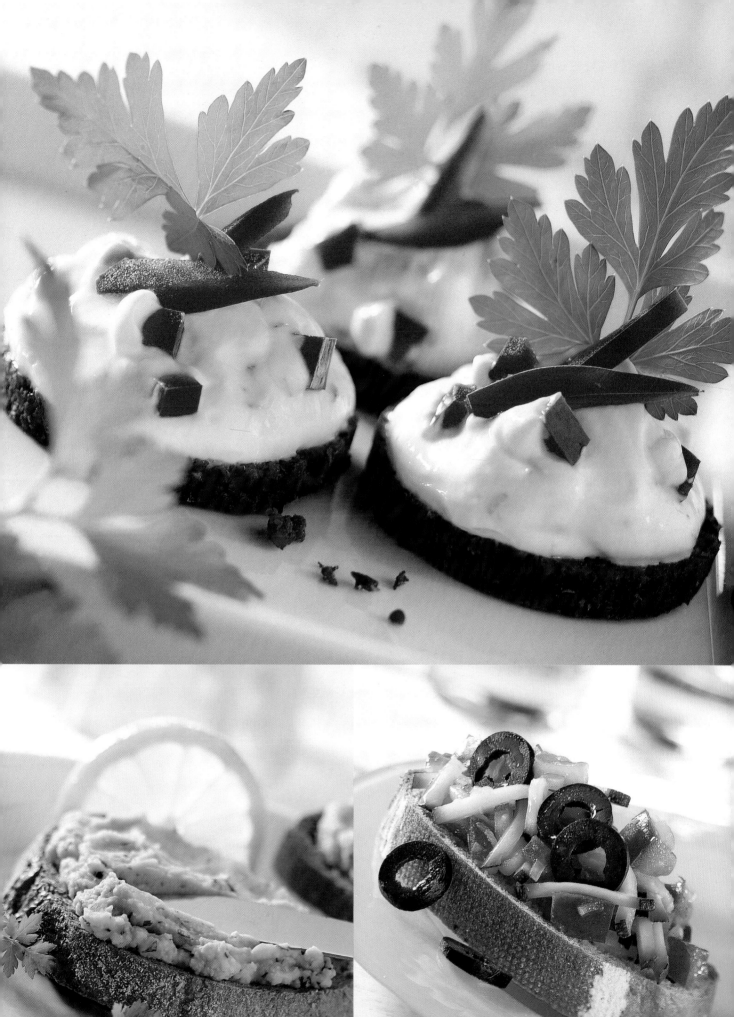

Vegetable–Ham Wraps

Carbohydrates	–	25 min.
Fat	●●●	
Fiber	●	

Per serving: approx. 168 calories
16 g protein · 10 g fat · 2 g carbohydrates

FOR 2 SERVINGS:
1 small red pepper
1 rib celery
2 small gherkins
4 slices cooked ham
Freshly ground pepper
½ bunch chives

1 Core the red pepper and cut away the inner membranes. Slice celery, red pepper and pickles into small finger-length sticks.

2 Remove rind from the ham, if necessary, and cut each slice in half. Divide the vegetable sticks among the pieces of ham and season with pepper.

3 Roll up the ham slices. Tie 2 or 3 chive stems around each wrap to garnish and hold it together.

!! **TIP:** These wraps make an ideal snack for the office. Roll each one in a lettuce leaf and store in a sealed container, and they will stay fresh for hours.

Shrimp and Dill Cream Baguettes

Carbohydrates	●●◖	20 min.
Fat	●●	
Fiber	●	

Per serving: approx. 222 calories
14 g protein · 7 g fat · 26 g carbohydrates

FOR 2 SERVINGS:
1 tbsp (15 mL) mayonnaise
2 tbsp (30 mL/30 g) low-fat yogurt
1 tsp (5 mL) lime juice
¼ tsp (1 mL) coarsely ground black pepper
Herbed salt
½ bunch fresh dill
2 to 3 leaves lettuce or other leafy greens
¼ cucumber
3 to 4 radishes
½ lime
3½ oz (100 g) cooked shrimp
2 baguette-style rolls

1 Combine mayonnaise and yogurt with the lime juice and pepper, and stir until creamy. Season with herbed salt. Finely chop the dill and stir it in.

2 Tear lettuce into large pieces. Thinly slice the cucumber, skin on or off, as desired. Thinly slice the radishes.

3 Cut very thin slices of lime and remove the peel. Rinse shrimp in cold water, dry thoroughly, then combine with ½ of the dill cream.

4 Slice the rolls lengthwise. Spread the remaining dill cream on the bottom half of each and cover with ½ of the lettuce leaves. Arrange the cucumber and radish slices on top of the lettuce leaves, then add the shrimp and the lime slices. Top with the rest of the lettuce, cover with the top half of the rolls, and serve immediately.

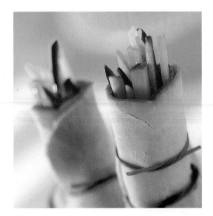

Shrimp and Dill Cream Baguettes, right

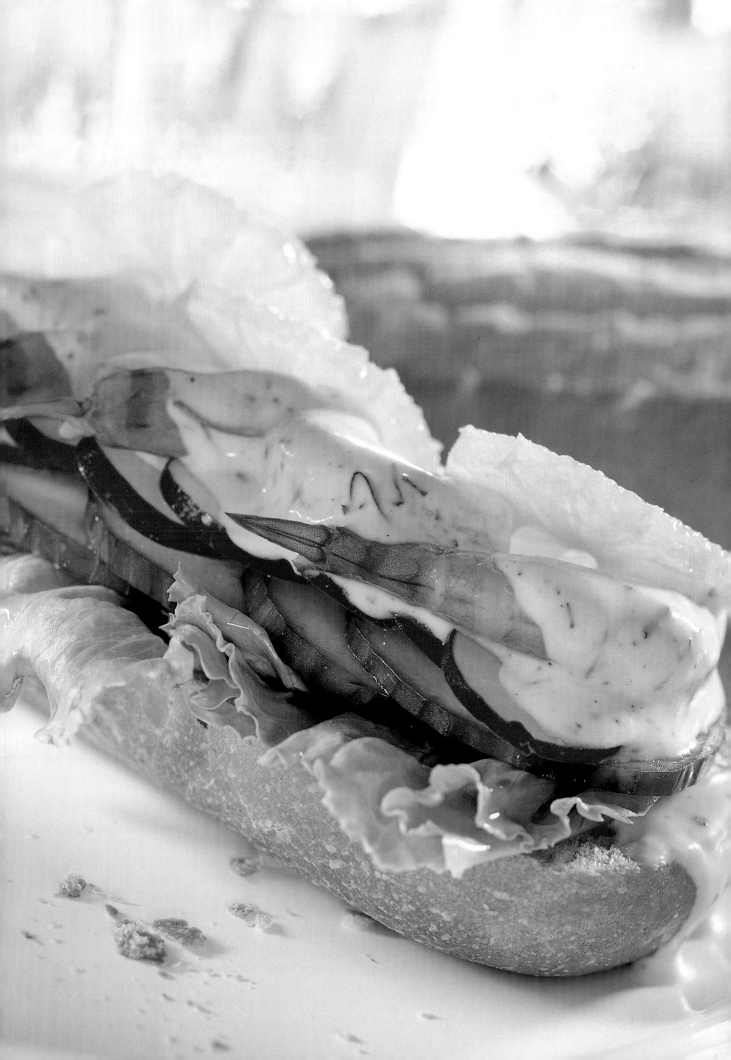

Rolls with Smoked Salmon, Chinese Cabbage and Green-Pepper Cream

Carbohydrates	●●◖	20 min.
Fat	●●	
Fiber	●●	

Per serving: approx. 233 calories
15 g protein · 8 g fat · 26 g carbohydrates

FOR 2 SERVINGS:
2 whole-grain rolls with pumpkin or sunflower seeds
4 to 5 leaves Chinese (Napa) cabbage
2 green (spring) onions
3 tbsp (45 mL) low-fat spreadable cream cheese
2 tbsp (30 mL) milk
½ tsp (2 mL) pickled green peppers or green-pepper relish
2 sprigs fresh dill
½ tsp (2 mL) lemon juice
Salt
2 oz (60 g) thinly sliced smoked salmon or gravlax

1 Toast the rolls in the oven at 300°F (150°C) and leave to cool. Wash, dry and cut the cabbage leaves into thin strips.

2 Remove any tough green part of the green onions, cut the remainder into quarters lengthwise, and then slice the quarters in half.

3 Stir the cream cheese into the milk. Using a fork, crush the pickled peppers and stir into the cheese mixture. Set aside 1 sprig of dill. Chop the remaining dill and stir in. Season with lemon juice and salt.

4 Cut the rolls in half and spread 1½ tsp (7 mL) of the cream mixture on the bottom of each. Arrange ½ the Chinese cabbage and green onions on top. Next, spread with 1½ tsp (7 mL) of the cream and a slice of salmon. Top with the remaining cabbage and cream. Garnish with the remaining dill. Cover with the upper half of each roll and serve immediately.

 TIP: Instead of rolls with seeds, you could use hearty onion rolls.

Tuna and Chive Cream Baguettes

Carbohydrates	●●●	20 min.
Fat	●●●	
Fiber	●●	

Per serving: approx. 307 calories
16 g protein · 12 g fat · 33 g carbohydrates

FOR 2 SERVINGS:
2 whole-grain baguette-style rolls
2 tbsp (30 mL) herbed crème fraîche or sour cream, divided
2 leaves iceberg lettuce
¼ English cucumber
½ tart apple
1 small (3½ oz/100 g) can water-packed tuna
2 tbsp (30 mL/30 g) sour cream
1 tbsp (15 mL) capers
¼ bunch chives
1 tsp (5 mL) lemon juice
Salt and freshly ground pepper

1 Core the apple, grate coarsely and set aside. Drain the tuna and crumble into a bowl.

2 Combine 1½ tsp (7 mL) of the crème fraîche with the sour cream in a small bowl and add the capers. Finely chop and stir in the chives. Add lemon juice and season with salt and pepper.

3 Cut the rolls in half and spread the remaining 1½ tsp (7 mL) crème fraîche on the bottom half of each. Place half a lettuce leaf on top. Thinly slice the cucumber, peeled or not, and arrange on top of the lettuce.

4 Fold ⅔ of the chive cream mixture into the tuna and spread over top of the cucumber. Garnish with the grated apple, the remaining chive cream and the lettuce. Cover with the top half of each roll and serve immediately.

 TIP: You can substitute coarsely chopped young herring for the tuna.

Rolls with Smoked Salmon, Chinese Cabbage and Green-Pepper Cream, top
Tuna and Chive Cream Baguettes, bottom

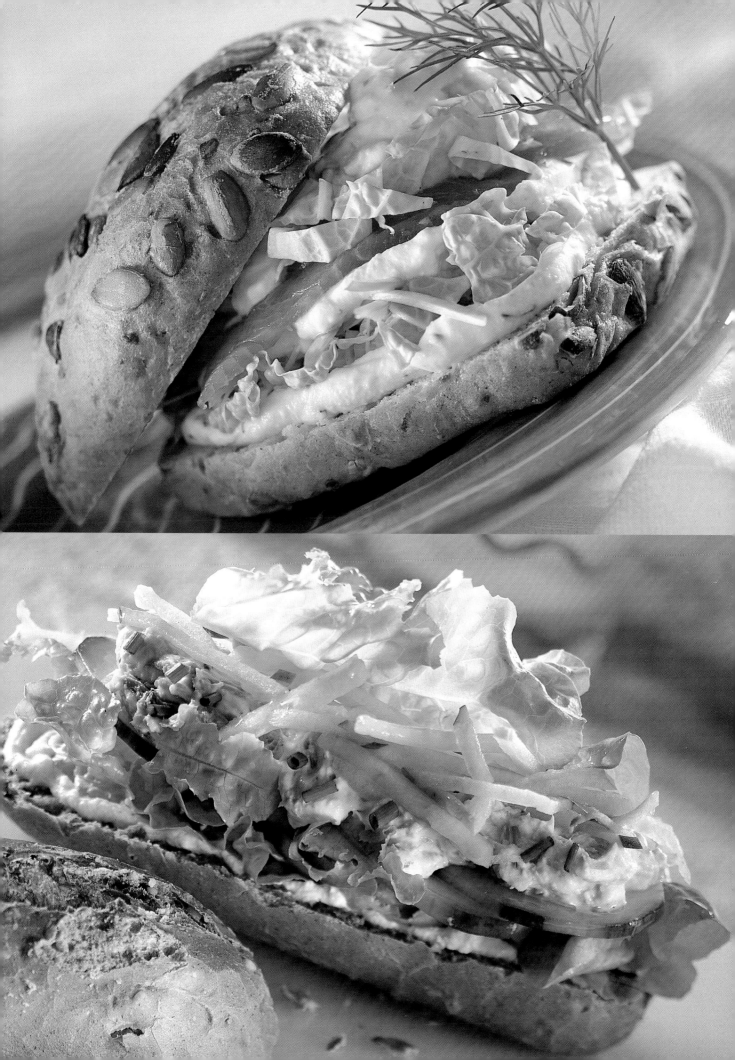

Vegetable Salad Sandwich

Carbohydrates ●●	20 min.
Fat ●●●	
Fiber ●	

Per serving: approx. 192 calories
11 g protein · 7 g fat · 22 g carbohydrates

FOR 2 SERVINGS:
1 small carrot
1 tender leek
½ bunch Italian (flat-leaf) parsley
1 tsp (5 mL) olive oil
Salt and freshly ground pepper
¼ tsp (1 mL) curry powder
4 slices whole-grain bread
4 tbsp (60 mL) cream cheese
2 leaves iceberg lettuce
2 tbsp (30 mL) low-fat yogurt
1 tbsp (15 mL) freshly grated Emmenthal cheese

1 Peel and finely grate carrot. Slice the leek lengthwise, wash thoroughly and cut into thin strips. Chop the parsley.

2 Using a pastry brush, coat a nonstick skillet with the oil and warm slightly. Add leek and cook on medium heat. Stir in the parsley, salt, pepper and curry powder and cook on low heat for 1 minute, stirring constantly. Leave to cool.

3 Add a little water to the cream cheese as needed and stir until creamy. Toast the bread, then spread with cream cheese. Shred the lettuce and arrange on the slices of toast.

4 Combine the vegetable mixture with the yogurt and cheese. Spread on two slices of toast and cover with the other two slices. Gently press down on the sandwiches and cut in half diagonally.

 TIP: The vegetable salad can easily make 3 servings, so you can save some for the next day.

Chicken and Curry Cream Sandwich

Carbohydrates ●●◖	40 min.
Fat ●●●	
Fiber ●●	

Per serving: approx. 288 calories
17 g protein · 12 g fat · 27 g carbohydrates

FOR 2 SERVINGS:
2 tbsp (30 mL) whipping (35%) cream
1 tsp (5 mL) mild curry powder
½ tsp (2 mL) lemon juice
Salt
Pinch cayenne
1 green (spring) onion
1 tbsp (15 mL/15 g) sour cream
3½ oz (100 g) skinless boneless chicken or turkey breast
1 tsp (5 mL) butter
Pinch ground ginger
½ ripe mango
2 whole-grain rolls
Lettuce leaves
Italian (flat-leaf) parsley leaves

1 Combine cream, curry powder and lemon juice, season with salt and cayenne, and set aside. Slice the white and light green parts of the onion into fine rings and combine with sour cream. Season with salt and pepper and set aside.

2 Cut the chicken in half crosswise. Heat butter in a nonstick skillet and brown the chicken on each side for 2 to 3 minutes. Season with salt and ginger.

3 Peel the mango and cut into thin slices, away from the pit. Cut the rolls in half and toast until golden brown.

4 Spread curry cream mixture on the lower half of each roll, cover with lettuce leaves, and arrange the onion mixture on top. Top with chicken. Arrange the mango slices over the chicken and garnish with parsley. Cover with the top half of each roll and serve immediately.

Vegetable Salad Sandwich, top
Chicken and Curry Cream Sandwich, bottom

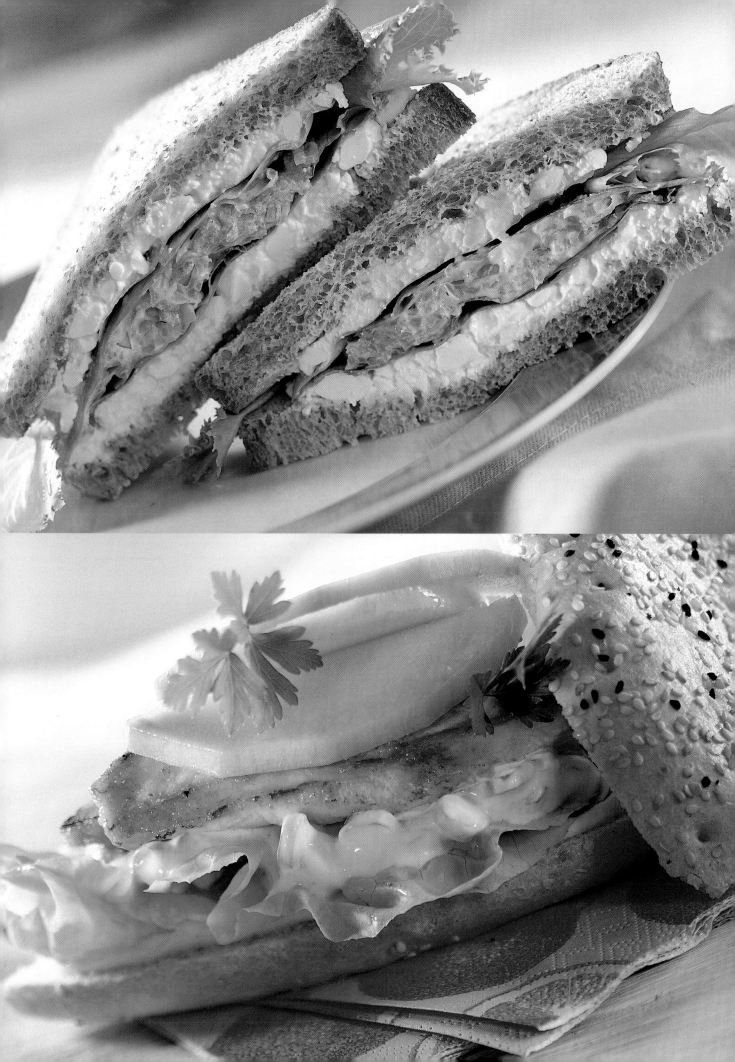

Pumpkin–Orange Jam

Carbohydrates	NA	40 min.
Fat	NA	(+ 30 min. resting)
Fiber	NA	

Per jar: approx. 310 calories
1 g protein · 0 g fat · 73 g carbohydrates

FOR ABOUT SIX 1-CUP (250 mL) JARS

1 lb (500 g) seeded, peeled pumpkin or squash (about 4 cups/1 L grated)
2 oranges (about 1½ cups/375 mL, peeled and sectioned)
3 or 4 pieces orange zest
4 tsp (20 mL/10 g) fresh ginger
3 tsp Pomona's Universal Pectin mixed with 1½ cups sugar, or 1½ cups gelling sugar 3:1
3 tsp (15 mL) calcium water (see instructions in pectin)
3 cups (750 mL) orange juice
3 tbsp (45 mL) orange liqueur or rum

1 Finely grate pumpkin. In a large saucepan, combine with orange sections, their juice and fairly large pieces of zest, scraped off with a vegetable peeler. Peel and finely grate ginger and combine. Stir in the sugar and pectin and calcium water. Leave the mixture to render its juices for 30 minutes.

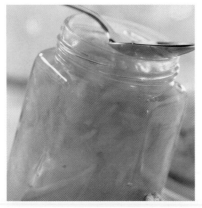

2 Mix in the orange juice and bring to a boil. Cook on medium heat for 5 minutes, stirring often. Remove orange zest and stir in the liqueur. Fill sterile jars with hot jam and seal with two-part preserving lids. Stand the jars upside down for 15 minutes, then turn upright and allow to cool.

!! **TIP:** Soak ½ cup (125 mL) currants for 20 minutes, drizzle with orange liqueur or orange flower water, and add to the jam before cooking.

Strawberry–Pineapple Jam

Carbohydrates	NA	30 min.
Fat	NA	(+ ½ to 2 hrs. resting)
Fiber	NA	

Per jar: approx. 434 calories
1 g protein · 2 g fat · 103 g carbohydrates

FOR ABOUT FOUR 1-CUP (250 mL) JARS:

4 heaping cups (1 L/700g) strawberries
¼ small ripe pineapple, or 1 cup (250 mL/200 g) drained canned pineapple pieces
2 tsp (10 mL/5 g) fresh ginger
1 piece lemon zest
2 tsp Pomona's Universal Pectin mixed with 1 cup (250 mL) sugar, or 1 cup gelling sugar 3:1
2 tsp (20 mL) calcium water (see instructions in pectin)

1 Hull and cut small strawberries in quarters or roughly chop larger ones (you should have about 3½ cups/875 mL prepared fruit). Place in a large saucepan.

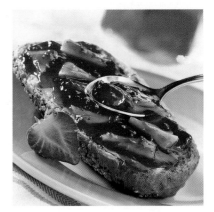

2 Peel, core and chop the pineapple and mix it in with the strawberries. Peel the ginger, chop finely and add to the fruit. Stir in a fairly large piece of zest, scraped off with a vegetable peeler, the pectin and sugar and calcium water. Leave the fruit to render its juices for ½ to 2 hours, stirring occasionally, until the sugar has dissolved.

3 Bring to a boil, stirring, then cook on medium heat for 3 to 4 minutes. Remove lemon zest.

4 Fill sterile jars with the hot jam and seal with two-part preserving lids. Stand the jars upside down for 15 minutes, then turn upright and allow to cool.

!! **TIP:** Use ½ cup maple syrup instead of the sugar.

Marmalades, Jellies and Jams

A breakfast with a low-sugar jam spread on thinly buttered whole-grain bread or rolls, or with low-fat quark or puréed cottage cheese, has very little effect on your blood glucose. Here are a few tips on preparing cooked jams with a low sugar content.

Choice of Fruit
The careful choice of fruit is essential to any good jam. The fresher and riper the fruit, the better the flavor. Prepare delicious spreads by using fruit from the garden, the farmer's market or the freezer. Whether you use one fruit or a combination is up to your imagination and taste.

Preparing the Fruit
Carefully wash the fruit and remove stems and flowers. Frozen fruit should be thawed in a sieve and the juice reserved. Since thawed fruit is already very soft, start with the juice, about ½ of the fruit and the other ingredients, then add the remaining fruit and cook the entire mixture once more.

Acidity of Fruit
Along with a fruit's natural pectin, a certain amount of acidity improves a jam's setting ability. Acid also reinforces the taste of the fruit and helps maintain its fresh color. You can increase acidity by adding a little fresh lemon juice. Depending on the amount being prepared, 2 to 3 tbsp (30 to 45 mL) is usually enough. Or you can combine low-acid with high-acid fruit.

Low acidity	High acidity
Banana	Gooseberry
Pear	Kiwi
Pineapple	Orange

Sugar—It Won't Work Without It
Sugar is the main ingredient in almost all types of marmalades, jams and jellies. Even in diabetic products, the amount of sugar is still fairly high. Table sugar is often replaced with fructose, but that doesn't really help control blood glucose levels. So forgo the fructose—you need to use sugar because it helps preserve the fruit by preventing the buildup of mold.

However, different combinations of sugar and pectin products can contain varying amounts of sugar. In Europe, a product called "gelling sugar" comes in three formulas:

Gelling Sugar 1:1
1 part fruit:	1 part gelling sugar
1 lb (500 g) fruit:	1 lb (500 g) gelling sugar

Gelling Sugar 2:1
2 parts fruit:	1 part gelling sugar
2 lb (1 kg) fruit:	1 lb (500 g) gelling sugar

Gelling Sugar 3:1
3 parts fruit:	1 part gelling sugar
3 lb (1.5 kg) fruit:	1 lb (500 g) gelling sugar

In North America, we can make similar blends of our own with such products as Pomona's Universal Pectin, which uses a calcium compound (monocalcium phosphate) to initiate gelling and thus permits a sugar content similar to gelling sugar 3:1—or less.

Because the shelf life of jam decreases with a lower concentration of sugar, low-sugar jams must be refrigerated. It's also better to produce sugar-reduced jams in small quantities. Once you've consumed these, you can make new ones with seasonal fruit. Freshly prepared jams have superior taste. The food industry uses preservatives such as sorbic acid, found on most lists of ingredients, to increase the shelf life of low-sugar jams.

Pectin
If you can't find gelling sugar or universal pectin, you need to add another pectin product to make the jam set. Pectins are sold in both liquid and powdered form, and in different formulas, such as Certo Light and Sure Jell for Low-Sugar Recipes. Follow the instructions closely. Test the firmness of the jam before you fill the jars: take a little jam, place it on a cold plate and refrigerate for a few minutes. If the jam is still runny, cook it for a few more minutes.

Other Ingredients
Herbs and spices can enhance the flavor of the fruit. The most widely used in some quarters are star anise, vanilla and allspice , but the following combinations of herbs and fruit work particularly well together:

Cinnamon: apple, plum, cherry
Anise: plum, black currant
Cloves: pear, apple, plum
Ginger: lemon jelly, orange, pineapple
Lemon balm: apple, lemon, red currant

If you don't have dental problems, you can enhance your jams with chopped or slivered almonds, roasted hazelnuts, walnuts, pistachios or macadamia nuts.

Foaming and Filling
Cooking fruit produces a layer of foam on the surface. Skim it off carefully. Use only clean, undamaged screw-top jars with two top parts for filling. If the upper rim of the jar is damaged, it can't be hermetically sealed. So-called twist-off lids have proven to be the most effective, but be sure to test the rubber seal to make sure it's not damaged. The most important criterion is cleanliness. Wash the jars in soapy water, rinse, and then sterilize by placing them in a large pot, filling it with water and boiling for 10 to 15 minutes. Leave in water until needed.

Fill the jars with the hot jam to roughly ½ inch (1 cm) below the rim and seal immediately with the two parts of the lid. Further processing in a hot-water bath is generally recommended. Once the jars have cooled, attach labels identifying the type of jam and the date prepared. Then store in a cool, dark place. Spreads that are very low in sugar are best kept in the refrigerator.

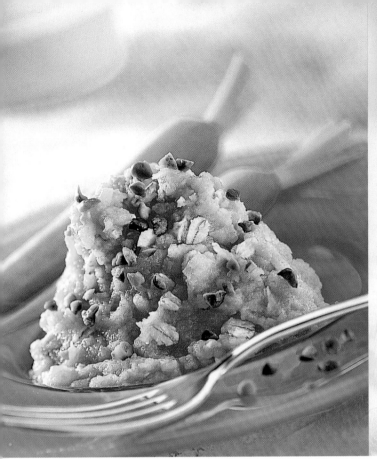

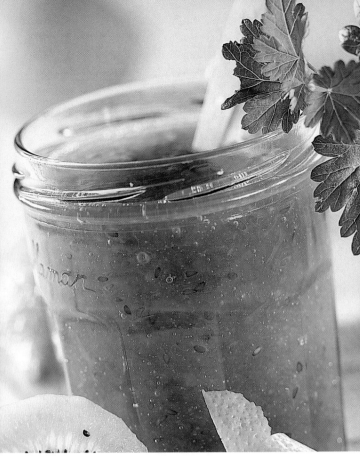

Sweet Creamed Carrots

Carbohydrates	◖	30 min.
Fat	–	
Fiber	●	

Per serving: approx. 49 calories
1 g protein · 2 g fat · 7 g carbohydrates

FOR 6 SERVINGS:
3 medium carrots (about 2 cups/500 mL/300 g diced)
½ cup (125 mL) water
1 apple
2 to 3 tbsp (30 to 45 mL) rolled oats
1 to 2 tbsp (15 to 30 mL) chopped pistachio nuts
A few drops liquid sweetener

1 Combine carrots and water in a medium saucepan, cover and cook on low heat for 10 minutes.

2 Meanwhile, core the apple, cut into quarters and dice. Add to the carrot and cook for 5 minutes.

3 Drain the carrot–apple mixture and mash with a potato masher. Stir in the oats and pistachios. Add sweetener to taste.

TIP: Store the creamed carrot in a screw-top or clamped jar in the refrigerator, where it will keep for about 5 days.

Gooseberry Jam

Carbohydrates	NA	30 min.
Fat	NA	
Fiber	NA	

Per jar: approx. 261 calories
3 g protein · 1 g fat · 57 g carbohydrates

FOR ABOUT FIVE 1-CUP (250 mL) JARS:
3¼ cups (800 mL/500 g) gooseberries
6 kiwi fruit (about 2 cups/500 mL/500 g, peeled and diced)
5 tbsp (75 mL) dry white wine
1¼ cup (300 mL/300 g) maple syrup
Zest of 1 lemon
1 package pectin for low-sugar jam

1 Wash and drain the gooseberries. Place in a large saucepan and stir in the kiwis. Crush with a potato masher. Add wine, maple syrup and lemon zest. Stir in pectin.

2 Bring the fruit to a boil on low heat, stirring occasionally. Cook for 3 minutes.

3 Fill jars with the hot jam and seal immediately with two-part preserving lids. Turn the jars upside down for 15 minutes, then turn upright and allow to cool.

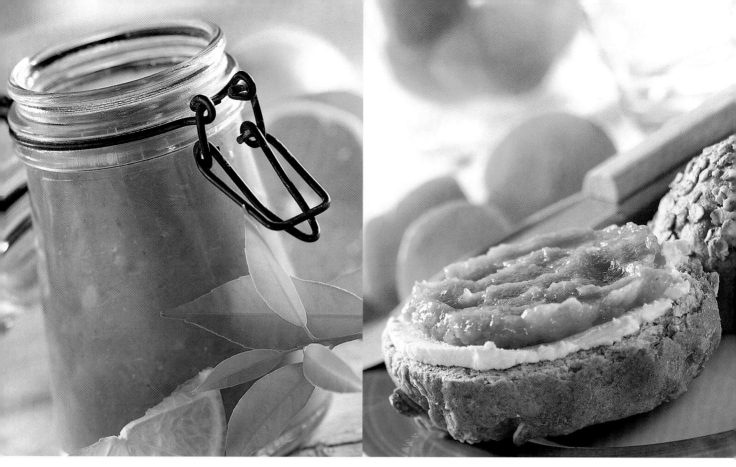

Orange–Pear Relish

Carbohydrates	NA	2 hrs.
Fat	NA	
Fiber	NA	

Per jar: approx. 215 calories
3 g protein · 1 g fat · 49 g carbohydrates

(500 mL) JARS
FOR ABOUT FOUR 2-CUP:

1½ lb (750 g) oranges (4 or 5)
1 lemon
1½ lb (750 g) pears (4 or 5)
1½ onions (about 1 cup/250 mL/150 g finely chopped)
2½ tbsp (37 mL/20 g) fresh ginger
¼ cup (50 mL/50 g) sugar
1 tsp (5 mL) liquid sweetener
1 tsp (5 mL) salt
¾ cup (175 mL) white-wine vinegar
1 small cinnamon stick
½ tsp (2 mL) mustard powder
2 tsp (10 mL) mild Madras curry powder

1 Peel the oranges, lemon and pears. Cut the citrus fruit in half crosswise and remove the pits. Core the pear. Finely dice the fruit.

2 Finely chop the onions and peeled ginger. Stir into the fruit. Stir in the sugar, sweetener, salt, vinegar, cinnamon, mustard and curry powder. Cover and bring to a boil.

3 Cook, partly covered, on low heat for 1½ hours, stirring occasionally. Fill clean jars that close with firm clamps, or screw-top preserving jars, and seal immediately. Stand upside down for 15 minutes, then turn upright and leave to cool.

Dried-Fruit Purée

Carbohydrates	NA	45 min.
Fat	NA	
Fiber	NA	

Per jar: approx. 418 calories
5 g protein · 1 g fat · 84 g carbohydrates

(250 mL) JARS
FOR ABOUT THREE 1-CUP:

3 cups (750 mL/500 g) unsulphured dried fruit: plums, apricots, apples, figs, etc.
⅓ cup (75 mL/100 g) dry white wine
2 tbsp (30 mL) lemon juice
1 tsp (5 mL) ground cinnamon
Pinch ground allspice

1 Soak the dried fruit overnight in just enough cold water to cover. Drain. Set aside the water.

2 Purée the fruit in a blender or with a potato masher. Combine with reserved water, wine, lemon juice, cinnamon and allspice in a saucepan. Cook on low heat for 15 to 20 minutes, stirring constantly, until the liquid evaporates.

3 Pour the hot mixture into clean jars and seal immediately with two-part preserving lids. Stand the jars upside down for 10 minutes, then turn upright and leave to cool.

TIP: The purée will keep for 2 to 3 months. The dried fruit is so sweet that no sugar is needed.

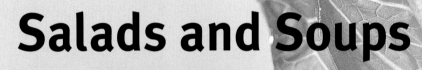

Salads and Soups

Cold and crunchy or hot and drinkable?

Soups and salads are classic appetizers. They stimulate the stomach and ensure that you'll soon feel full. But salad isn't just salad, and soup isn't just soup. In this chapter, you'll find not only simple small appetizers but also a variety of good solid alternatives to satisfy a huge hunger. And if you eat these with a slice of whole-grain bread and a healthy dessert, you'll have a nutritious meal that's easy to prepare.

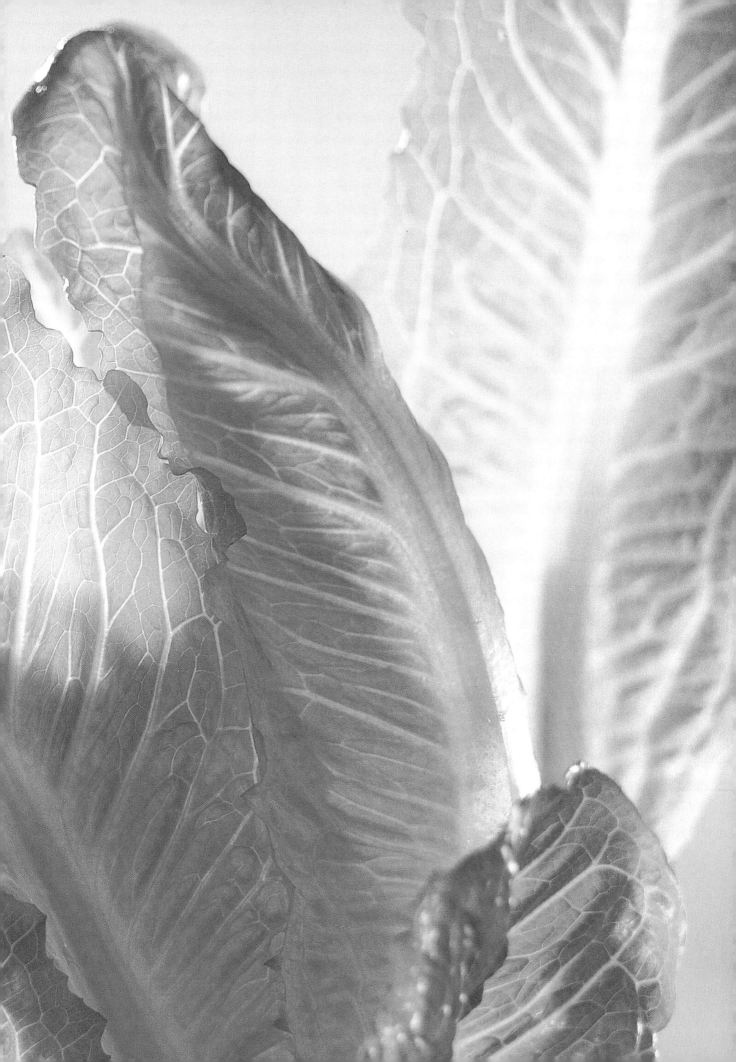

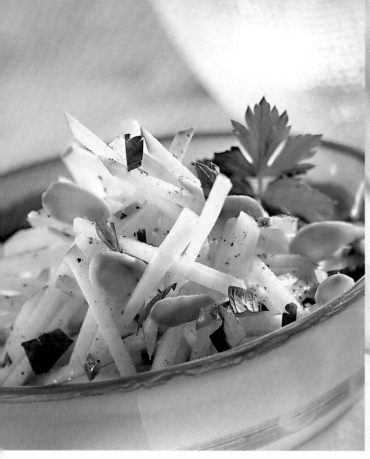

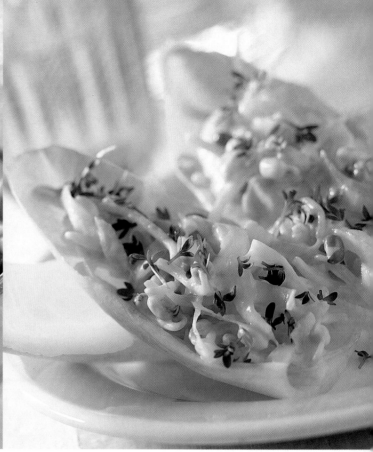

Apple–Celery Root Salad

Carbohydrates ●◖		**25 min.**
Fat ●●		
Fiber ●●●		

Per serving: approx. 154 calories
4 g protein · 7 g fat · 18 g carbohydrates

FOR 2 SERVINGS:
2 small apples
1 small celery root
Juice of ½ lemon
1 tsp (5 mL) cider vinegar
1 tsp (5 mL) walnut oil
2 tbsp (30 mL) slivered
  almonds

1 Halve and core the apples. Peel the celery root and remove any tough parts. Set aside a few leaves from the top for garnishing. Coarsely grate or julienne the apples and celery root.

2 Combine lemon juice, vinegar and walnut oil, and drizzle over the apples and celery.

3 Toast the almonds in a dry nonstick skillet on medium heat until golden. Coarsely chop the celery leaves. Sprinkle both over the salad and let stand for 10 minutes.

TIP: The salad will taste better if you use tart or spicy apples such as Granny Smith, Golden Delicious or russet.

Belgian Endive–Sprout Salad

Carbohydrates ●		**15 min.**
Fat ●		
Fiber ●		

Per serving: approx. 107 calories
7 g protein · 5 g fat · 12 g carbohydrates

FOR 2 SERVINGS:
Juice of 1 lime
1 tbsp (15 mL) walnut oil
⅔ cup (150 mL/150 g) fat-
  free yogurt
½ small bunch watercress
3 heads Belgian endive
1 cup (250 mL/100 g) mung
  bean sprouts
Salt and freshly ground
  pepper

1 Stir the lime juice and walnut oil into the yogurt. Rinse the watercress and stir into the mixture.

2 Wash and core the endives. Set aside 6 outside leaves. Finely chop the remaining endive and combine with the cress–yogurt dressing. Add sprouts. Season with salt and pepper and spoon the mixture into the reserved endive leaves.

TIP: If you don't want to serve the salad in the endive leaves, use 2 heads of endive and the sections of a small grapefruit. For a sweeter salad, use an orange instead of grapefruit.

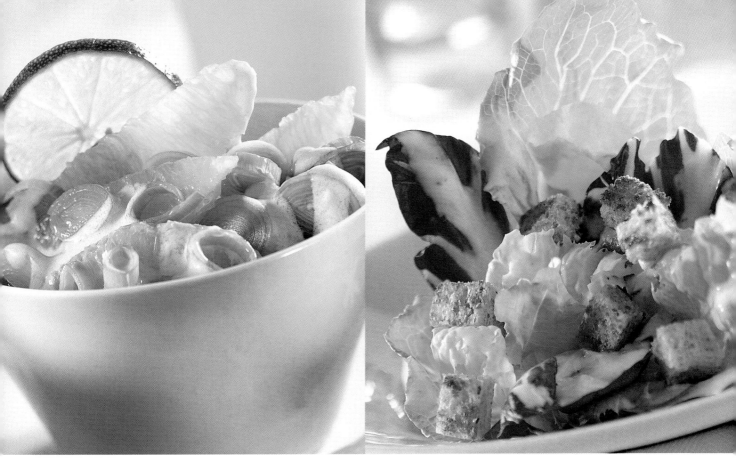

Orange–Leek Salad

Carbohydrates	●◖	15 min.
Fat	—	
Fiber	●	

Per serving: approx. 84 calories
3 g protein · 2 g fat · 15 g carbohydrates

FOR 2 SERVINGS:

1 small leek

2 oranges

Juice of 1 lime

3 tbsp (45 mL/40 g) low-fat yogurt

1 tsp (5 mL) walnut oil

2 tsp (10 mL) mild curry powder

1 Clean the leek, slice lengthwise and wash thoroughly. Slice the white and light green parts into thin strips.

2 Peel the oranges and remove the white pith. Combine orange sections with the leek.

3 Combine the lime juice with the yogurt and walnut oil. Season with curry powder. Arrange the oranges and leek on plates, drizzle with dressing and serve immediately.

TIP: On hot days, if you don't have much of an appetite, or if you want something light at the office, create a balanced meal by eating this salad with a slice of whole-grain bread and a protein-rich dessert.

Lettuce Salad with Croutons

Carbohydrates	●◖	20 min.
Fat	—	
Fiber	●	

Per serving: approx. 104 calories
4 g protein · 3 g fat · 14 g carbohydrates

FOR 2 SERVINGS:

2 tsp (10 mL) apple juice

½ cup (125 mL/100 g) low-fat yogurt

3½ tsp (17 mL) cider vinegar

Salt and freshly ground pepper

1 small red onion

2¼ cups (550 mL/125 g) mixed lettuce leaves

2 slices whole-grain bread

1 tsp (5 mL) olive oil

1 small clove garlic

1 Combine the apple juice, yogurt and vinegar in a small bowl and stir until smooth. Season with salt and pepper. Finely dice and stir in the onion. Tear the lettuce into bite-size pieces.

2 Remove the crusts from the bread and cut into cubes. Heat the oil in a small nonstick skillet. Peel and crush the garlic and lightly sauté to flavor the oil. Add bread cubes and brown lightly.

3 Arrange the lettuce on two plates, drizzle the dressing on top and garnish with croutons. Serve immediately.

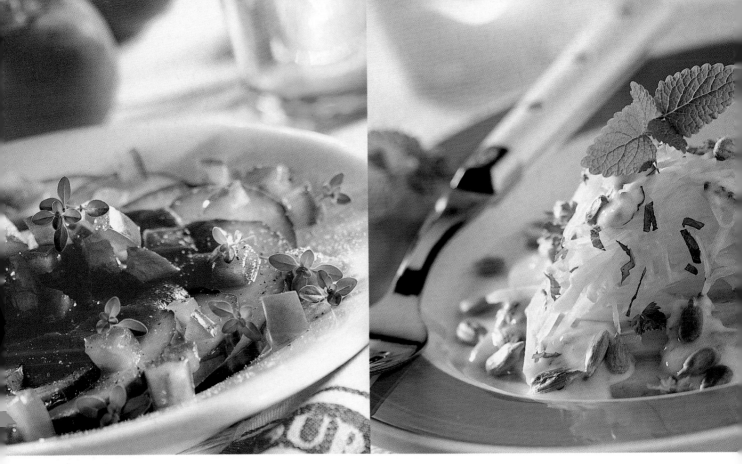

Cucumber Carpaccio with Tomato Dressing

Carbohydrates ●	30 min.
Fat —	
Fiber ●	

Per serving: approx. 72 calories
3 g protein · 2 g fat · 9 g carbohydrates

FOR 2 SERVINGS:
3 firm tomatoes
1 onion
1 tsp (5 mL) olive oil
Salt and white pepper
Ground cumin
1 tbsp (15 mL) tomato paste
3/4 English cucumber
2 tsp (10 mL) balsamic
    vinegar
2 sprigs lemon thyme

1 Lightly score the tomatoes crosswise, blanch, peel and dice coarsely. Set some aside.

2 Chop the onion and lightly sauté in hot olive oil on low heat until translucent. Stir in the tomato, salt, pepper, cumin and tomato paste. Cook on low heat for 10 minutes, then purée.

3 Finely slice the cucumber and arrange on two plates. Drizzle tomato sauce and balsamic vinegar over top. Garnish with remaining diced tomato and thyme leaves.

Kohlrabi with Grainy Mustard Dressing

Carbohydrates ◖	25 min.
Fat —	
Fiber ●	

Per serving: approx. 86 calories
5 g protein · 3 g fat · 8 g carbohydrates

FOR 2 SERVINGS:
1 tbsp (15 mL) sunflower
    seeds
1 cup (250 mL/300 g)
    peeled, grated kohlrabi
1/2 handful fresh chervil
4 to 5 lemon balm leaves
1/4 apple (30 g)
1/2 cup (125 mL/100 g) low-
    fat yogurt
1 tsp (5 mL) grainy mustard
Herbed salt

1 Toast the sunflower seeds in a dry non-stick skillet on medium heat until golden. Leave to cool on a plate.

2 Finely chop the chervil and lemon balm, and combine with the grated kohlrabi and sunflower seeds. Finely slice the apple and arrange on two plates. Top with kohlrabi mixture.

3 Combine yogurt and mustard in a small bowl and season with 2 pinches of herbed salt. Drizzle over the salad.

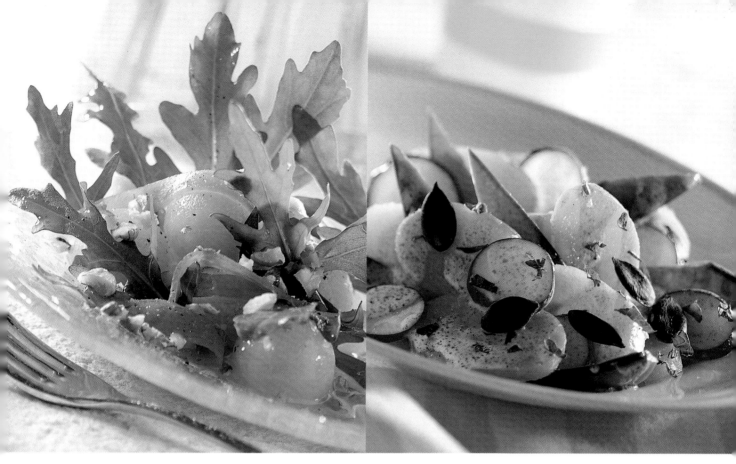

Arugula Salad with Melon

Carbohydrates	●●◖	25 min.
Fat	●●●	
Fiber	●	

Per serving: approx. 256 calories
13 g protein · 12 g fat · 26 g carbohydrates

FOR 2 SERVINGS:
1 bunch (150 g) arugula
2 oz (60 g) smoked ham, rind removed
½ Galia, honeydew or other melon
Salt and freshly ground pepper
2 tsp (10 mL) walnut oil
2 tbsp (30 mL) white-wine vinegar
2 tbsp (30 mL) chopped walnuts

1 Wash, stem and drain the arugula. Cut ham into thin strips.

2 Remove the seeds from the melon with a spoon and shape the flesh into balls with a melon baller. Combine melon balls, ham and arugula, and toss lightly.

3 Stir salt, pepper and walnut oil into the vinegar.

4 Arrange the salad on plates, drizzle the dressing over top and leave for the flavors to mingle. Sprinkle with walnuts and serve.

TIP: When you're buying melons, take a good sniff. A fully ripe melon should smell sweet.

Light Potato Salad with Snow (Mange-Tout) Peas

Carbohydrates	●●●●	40 min.
Fat	●●●	
Fiber	●●	

Per serving: approx. 239 calories
20 g protein · 11 g fat · 27 g carbohydrates

FOR 2 SERVINGS:
2 firm potatoes (300 g)
1¼ cup (300 mL/100 g) snow peas
3 tbsp (45 mL/40 g) low-fat yogurt
1 tsp (5 mL) mustard
2 tsp (10 mL) pumpkin seed oil
3 tbsp (45 mL) vegetable stock
Salt and white pepper
½ bunch radishes
2 tbsp (30 mL) pumpkin seeds

1 Boil the potatoes for approximately 20 minutes in a little water. Drain, leave to cool slightly, peel and slice.

2 Slice the snow peas diagonally into thirds. Steam or boil briefly (not more than 5 minutes) in a little salted water. Drain well.

3 Whisk together yogurt, mustard, oil, stock, salt and pepper. Slice the radishes and lightly toss with the potatoes and peas. Sprinkle with pumpkin seeds and serve.

Tuna–Mushroom Salad

Carbohydrates ◀		20 min.
Fat ●		
Fiber ●		

Per serving: approx. 112 calories
12 g protein · 5 g fat · 5 g carbohydrates

FOR 2 SERVINGS:
1 red onion
½ lb (250 g) mushrooms
1 sprig fresh oregano
1 sprig fresh thyme
3 fresh sage leaves
2 tsp (10 mL) olive oil
Salt and freshly ground pepper
½ (6 oz/170 g) can water-packed tuna
½ cup (125 mL/100 g) low-fat yogurt
1 tbsp (15 mL) wine vinegar
1 tbsp (15 mL) ketchup
A few lettuce leaves
2 tbsp (30 mL) small capers

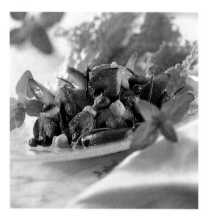

1 Peel the onion and cut into small wedges. Halve or quarter the larger mushrooms; leave the small ones whole. Finely chop the oregano, thyme and sage.

2 Heat the oil. Stir in the onion and sauté until translucent. Add mushrooms and cook for 2 to 3 minutes on high heat. Season with the herbs, salt and pepper, and leave to cool slightly.

3 Drain the tuna and place in a small bowl. Combine with the yogurt, vinegar and ketchup, and mix well or purée. Season with salt and pepper.

4 Tear lettuce into bite-size pieces. Arrange on two plates and cover with the mushrooms. Drizzle with the tuna dressing and sprinkle the capers on top.

Asparagus, Strawberry and Avocado Salad

Carbohydrates ◀		20 min.
Fat ●●●		
Fiber ●●		

Per serving: approx. 167 calories
6 g protein · 12 g fat · 13 g carbohydrates

FOR 2 SERVINGS:
4 spears green asparagus
Salt
1 cup (250 mL/150 g) strawberries
½ ripe avocado
1 oz (30 g) smoked turkey breast
3 tbsp (45 mL/40 g) buttermilk
3 tbsp (45 mL/40 g) low-fat sour cream
Pinch grated lemon zest
2 tsp (10 mL) lemon juice
5 fresh basil leaves
Salt
Liquid sweetener

1 Remove the tough end of each asparagus spear. Cook in lightly salted boiling water for 3 minutes. Remove and immerse immediately in ice water. Drain on a paper towel.

2 Halve or quarter the strawberries, depending on their size. Remove the pit of the avocado, then peel and dice the flesh. Slice the asparagus spears diagonally and julienne the turkey meat. Arrange the asparagus, strawberries, avocado and turkey on two plates. Finely chop the basil.

3 Combine buttermilk and sour cream in a small bowl. Add the lemon zest, lemon juice and basil. Season with a pinch of salt and a dash of sweetener. Drizzle over the salad plates.

!! **TIP:** Next to olives, avocados are the fattiest fruit, but they provide the nutritious unsaturated fatty acids we usually don't get enough of.

Asparagus, Strawberry and Avocado Salad, right

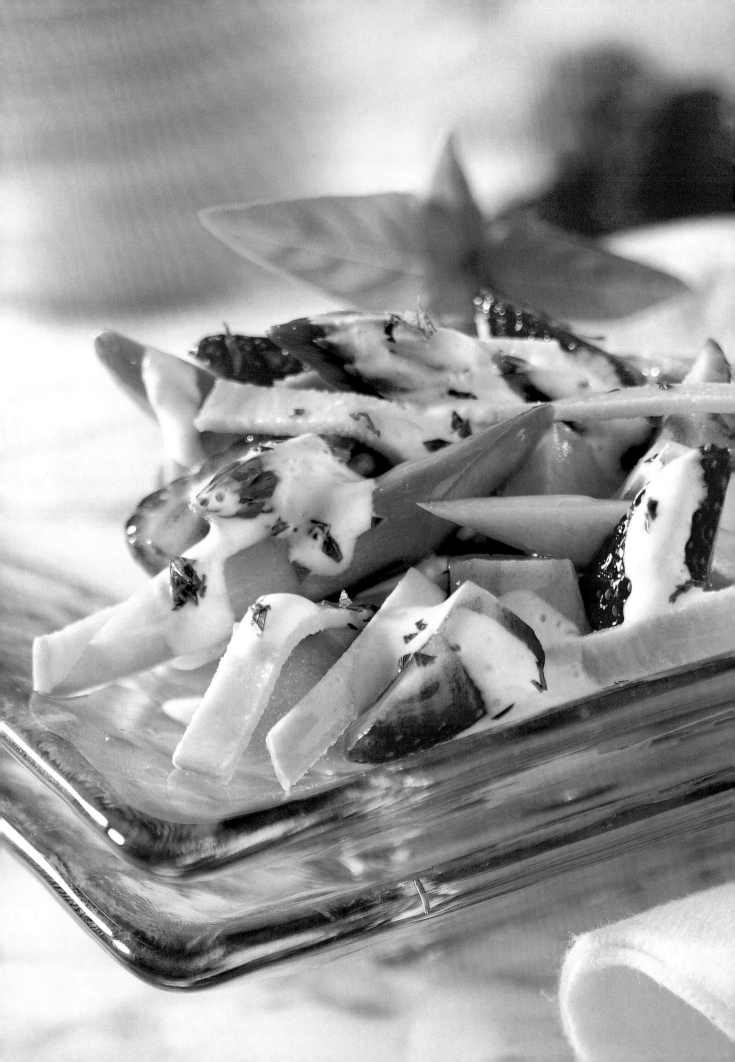

Green-Cabbage Salad with Shiitakes

Carbohydrates ◖		40 min.
Fat ●●		
Fiber ●●●		

Per serving: approx. 292 calories
10 g protein · 8 g fat · 5 g carbohydrates

FOR 2 SERVINGS:
½ small green cabbage
3½ oz (100 g) shiitakes
1 tbsp (15 mL) sesame oil
Salt
2 tsp (10 mL) lemon juice, divided
½ cup (125 mL/100 g) buttermilk
Liquid sweetener
½ handful parsley
½ red pepper
Freshly ground pepper

1 Cut the cabbage in half lengthwise, core and cut diagonally into fine strips. Remove the mushroom stems and slice the caps thinly.

2 Heat the oil in a nonstick skillet, stir in the mushrooms and lightly sauté on medium heat. Remove from heat. Add a little salt and sprinkle with 1 tsp (5 mL) lemon juice.

3 Whisk together the buttermilk, remaining lemon juice, salt and a dash of sweetener until smooth. Finely chop the parsley and stir it in. Dice the red pepper.

4 Arrange the cabbage, red pepper and mushrooms on two plates and drizzle with dressing. Season with pepper.

 TIP: If you can't digest raw cabbage, blanch it lightly ahead of time.

 TIP: You can use button mushrooms instead of shiitakes.

Lentils and Celery Root

Carbohydrates ●◖		1 hr.
Fat –		
Fiber ●●		

Per serving: approx. 88 calories
5 g protein · 2 g fat · 13 g carbohydrates

FOR 2 SERVINGS:
2½ tbsp (37 mL/30 g) uncooked lentils
⅔ (150 mL) cup water
Salt
1 tsp (5 mL) + 1 tbsp (15 mL) fruit vinegar
¾ cup (175 mL/100 g) celery root
⅓ pear
4 lettuce leaves (oakleaf preferred)
2 tbsp (30 mL) freshly squeezed orange juice
1 tbsp (15 mL) canola or vegetable oil
½ tsp (2 mL) medium mustard
1 tbsp (15 mL) chopped fresh marjoram
1 tbsp (15mL) chopped chives

1 Add lentils and 2 pinches of salt to water and bring to a boil. Cover and cook on low heat for 15 minutes. Drain and add the 1 tsp (5 mL) of vinegar. Leave to cool slightly.

2 Meanwhile, peel and finely grate the celery root. Thinly slice the pear. Place 2 lettuce leaves on each plate. Lightly toss together celery root, pear slices and lentils and arrange on the lettuce leaves.

3 Combine orange juice, oil, the 1 tbsp (15 mL) of fruit vinegar, mustard and marjoram. Drizzle over the salad, garnish with chives and serve.

TIP: Lentils contain a high amount of magnesium—the anti-stress mineral. A meal that includes ½ cup (125 mL) of dry lentils provides up to ⅓ of your daily magnesium requirement.

Green-Cabbage Salad with Shiitakes, top
Lentils and Celery Root, bottom

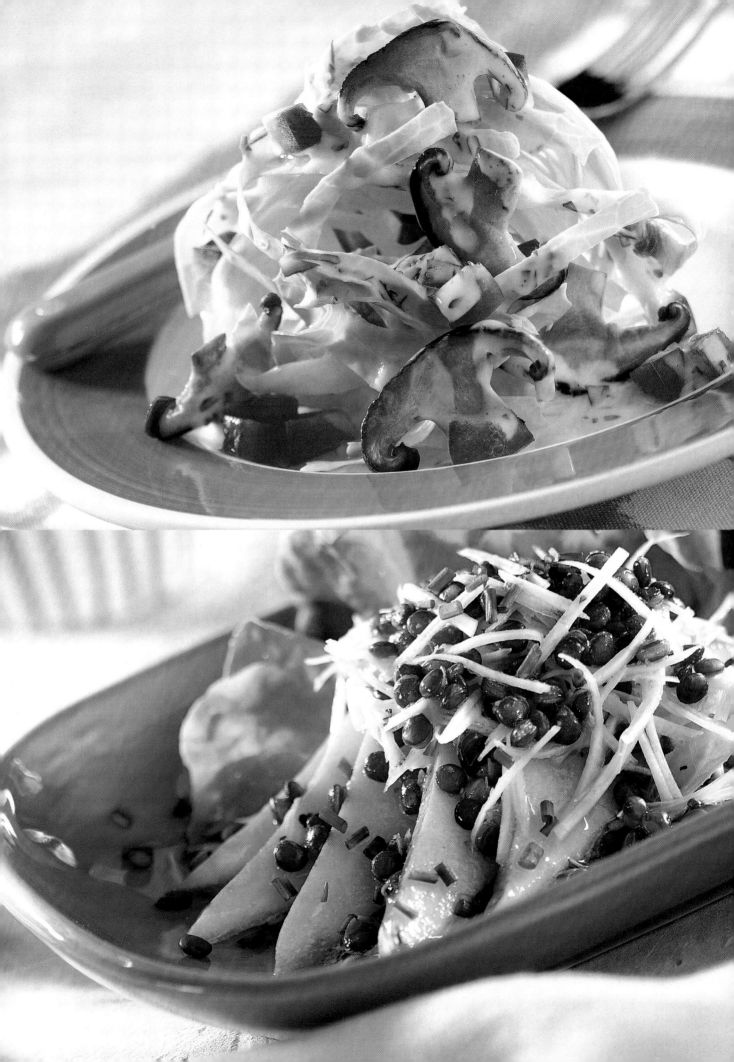

Exotic Fruit Salad with Chicken Breast

Carbohydrates	●●◖	35 min.
Fat	●●	
Fiber	●	

Per serving: approx. 135 calories
15 g protein · 5 g fat · 25 g carbohydrates

FOR 2 SERVINGS:
1 tsp (5 mL) flaked coconut
4 oz (125 g) skinless boneless chicken breast
Salt
½ tsp (2 mL) curry powder
2 tsp (10 mL) sunflower oil, divided
1 ripe kiwi fruit
½ very ripe papaya
1 tbsp (15 mL) fruit vinegar
½ tsp (2 mL) grated fresh ginger
2 pinches sambal oelek or other hot chili-based sauce
Liquid sweetener

1 Toast the coconut in a dry nonstick skillet until golden, being careful not to burn it. Leave to cool on a plate.

2 Season the chicken breast with 2 pinches of salt and the curry powder. Heat 1 tsp (5 mL) oil in a skillet (frying pan). Add chicken and cook on medium heat for 3 minutes. Turn and cover; cook on low heat for another 4 minutes. Remove and set aside on a plate.

3 Peel the kiwi, cut in half lengthwise and slice thinly. Peel the papaya, remove the seeds with a spoon and slice thinly.

4 While the chicken breast is still warm, slice and arrange on a plate with the fruit.

5 Combine the vinegar and 1 tsp (5 mL) oil in a small bowl. Stir in ginger, sambal oelek and 2 pinches of salt. Season with 2 to 3 dashes of sweetener and drizzle over the salad. Sprinkle with coconut and serve immediately.

Brussels Sprout, Pear and Prosciutto Salad

Carbohydrates	●◖	40 min.
Fat	●●●	
Fiber	●●●	

Per serving: approx. 214 calories
16 g protein · 11 g fat · 15 g carbohydrates

FOR 2 SERVINGS:
½ lb (250 g) Brussels sprouts
½ cup (125 mL) vegetable juice
1 small pear
1 tbsp (15 mL) lemon juice
2 oz (60 g) paper-thin prosciutto
½ cup (125 mL/100 g) low-fat yogurt
2 tbsp (30 mL) low-fat quark or puréed cottage cheese
1 tsp (5 mL) grated fresh horseradish
Salt and freshly ground pepper

1 Carefully remove most of the leaves from the Brussels sprouts and set aside. Score the stems of what's left of the Brussels sprouts crosswise.

2 In a medium saucepan, bring the stock to a boil. Place the Brussels sprouts in a steamer over it, cover, and cook on medium heat for 5 minutes. Add the leaves and steam for 1 to 2 minutes.

3 Peel the pear, quarter, core, cut into sections and sprinkle with lemon juice. Combine with the warm Brussels sprouts. Arrange on plates with prosciutto.

4 Combine yogurt, quark, horseradish, salt and pepper, and drizzle over the salad.

 TIP: You can use vegetable stock instead of vegetable juice.

Exotic Fruit Salad with Chicken Breast, top
Brussels Sprouts, Pear and Prosciutto Salad, bottom

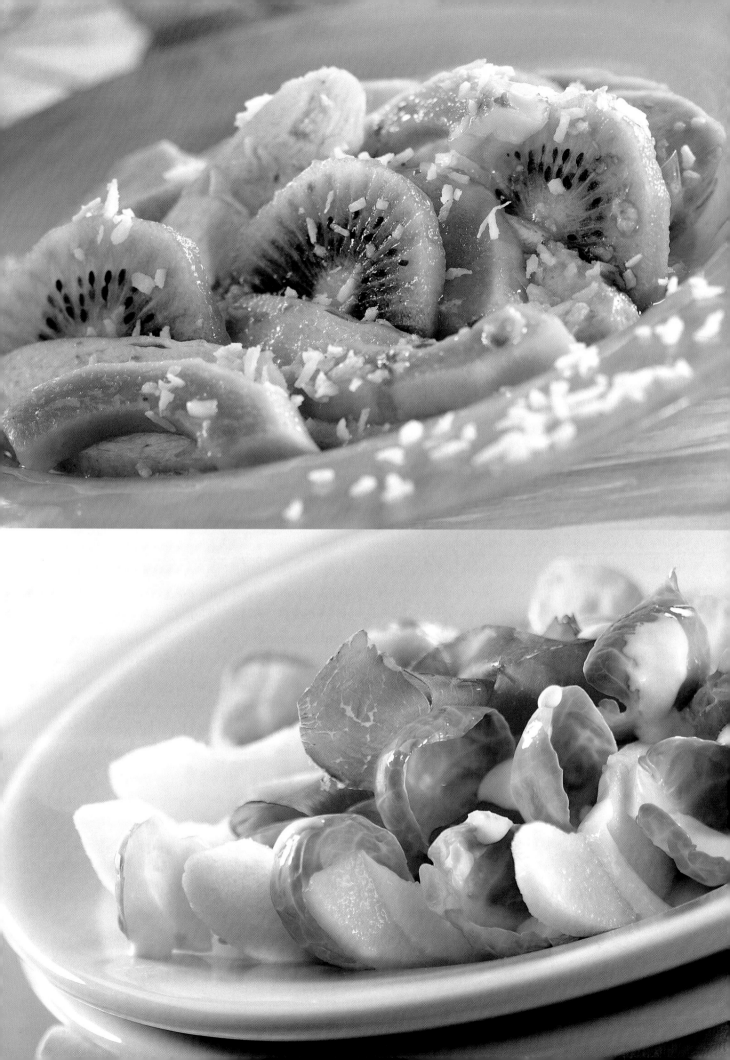

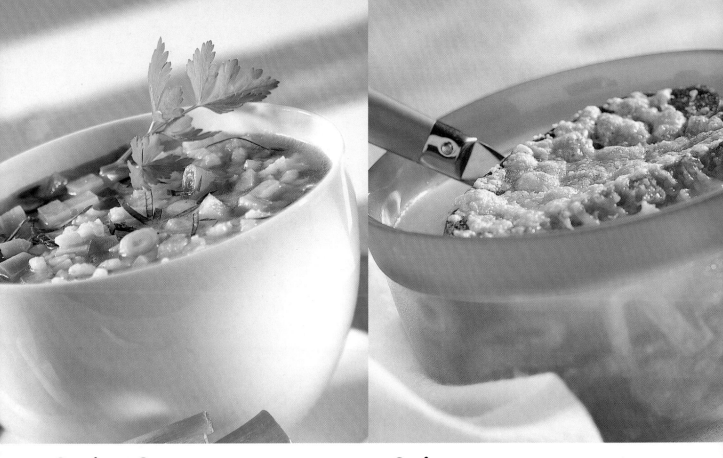

Spring Soup with Rice

Carbohydrates	●◀	40 min.
Fat	●●	
Fiber	●●●	

Per serving: approx. 127
4 g protein · 7 g fat · 13 g carbohydrates

FOR 2 SERVINGS:
1 medium carrot
1 small kohlrabi
1 bunch green (spring)
  onions
2 tsp (10 mL) olive oil
Curry powder to taste
2 tbsp (30 mL) short-grain
  rice
2½ cups (625 mL)
  vegetable stock
Freshly grated nutmeg
Salt and freshly ground
  pepper
½ bunch parsley

1 Peel carrot and kohlrabi and dice. Finely slice the green onions.

2 Heat the oil, stir in the curry powder and rice, and cook on low heat until the spices are fragrant and the rice is translucent. Stir in onions and cook briefly. Pour in the stock and stir in the vegetables. Cook for 20 minutes, or until rice and vegetables are soft and cooked through but not mushy.

3 Season with nutmeg, salt and pepper. Finely chop the parsley to use as a garnish and serve.

!! TIP: For a satisfying main meal, double the quantities and add 5 oz (150 g) frozen cooked shrimp just before the end of the cooking time.

Onion Soup

Carbohydrates	●●●	50 min.
Fat	●●●	
Fiber	●●●	

Per serving: approx. 276 calories
7 g protein · 14 g fat · 30 g carbohydrates

FOR 2 SERVINGS:
2 large cooking onions
1 tbsp (15 mL) olive oil
2 cups (500 mL) vegetable
  stock
½ tsp (2 mL) cornstarch
5 tbsp (75 mL) cream
2 thin slices rye bread
Salt and freshly ground
  pepper
1 tbsp (15 mL) chopped
  fresh marjoram
3 tbsp (45 mL) freshly
  grated Parmesan cheese

1 Thinly slice the onions. Heat the oil in a medium saucepan, add onions and cook on low heat until translucent. Pour in the stock and cook for another 30 minutes on low.

2 Preheat the oven to 400°F (200°C) or turn on the broiler (grill). Combine cornstarch and cream and stir into the soup.

3 Toast the bread. Season the soup with salt, pepper and marjoram, and pour into two ovenproof bowls. Cover each with a slice of toast. Sprinkle with Parmesan and heat in the oven or under the broiler until the cheese melts and browns slightly.

!! TIP: To reduce the fat content of this soup, use only 2 tbsp (30 mL) Parmesan.

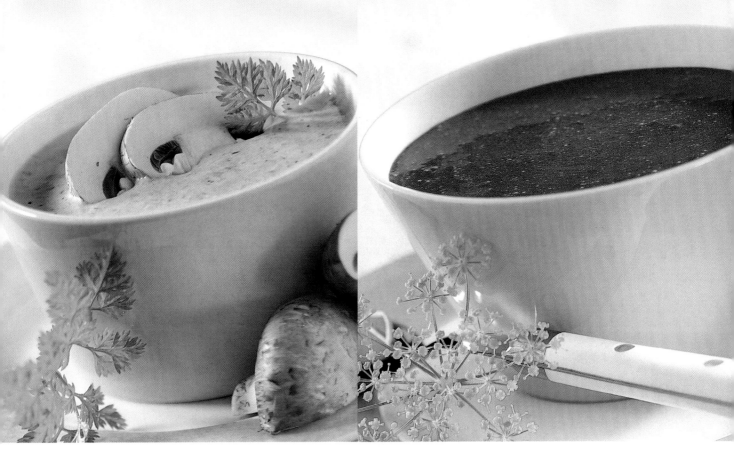

Mushroom–Leek Soup

Carbohydrates	◀	35 min.
Fat	●●●	
Fiber	●	

Per serving: approx. 146 calories
8 g protein · 13 g fat · 6 g carbohydrates

FOR 2 SERVINGS:
1 small leek
1 tbsp (15 mL) canola or vegetable oil
1 ⅔ cups (400 mL) chicken stock
5 oz (150 g) small mushrooms
½ cup (125 mL/100 g) sour cream
1 tbsp (15 mL) chopped almonds
1 bunch chervil or parsley
Salt and freshly ground pepper

1 Slice the leek lengthwise and wash thoroughly. Cut the white and light green parts into fine strips. Heat the oil, add the leek and cook on low heat until wilted. Pour in the stock and bring to a boil.

2 Slice the mushrooms. Set a few aside and sauté the rest on low heat for 10 minutes. Add leek, stock, sour cream, almonds and most of the chervil. Purée.

3 Season with salt and pepper, garnish with the remaining mushroom slices and chervil, and serve.

Creamed Beet Juice Soup

Carbohydrates	●◀	35 min.
Fat	–	
Fiber	–	

Per serving: approx. 74 calories
3 g protein · 2 g fat · 14 g carbohydrates

FOR 2 SERVINGS:
1 mealy (floury) potato
2 cups (500 mL) red-beet juice
½ tsp (2 mL) ground cinnamon
Ground cloves
Salt and freshly ground pepper
1 tbsp (15 mL) sour cream

1 Peel and dice the potato. Combine with the beet juice in a medium saucepan. Bring to a boil and cook on low heat for 15 minutes.

2 Purée potato and juice in a blender or food processor or with a potato masher. Reheat gently. Season with cinnamon, cloves, salt and pepper. Stir in the sour cream and serve immediately.

TIP: To make creamed carrot soup, simply use carrot juice instead of beet juice and curry powder instead of cinnamon and cloves.

Cream of Carrot Soup with Pistachios

Carbohydrates	●	25 min.
Fat	●●●	
Fiber	●●	

Per serving: approx. 148 calories
3 g protein · 10 g fat · 10 g carbohydrates

FOR 2 SERVINGS:
5 medium carrots
1 parsley root or small kohlrabi
1 tbsp (15 mL) butter, divided
1½ cups (375 mL) hot water
2 green (spring) onions
Salt and freshly ground pepper
Pinch ground coriander seeds
Pinch freshly grated nutmeg
Pinch ground ginger
Pinch cayenne
4 tbsp (60 mL) cream
1 tbsp (15 mL) chopped pistachios

1 Peel and dice the carrots and parsley root. Heat ½ the butter in a medium saucepan, stir in carrots and parsley root, and cook on medium heat for 1 minute. Add water and cook for 15 minutes.

2 Finely slice the white and light green parts of the onions. Heat remaining butter in a skillet (frying pan), add onions and cook on low heat until translucent. Set aside.

3 Purée the carrot and parsley root mixture. Season with salt, pepper, ground coriander, nutmeg, ginger and cayenne. Stir in the onions and cook on low heat for 5 minutes. Using a fork, whisk the cream until frothy and fold into the soup. Garnish with pistachios and serve.

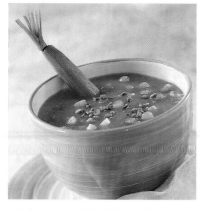

Broccoli Soup with Thyme Cream

Carbohydrates	●●	45 min.
Fat	●	
Fiber	●●●	

Per serving: approx. 187 calories
9 g protein · 6 g fat · 22 g carbohydrates

FOR 2 SERVINGS:
1 firm potato
1 (1 lb/500 g) bunch broccoli
1 medium onion
1 tsp (5 mL) olive oil
2 cups (500 mL) vegetable stock
Salt
1 tbsp (15 mL) sour cream
½ lime
½ tsp (2 mL) chopped fresh thyme
Freshly ground pepper
Pinch freshly grated nutmeg

1 Peel and finely dice the potato. Separate the broccoli florets. Cut off stems, peel and slice coarsely.

2 Heat the oil in a medium saucepan and lightly brown the onion on medium heat. Stir in the potato and cook slightly. Pour in the vegetable stock. Set aside about 3 cups (750 mL) of the broccoli florets and add what remains to the soup. Bring to a boil and cook, covered, on low heat for 25 minutes.

3 Meanwhile, place the broccoli florets set aside earlier in another saucepan or a steamer. Cook on low heat, covered, in a little salted water or steam for 10 minutes. Drain off the cooking water and keep the broccoli warm in the covered saucepan or steamer.

4 Stir the sour cream in a small bowl until smooth. Grate and stir in a little of the lime zest. Squeeze out 2 tbsp (30 mL) lime juice and stir into the cream with the thyme.

5 Purée the soup and season with salt, pepper and nutmeg. Stir in the broccoli florets. Ladle the soup into two bowls and serve with a dollop of thyme cream, and thin slices of lime, if desired.

Broccoli Soup with Thyme Cream, right

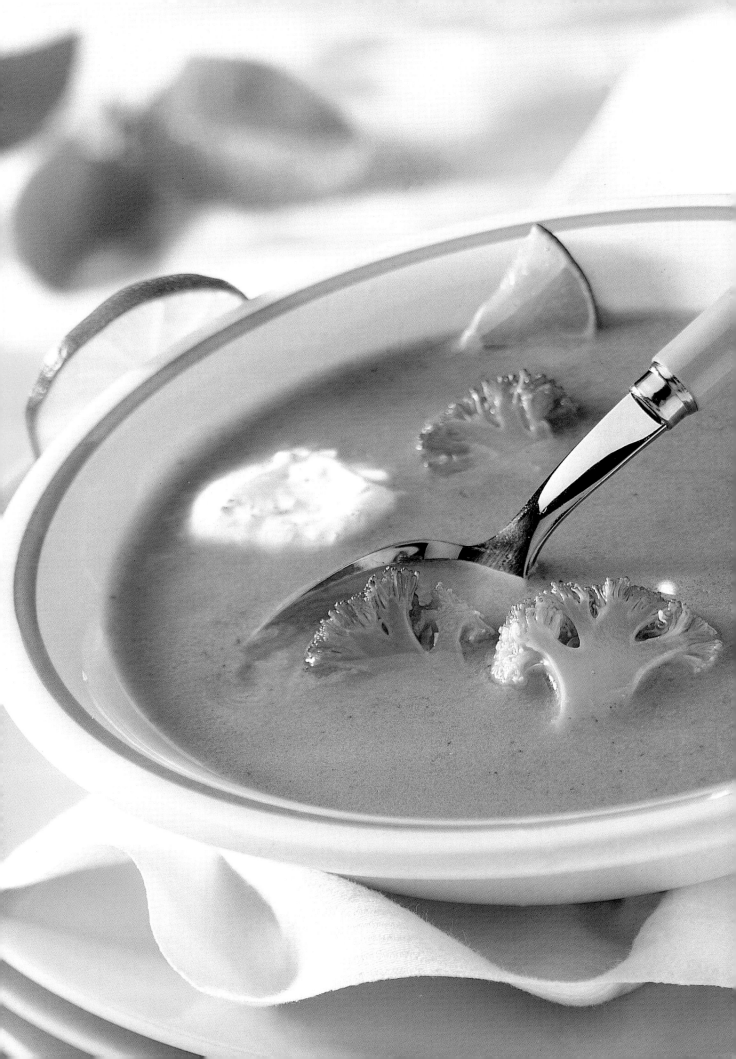

Barley Soup with Parmesan Cheese

Carbohydrates ●●●◖		1 hr.
Fat ●●●		
Fiber ●●●		

Per serving: approx. 317 calories
14 g protein · 12 g fat · 37 g carbohydrates

FOR 2 SERVINGS:
1 tbsp (15 mL) olive oil
1 small clove garlic
½ cup (125 mL/80 g) pearl barley
2 cups (500 mL) vegetable stock
½ bunch green (spring) onions
1 small zucchini (courgette)
2 small tomatoes
⅓ cup (75 mL/50 g) green peas
1 small sprig fresh rosemary
1 small sprig fresh thyme
½ tsp (2 mL) salt
1 to 2 tsp (5 to 10 mL) lemon juice
1 handful fresh basil leaves
¼ cup (50 mL/30 g) finely grated Parmesan cheese

1 Heat the oil in a medium-sized saucepan. Finely chop the garlic and cook on low heat. Rinse barley in cold water and drain. Stir into the saucepan and cook slightly, stirring constantly. Add vegetable stock and stir once. Cover and cook on low heat for 30 minutes.

2 Meanwhile, finely slice the white and light green parts of the onions. Finely dice the zucchini. Crush the tomatoes with a potato masher or chop finely.

3 Add onions, tomatoes, zucchini, peas, rosemary and thyme to the barley. Cook, covered, on low heat for 20 minutes.

4 Season with salt and lemon juice. Finely chop and garnish with basil. Serve with Parmesan on the side

Potato Soup with Smoked Salmon

Carbohydrates ●●●◖		35 min.
Fat ●●●		
Fiber ●●●		

Per serving: approx. 342 calories
13 g protein · 13 g fat · 36 g carbohydrates

FOR 2 SERVINGS:
3 mealy (floury) potatoes
3 green (spring) onions
1 clove garlic
1 bunch soup greens: spinach, collard greens, etc.
2 tsp (10 mL) butter
2½ cups (625 mL) vegetable stock
1 bay leaf
Pinch ground caraway
Salt and freshly ground pepper
2 tbsp (30 mL) sour cream
3 to 4 sprigs Italian (broad-leaf) parsley
2 oz (60 g) smoked salmon

1 Peel and dice the potatoes. Coarsely chop the white parts of the onions. Finely slice the light green parts and set aside. Finely chop the garlic. Chop the soup greens.

2 In a large saucepan, heat the butter and add the onions (white parts), garlic and soup greens. Sauté gently on medium heat, stirring constantly. Add potatoes and brown slightly.

3 Pour in the vegetable stock and add bay leaf and caraway. Cover and cook on medium heat for 15 minutes.

4 Finely chop the parsley. Purée the soup coarsely and season with salt and pepper. Stir in ½ of the parsley.

5 Slice the smoked salmon into thin strips. Ladle the soup into soup bowls and garnish with the sour cream and salmon. Sprinkle onion greens and remaining parsley on top.

Barley Soup with Parmesan Cheese, top
Potato Soup with Smoked Salmon, bottom

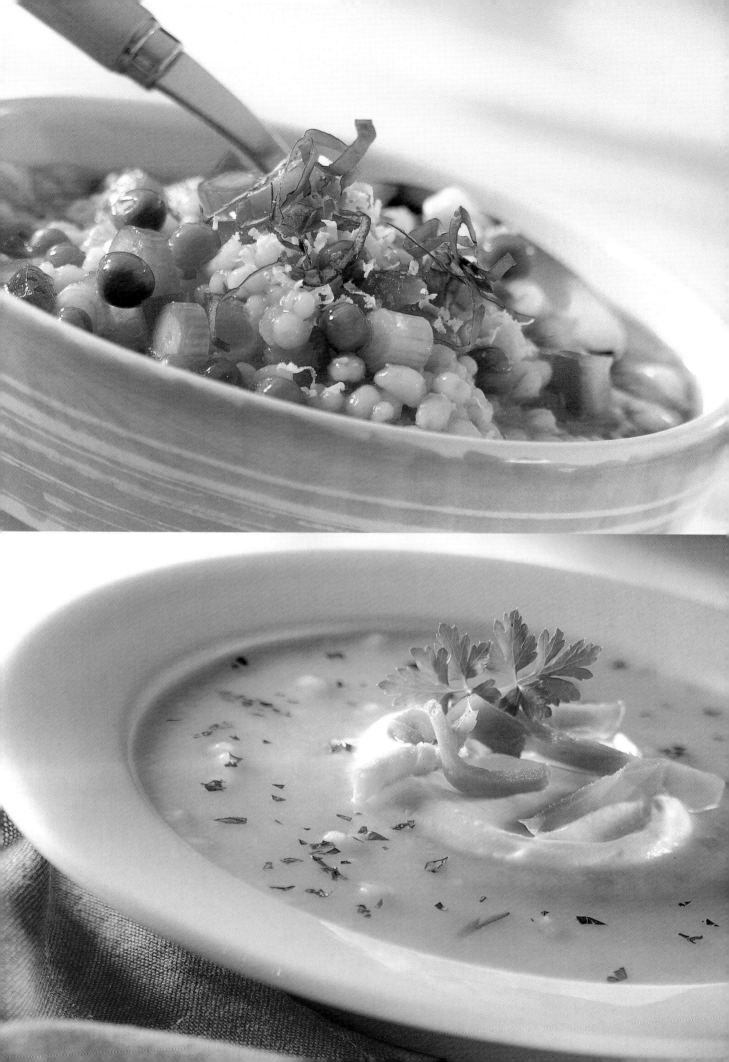

Lean Pea Soup

Carbohydrates ●●●		**2 hrs.**
Fat –		**(+ overnight soaking)**
Fiber ●●●		

Per serving: approx. 213 calories
17 g protein · 3 g fat · 31 g carbohydrates

FOR 2 SERVINGS:
½ cup (125 mL/125 g) dried yellow peas
2 cups (500 mL) cold water
⅔ cup (150 mL/80 g) celery root
1½ medium carrots
1 small leek
½ bunch parsley
½ tsp (2 mL) salt
1 tsp (5 mL) dried marjoram
1 tsp (5 mL) canola or vegetable oil
1 small onion

1 Soak the peas in cold water for 8 to 12 hours, or overnight.

2 Peel and finely dice the celery root. Peel the carrots, cut in half lengthwise and slice. Slice the leek lengthwise, wash thoroughly and slice thinly. Remove the larger stems of the parsley and tie the sprigs together with kitchen twine.

3 Add the vegetables, parsley stems, salt and marjoram to the peas and water, and bring to a boil. Cover and cook on low heat for 1 hour and 20 minutes. Remove the parsley. Stir in additional water as needed.

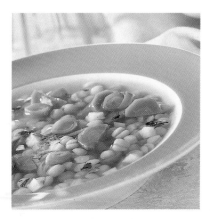

4 Heat the oil and brown the onion on medium heat. Finely chop the remaining parsley and stir into the onion. Ladle soup into bowls, garnish with onion and parsley mixture and serve.

Quick and Easy Tomato Soup

Carbohydrates ◖		**15 min.**
Fat ●●		
Fiber ●		

Per serving: approx. 170 calories
4 g protein · 9 g fat · 8 g carbohydrates

FOR 2 SERVINGS:
1 tbsp (15 mL) olive oil
1 onion
1 small clove garlic
14-oz (398 mL) can tomatoes
1 tbsp (15 mL) tomato paste
¼ cup (50 mL) dry red wine
1 cup (250 mL) vegetable stock
1 bay leaf
Salt and freshly ground pepper
¼ tsp (1 mL) sweet paprika
Pinch cayenne
2 sprigs fresh basil
2 tbsp (30 mL) freshly grated pecorino or Gouda cheese

1 Chop the onion and garlic. Heat the oil in a medium saucepan, stir in the onion and garlic, and cook on low heat until translucent.

2 Drain the tomatoes, reserving the juice. Chop coarsely and stir into the saucepan. Mix in the tomato paste and cook briefly. Add reserved tomato juice, wine, stock and bay leaf, and cook the soup, covered, on medium heat for 10 minutes.

3 Season with salt, pepper, paprika and cayenne. Purée.

4 Cut the basil into fine strips and stir through the soup. Ladle into warmed bowls and sprinkle with the cheese.

‼ TIP: According to many gourmets, grated cheese is essential as a topping for casseroles or the finishing touch in a soup or a salad. In the case of this soup, the flavor won't suffer if you decide to omit the cheese, but your fat intake will be significantly lower.

Quick and Easy Tomato Soup, right

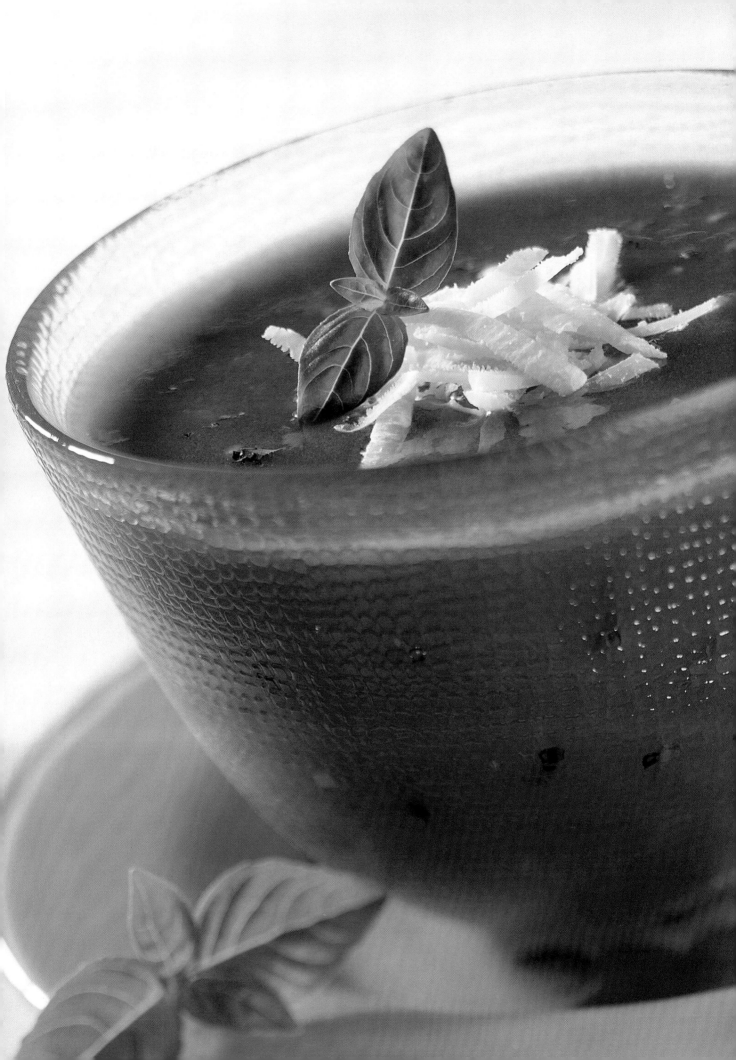

Vegetables

A meal with plenty of crunchy fresh vegetables leaves you feeling fit and full of energy.

Colorful vegetable dishes are not just a feast for the eyes. Since vegetables can be prepared in a variety of ways and combinations, the possibilities are endless and always interesting. In addition, you can enjoy them as often as you want—raw or cooked—without affecting your blood glucose levels.

And the big plus? You also get a lot of energy-boosting vitamins and minerals.

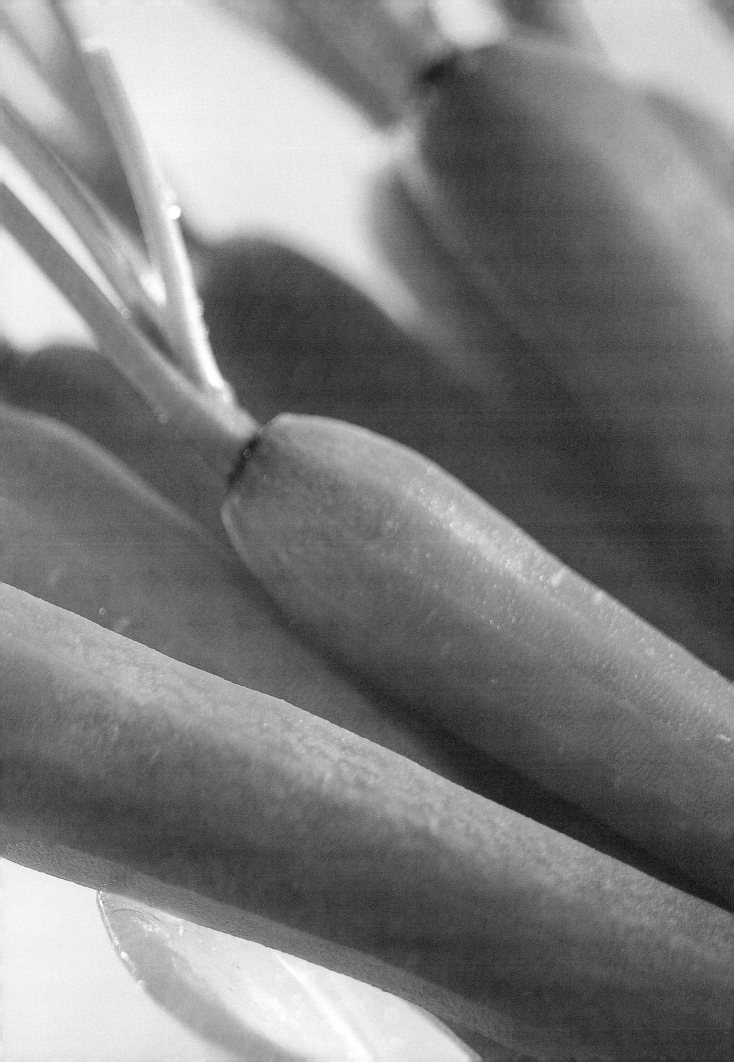

White Asparagus with New Potatoes and Chervil Sauce

Carbohydrates	●●●◖	1 hr.
Fat	●●●	
Fiber	●●●	

Per serving: approx. 348 calories
15 g protein · 13 g fat · 42 g carbohydrates

FOR 2 SERVINGS:
14 oz (400 g) small new potatoes
Salt
Sugar
2 lb (1 kg) white asparagus
2 tbsp (30 mL/20 g) margarine
1 heaping tsp (5 mL/10 g) flour
1 cup (250 mL) whole milk
Pinch nutmeg
1 to 2 tsp (5 to 10 mL) lemon juice
Pinch lemon zest
½ handful fesh chervil

1 Barely cover potatoes with salted water and cook for 20 minutes.

2 In a large saucepan, combine about 4 cups (1 L) water, 1 tsp (5 mL) salt and 2 pinches sugar, and bring to a boil. Add asparagus and cook on low heat for 15 minutes.

3 Meanwhile, melt margarine in a small saucepan on low heat. Whisk in the flour and brown slightly. Whisk the milk into the roux and cook on low heat for 10 minutes, stirring occasionally.

4 Just before the asparagus is cooked, add ½ cup (50 mL) of the cooking water to the white sauce. Remove from heat and season with salt, nutmeg, lemon zest, lemon juice and a little sugar. Finely chop most of the chervil and stir into the sauce. Keep warm over low heat.

5 Drain the potatoes and leave to steam dry for a few minutes. Drain the asparagus and serve immediately with potatoes and sauce, garnished with the remaining chervil leaves.

Vegetable Ragout with Saffron Gnocchi

Carbohydrates	●●●	30 min.
Fat	–	
Fiber	●●●	

Per serving: approx. 278 calories
7 g protein · 3 g fat · 35 g carbohydrates

FOR 2 SERVINGS:
4 cups (1 L/400 g) mixed spring vegetables: carrots, green (spring) onions, snow (mange-tout) peas, etc.
1 cup (250 mL) vegetable stock
⅔ cup (150 mL) skim milk
⅓ cup (75 mL/40 g) whole wheat semolina
Salt
Pinch ground saffron
1 tbsp (15 mL) chopped fresh parsley
1 handful fresh chervil leaves
Freshly ground pepper

1 Finely slice the vegetables and stir into a large saucepan with the stock. Bring to a boil, cover and cook on low heat for 10 to 15 minutes.

2 Meanwhile, heat the milk in a small saucepan. Gradually add the semolina, stirring constantly, and cook on low heat until thick. Stir in salt, saffron and parsley.

3 Finely chop the chervil and mix with the vegetables. Season with salt and pepper.

4 Using two spoons, form the semolina mixture into gnocchi shaped like quenelles, or small footballs. Arrange on a plate and serve immediately with vegetables.

!! **TIP:** The saffron gives the gnocchi a sophisticated flavor, as well as the golden color usually obtained with an egg yolk. This version is low in fat and cholesterol-free.

White Asparagus with New Potatoes and Chervil Sauce, top
Vegetable Ragout with Saffron Gnocchi, bottom

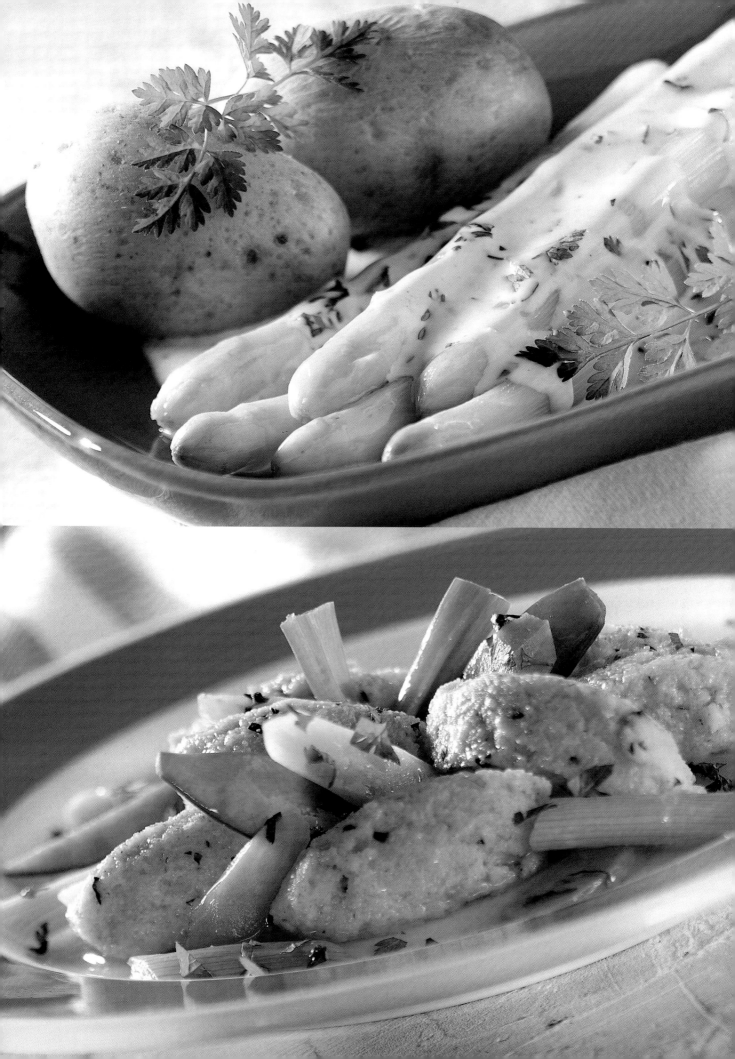

Twice-Cooked Potatoes with Quark and Tomato Salad

Carbohydrates	●●●◖	50 min.
Fat	—	(+ 10 to 15 min. baking)
Fiber	●●	

Per serving: approx. 267 calories
23 g protein · 2 g fat · 38 g carbohydrates

FOR 2 SERVINGS:
2 large firm potatoes (about 1 lb/500 g)
Salt
1 cup (250 mL/250 g) low-fat quark or puréed cottage
   cheese
1 tbsp (15 mL) mineral water
½ handful watercress
Freshly grated nutmeg
Liquid sweetener
1 tbsp (15 mL) olive oil
1 tsp (5 mL) balsamic vinegar
2 small tomatoes
1 small onion

1 Barely cover the potatoes with salted water, bring to a boil, then cover and cook on low heat for 30 minutes.

2 Meanwhile, stir the quark and the mineral water together in a bowl until smooth. Finely chop the watercress and stir it in along with 2 or 3 pinches of salt, a little nutmeg and a dash of sweetener. Set aside.

3 Whisk oil and vinegar together in a salad bowl and season with a pinch of salt. Cut the tomatoes into bite-size pieces and add to the dressing. Finely slice and add the onion. Toss lightly.

4 Preheat the oven broiler (grill). Drain the potatoes, cut in half lengthwise and arrange on a sheet of aluminum foil about 8 x 12 inches (20 x 30 cm). Sprinkle a little salt on each half of potato. Place on a rack in the middle of the oven and broil (grill) for 10 to 15 minutes, until lightly browned. Serve with quark, garnished with watercress leaves, and tomato salad.

Eggplant (Aubergine) with Tomatoes and Mint Yogurt

Carbohydrates	●◖	45 min.
Fat	●●●	
Fiber	●●●	

Per serving: approx. 268 calories
17 g protein · 14 g fat · 16 g carbohydrates

FOR 2 SERVINGS:
2 medium eggplants
1 tbsp (15 mL) olive oil
2 tomatoes
Salt and freshly ground pepper
½ tsp (2 mL) dried oregano
½ cup (125 mL/50 g) freshly grated Parmesan cheese
¾ cup (175 mL/200 g) low-fat yogurt
1 tsp (5 mL) lemon juice
1 small clove garlic
2 sprigs fresh mint or ½ tsp (2 mL) dried

1 Preheat the oven to 400°F (200°C). Cut the eggplant into ½-inch (1 cm) slices. Heat the oil in a nonstick skillet (frying pan), add eggplant and brown lightly on both sides on medium heat. Leave to cool. Set aside.

2 Slice the tomatoes. Alternate eggplant and tomato slices in an ovenproof dish. Season with salt, pepper and oregano. Sprinkle with the Parmesan and bake in the preheated oven for 20 minutes.

3 Meanwhile, combine yogurt and lemon juice. Peel and crush the garlic and stir into the yogurt. Stir in salt, pepper and mint, and serve on the side, garnished with additional mint leaves.

!! TIP: You can substitute zucchini (courgettes) for the eggplant in this recipe. Slice the zucchini into rounds and brown on both sides in a little oil in a nonstick skillet. Alternate with the tomatoes in a baking dish and bake as indicated.

Twice-Cooked Potatoes with Quark and
Tomato Salad, top
Eggplant with Tomatoes and Mint Yogurt, bottom

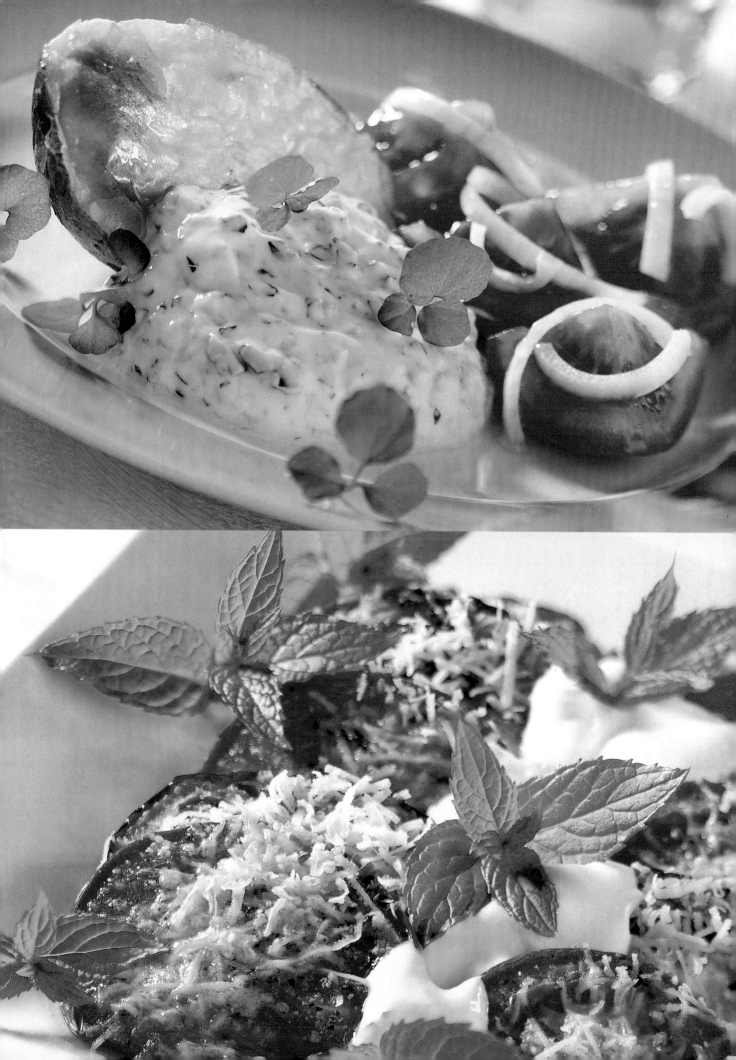

Spanish Omelet with Vegetables

Carbohydrates	●◖	40 min.
Fat	+	
Fiber	●●●	

Per serving: approx. 221 calories
11 g protein · 17 g fat · 18 g carbohydrates

FOR 2 SERVINGS:
2 tbsp (30 mL) olive oil, divided
2 firm medium potatoes
1 red pepper
1 small eggplant (aubergine)
1 onion
1 clove garlic
2 eggs
Salt and freshly ground pepper
2 tbsp (30 mL) chopped fresh parsley

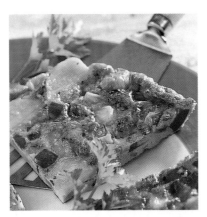

1 Slice the potatoes. Heat 1 tbsp (15 mL) of the olive oil in a skillet (frying pan). Add the potatoes and brown on medium heat, turning often. Dice the red pepper and eggplant. Chop the onion and garlic. Combine the vegetables and garlic with the potatoes and sauté for 10 minutes, stirring often. Season lightly with salt and pepper. Leave to cool.

2 Whisk the eggs with a little salt, a pinch of pepper and the parsley. Stir in the potato–vegetable mixture. Heat 1 tsp (5 mL) of the oil in the skillet. Pour in the egg mixture and spread smooth. Let it set on low heat. Gently shake the skillet back and forth, adding a little oil if necessary, and flip it over. Cook until golden on both sides, divide into quarters and serve immediately.

 TIP: A green salad goes well with this dish.

Pan-Fried Vegetables with Eggs

Carbohydrates	●	30 min.
Fat	●●●	
Fiber	●●●	

Per serving: approx. 199 calories
14 g protein · 11 g fat · 11 g carbohydrates

For 2 servings:
³⁄₄ cup (175 mL/75 g) bean sprouts
1 tsp (5 mL) olive oil
1 tsp (5 mL) grated fresh ginger
1 clove garlic
2 green (spring) onions
1 zucchini (courgette)
1 small eggplant (aubergine)
1 small red pepper
¹⁄₂ cup (125 mL) vegetable stock
1 to 2 tbsp (15 to 30 mL) soy sauce
Black pepper
2 eggs
2 tbsp (30 mL) freshly grated Parmesan cheese
1 sprig fresh basil

1 Rinse and drain the bean sprouts. Chop the garlic and slice the green onions. Dice the zucchini, eggplant and red pepper.

2 Heat the oil, add ginger, garlic and green onions, and sauté on low heat for 1 minute. Stir in the zucchini, eggplant and red pepper, and sauté for 6 minutes. Add stock, soy sauce and pepper to taste and cook for 1 minute.

3 Using a big spoon, make two wells in the center of the vegetables and carefully crack 1 egg into each. Sprinkle with Parmesan. Cover and cook for 5 minutes, until the egg white sets. Finely chop and sprinkle basil on top.

TIP: Eggs are rich in vitamins and protein, but they are also high in fat and cholesterol. That's why egg dishes should only be eaten once or twice a week.

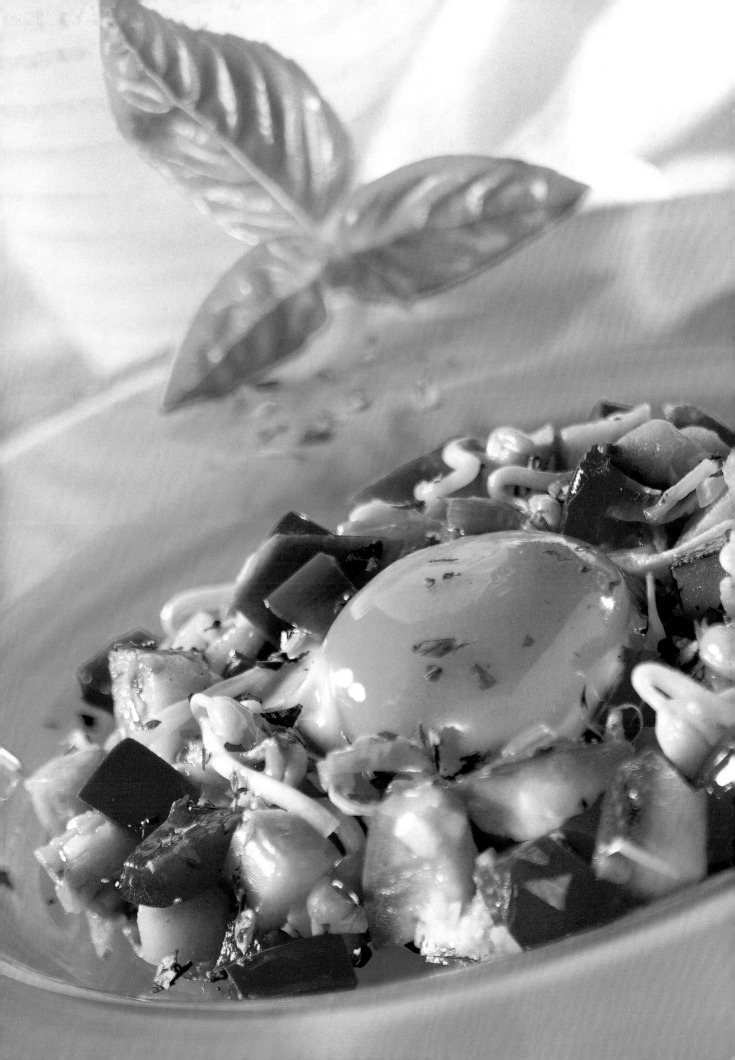

Spinach Gratin

Carbohydrates	◖	25 min.
Fat	●●	(+ 10 min. baking)
Fiber	–	

Per serving: approx. 164 calories
15 g protein · 8 g fat · 8 g carbohydrates

FOR 2 SERVINGS:
1 tbsp (15 mL) chopped pine nuts
6 to 8 fresh basil leaves
1 clove garlic
Salt
1 tsp (5 mL) lemon juice
1 lb (500 g) spinach
2 tomatoes
Freshly grated nutmeg
2½ oz (75 g) mozzarella cheese

1 Toast the pine nuts in a nonstick skillet (frying pan) on medium heat, being careful not to burn them. Finely chop the basil and garlic and combine with the pine nuts. Season with a pinch of salt and the lemon juice.

2 Wash the spinach and remove large stems. Place the wet spinach in a large saucepan and steam on medium heat for 4 minutes, until wilted. Drain and chop coarsely.

3 Preheat oven to 350°F (180°C). Grease an ovenproof dish. Slice the tomatoes and arrange in one half of the dish. Season with a little salt and cover with the seasoned pine nuts. Arrange the spinach in the other half. Season with 2 pinches of salt and the nutmeg. Cut the mozzarella into 4 slices and arrange on top of the spinach. Bake for 10 minutes. Serve with Spelt Brioche (recipe on page 184).

 TIP: You can use frozen spinach instead of fresh. Simply thaw a 10-oz (300 g) package before following the directions above.

Olive Omelet

Carbohydrates	●	15 min.
Fat	++	
Fiber	●●	

Per serving: approx. 335 calories
17 g protein · 25 g fat · 10 g carbohydrates

FOR 2 SERVINGS:
1 tbsp + 2 tsp canola or vegetable oil
1 clove garlic
1 onion
1 small eggplant (aubergine)
1 zucchini (courgette)
¾ cup (175 mL) tomato juice
½ bunch parsley
Salt and freshly ground pepper
4 eggs
2 tbsp (30 mL) milk
Curry powder
10 pitted green olives

1 Finely slice the garlic and onion. Heat the 1 tbsp (15 mL) of oil, add garlic and onion, and gently sauté on low heat until translucent.

2 Dice the eggplant and zucchini, stir them in and cook slightly. Add the tomato juice and cook on medium heat for 15 minutes. Chop the parsley and stir it in. Season with salt and pepper.

3 Slice the olives. Beat the eggs with the milk until frothy. Stir in salt, pepper, curry powder and olives.

4 Cook the omelets one at a time. For each omelet, heat 1 tsp (5 mL) oil in a skillet (frying pan), pour ½ the egg mixture into the skillet, and cook until set and lightly browned. Set aside and keep warm. Spread the vegetables over half of each omelet, fold once, arrange on two plates and serve.

VEGETABLES

Spinach Gratin, top
Olive Omelet, bottom

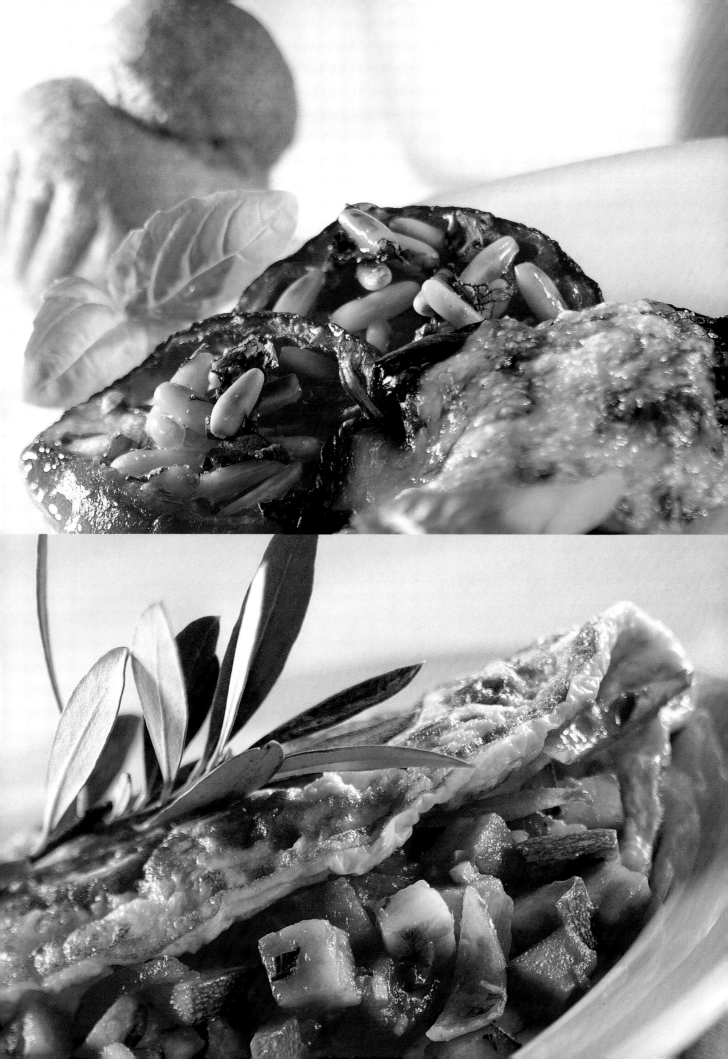

Vegetable Ragout with Poached Eggs

Carbohydrates	●◖	50 min.
Fat	●●●	
Fiber	●●	

Per serving: approx. 201 calories
11 g protein · 12 g fat · 13 g carbohydrates

FOR 2 SERVINGS:
1 leek
2 cups (500 mL/100 g) trimmed leaf spinach
2 carrots
1 kohlrabi
1 clove garlic
1 tbsp (15 mL) olive oil
½ cup (125 mL) vegetable stock
4 cups (1 L) water
½ cup (125 mL) vinegar
2 eggs
Salt and freshly ground pepper
Freshly grated nutmeg

1 Cut the leek lengthwise, wash thoroughly and cut into thin strips. Peel the carrots and kohlrabi and slice into strips. Finely chop the garlic.

2 Heat the oil. Add garlic and leek and lightly sauté on medium heat. Add the spinach, cover and cook for 5 minutes, until wilted. Add carrots, kohlrabi and stock, and cook for 15 minutes more.

3 In a medium saucepan, bring water and vinegar to a light boil. Crack each egg individually, slide it into the water–vinegar mixture, and cook for about 4 minutes. Remove with a slotted spoon.

4 Season the vegetables with salt, pepper and nutmeg. Ladle onto plates and serve with the poached eggs alongside.

!! **TIP:** Fried tofu also tastes good with vegetable ragout. Finely dice 5 oz (150 g) firm tofu, fry in 1 to 2 tsp (5 to 10 mL) olive or peanut oil until crisp on the outside, and add to the vegetables before serving. This combination will significantly increase your calcium intake.

Vegetable Casserole with Pasta and Pesto

Carbohydrates	●●●●◖	40 min.
Fat	+	
Fiber	●●●	

Per serving: approx. 422 calories
19 g protein · 16 g fat · 50 g carbohydrates

FOR 2 SERVINGS:
2 tbsp (30 mL) olive oil, divided
1 oz (30 g) cooked ham
1 onion
3 ribs celery
1 small fennel bulb
4 cups (1 L/200 g) broccoli florets
1 red pepper
2 thin carrots
10-oz (284 mL) can tomatoes
2 cups (500 mL) vegetable stock
1 cup (250 mL) durum wheat pasta (shells or bow ties)
½ bunch parsley
2 sprigs fresh basil
1 clove garlic
1 tbsp (15 mL) freshly grated Parmesan or old pecorino
1 tsp (5 mL) lemon juice
Salt
1 tbsp (15 mL) pine nuts
Pepper

1 Dice the ham and onion and finely slice the celery, fennel, red pepper and carrots. Heat 1 tbsp (15 mL) of the oil. Brown the ham and onion. Add celery, fennel, broccoli, red pepper and carrots, and sauté for 1 minute. Add the tomatoes and juice, breaking the tomatoes into smaller pieces. Add the stock, cover, and cook for 10 to 15 minutes on medium heat.

2 Cook the pasta according to the package directions, just until al dente, and drain.

3 To prepare the pesto, purée the herbs with garlic, cheese, lemon juice, the remaining 1 tbsp (15 mL) of oil, salt and pine nuts.

4 Combine pasta and vegetables and season with salt and pepper. Serve in bowls, garnished with a dollop of pesto.

Vegetable Ragout with Poached Eggs, top
Vegetable Casserole with Pasta and Pesto, bottom

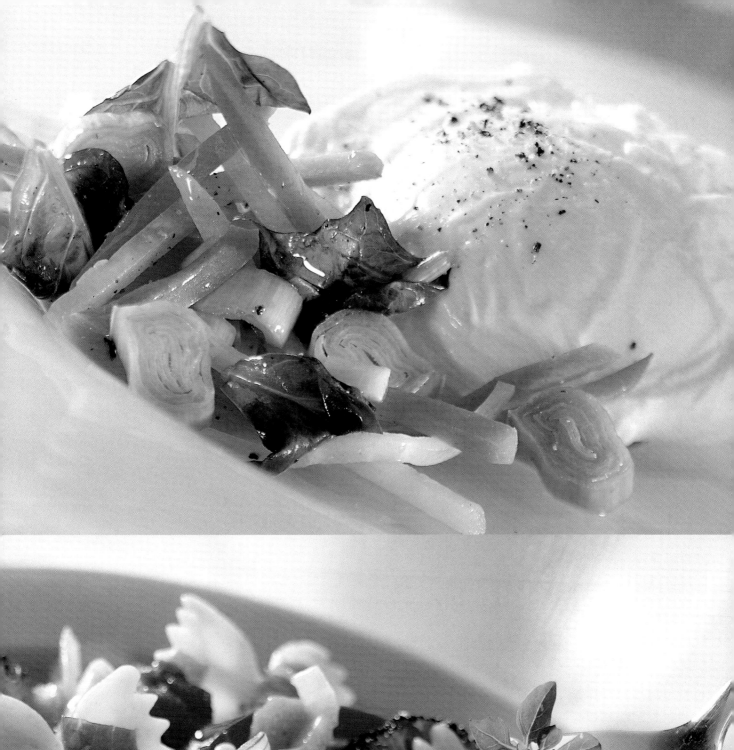
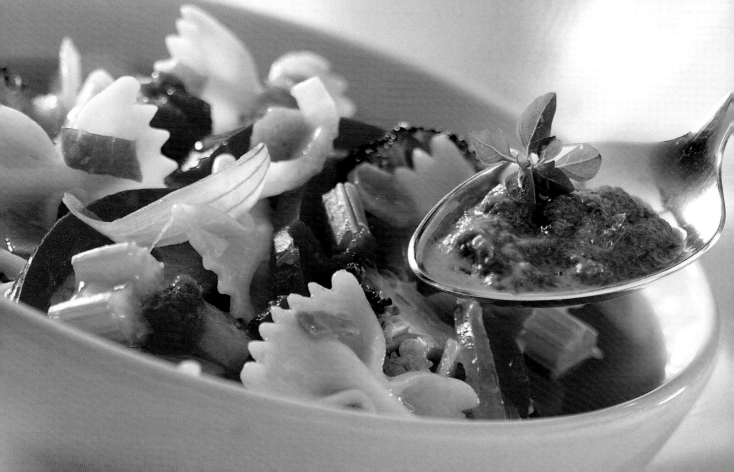

Thai Vegetables

Carbohydrates	●●◖	35 min.
Fat	●	
Fiber	●●●	

Per serving: approx. 168 calories
7 g protein · 6 g fat · 25 g carbohydrates

FOR 2 SERVINGS:

2½ cups (625 mL/250 g) broccoli
1 tsp (5 mL) oil
1 clove garlic
1 tbsp (15 mL) chopped fresh ginger
1 small red chili pepper
1 carrot
2 green (spring) onions
1 to 2 tsp (5 to 10 mL) sugar
½ cup (125 mL) vegetable stock
1¼ cups (300 mL/75 g) sliced bok choy or Chinese (Napa) cabbage
2 slices fresh pineapple
2 tbsp (30 mL) fish sauce
Squeeze of lime juice
A few sprigs Thai basil

1 Separate the broccoli florets; peel and dice the stems finely. Finely chop the garlic and thinly slice the chili pepper, carrot and green onions.

2 Heat the oil in a wok. Add garlic, ginger and chili pepper, and brown lightly. Add carrot and broccoli, and stir-fry for 2 minutes. Add the green onions and stir-fry for 1 minute. Add sugar and vegetable stock.

3 Dice the pineapple and stir in with the bok choy, fish sauce and lime juice. Cook until all is crisp-tender. Finely slice the Thai basil, sprinkle over the vegetables and serve.

Stuffed Eggplant (Aubergine) with Bulgur

Carbohydrates	●●●◖	45 min.
Fat	+	
Fiber	●●●	

Per serving: approx. 353 calories
17 g protein · 15 g fat · 37 g carbohydrates

FOR 2 SERVINGS:

1 large eggplant
Juice of 1 lemon
2 tbsp (30 mL) olive oil
⅓ cup (75 mL/60 g) bulgur
1 onion
½ cup (125 mL) vegetable stock
2 red peppers
1 zucchini (courgette)
7 oz (200 g) tomato paste
Salt and freshly ground pepper
¼ cup (50 mL/30 g) freshly grated Parmesan cheese

1 Cut the eggplant in half lengthwise. Remove the flesh, leaving a shell on the skin. Dice the flesh and set aside. Brush the shells with lemon juice.

2 Preheat the oven to 400°F (200°C). Place the eggplant shells in an ovenproof dish and bake for 15 minutes.

3 Chop the onion and dice the red peppers and zucchini. Heat the oil, stir in the bulgur and brown slightly. Mix in the onion and cook briefly. Add vegetable stock, red peppers, zucchini and eggplant flesh. Simmer for 15 minutes. Stir in the tomato paste and season with salt and pepper.

4 Stuff eggplant shells with mixture, sprinkle cheese on top, and bake for another 15 minutes.

Curried Lentil Casserole

Carbohydrates	●●●●◖	1 hr.
Fat	●●	
Fiber	●●●	

Per serving: approx. 371 calories
19 g protein · 8 g fat · 51 g carbohydrates

FOR 2 SERVINGS:

⅔ cup (150 mL/120 g) green lentils
2 cups (500 mL) vegetable stock
1 red pepper
14-oz (398 mL) can tomatoes
1 tbsp (15 mL) olive oil
1 onion
1 clove garlic
¼ cup (50 mL) red wine or tomato juice
1 tbsp (15 mL) chopped fresh coriander leaves
1 tsp (5 mL) curry powder
Pinch cayenne
Salt and freshly ground pepper
A few whole coriander leaves

1 Rinse the lentils in cold water and drain. Bring the stock to a boil. Add lentils and cook on low heat for 45 minutes.

2 Finely dice the red pepper. Drain the tomatoes, reserving the juice, and chop coarsely. Chop the onion and garlic.

3 Heat the oil. Add onion and garlic and sauté on low heat until translucent. Stir in the tomatoes and reserved juice, additional juice or the wine and chopped coriander. Bring to a boil. Stir in the lentils and stock, cover and cook for 15 minutes. Add curry powder, cayenne, salt and pepper. Garnish with whole coriander leaves and serve.

Thai Vegetables, top
Stuffed Eggplant with Bulgur,
bottom left
Curried Lentil Casserole,
bottom right

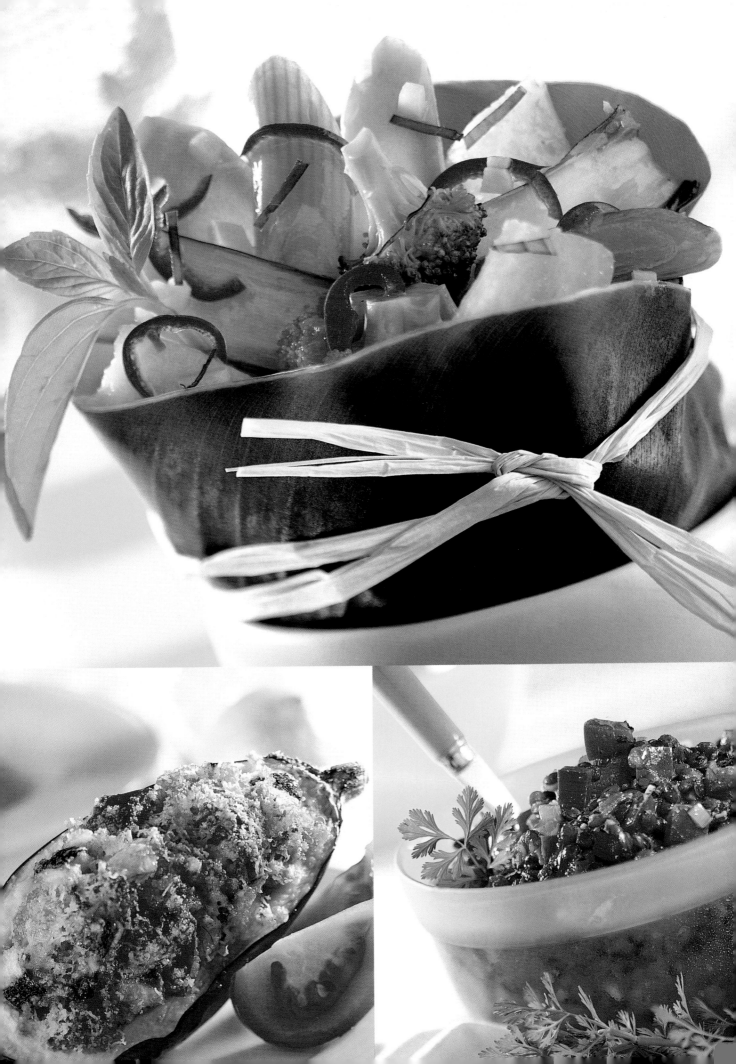

Zucchini (Courgette) Boats with Rice Stuffing

Carbohydrates ●●●	1 hr. 5 min.
Fat ●●●	(+ 30 min. baking)
Fiber ●●	

Per serving: approx. 333 calories
15 g protein · 14 g fat · 36 g carbohydrates

FOR 2 SERVINGS:
¾ cup (175 mL) vegetable stock
⅓ cup (75 mL/65 g) brown rice
2 large zucchini
2 tsp (10 mL) olive oil
2 onions
14-oz (398 mL) can tomatoes
Salt and pepper
Tabasco
½ cup (125 mL) finely diced mozzarella (about 2 oz/60 g)
2 tbsp (30 mL) chopped pine nuts
½ bunch basil

1 Bring stock to a boil, add the rice and cook, covered, on low heat for 20 to 40 minutes, just until done but still firm.

2 Cut the zucchini in half lengthwise. Using a small knife, loosen the flesh all the way around, leaving an edge ¼ to ½ inch (0.5 to 1 cm) wide. Chop the flesh and set aside. Chop the onions.

3 Heat the oil, add onions, and lightly sauté on low heat until translucent. Stir in the tomatoes and juice, coarsely crushing the tomatoes. Add the zucchini flesh, season with salt, pepper and a few drops of Tabasco, and simmer, covered, for 15 minutes.

4 Preheat the oven to 350°F (180°C). Finely slice the basil and combine with the rice, mozzarella and pine nuts. Season with salt and pepper, and fill the zucchini shells with the rice mixture.

5 Pour the tomato mixture into an ovenproof dish. Place the zucchini halves in the dish and bake for 30 minutes.

Red Peppers with Polenta Stuffing

Carbohydrates ●●●◖	20 min.
Fat ●●●	(+ 45 min. baking)
Fiber ●●	

Per serving: approx. 311 calories
12 g protein · 12 g fat · 37 g carbohydrates

FOR 2 SERVINGS:
Salt
⅔ cup (150 mL/75 g) cornmeal
2 (500 mL) cups water
½ tsp (2 mL) salt
2 large red peppers
1 tbsp (15 mL) olive oil
3 tomatoes
1 tbsp (15 mL) chopped fresh parsley
Freshly ground pepper
⅔ cup (150 mL) vegetable stock
¼ cup (50 mL/30 g) freshly grated Gruyère or Emmenthal

1 In a medium saucepan, combine water and salt and bring to a boil. Slowly stir in the cornmeal and cook on low heat, stirring constantly, until thick. Remove from the heat.

2 Halve the red peppers lengthwise, seed and core.

3 Preheat the oven to 350°F (180°C). Brush a medium gratin dish with olive oil. Dice the tomatoes finely and arrange in the dish. Season with parsley, salt and pepper. Stuff the peppers with the polenta and arrange on top of the tomatoes. Pour in the vegetable stock and bake for 20 minutes.

4 Remove the dish from the oven and stir the tomatoes. Drizzle tomato mixture over the peppers and bake for a further 20 minutes, basting twice more.

5 Sprinkle the cheese on top and bake for 5 minutes more, or until the cheese melts and browns slightly.

Zucchini (Courgette) Boats with Rice Stuffing, top
Red Peppers with Polenta Stuffing, bottom

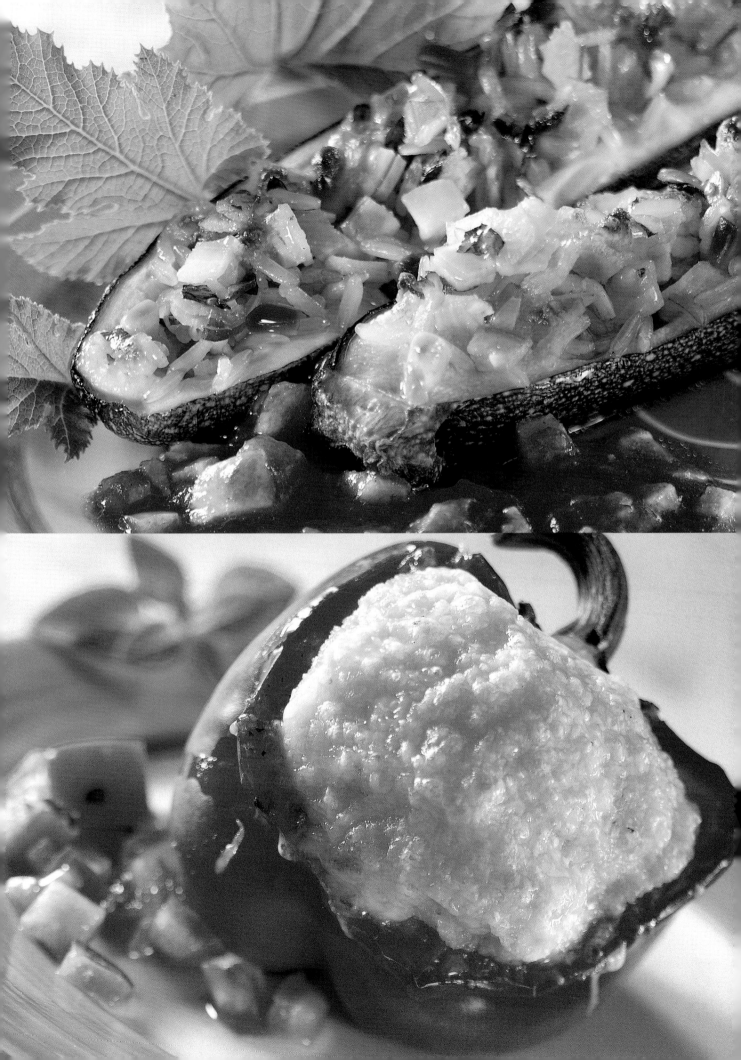

Savoy Cabbage Rolls with Semolina–Carrot Stuffing

Carbohydrates	●●●◖	55 min.
Fat	●●●	
Fiber	●●●	

Per serving: approx. 431 calories
20 g protein · 20 g fat · 41 g carbohydrates

FOR 2 SERVINGS:
1 small Savoy cabbage
2 tbsp (30 mL) canola or vegetable oil, divided
1²⁄₃ cups (400 mL) vegetable stock, divided
1 onion
1 carrot
1¼ cups (300 mL) low-fat milk
½ cup (125 mL/75 g) durum wheat semolina
1 egg, lightly beaten
1 tsp (5 mL) crumbled dried rosemary
Salt and freshly ground pepper
Freshly grated nutmeg
¼ cup (50 mL/50 g) sour cream
2 tbsp (30 mL) chopped fresh parsley

1 Wash the cabbage. Remove the 4 outside leaves. Finely slice the remainder. Heat 1 tbsp (15 mL) of the oil, add the sliced cabbage and cook on medium heat for 5 minutes. Pour in ½ cup (175 mL) of the stock and simmer, covered, for 30 minutes. Meanwhile, blanch the whole cabbage leaves in boiling salted water, plunge into ice water and drain well.

2 Chop the onion and finely dice the carrot. Heat the remaining 1 tbsp (15 mL) of oil and sauté the onion until translucent. Stir in the carrot and cook for 10 minutes.

3 Heat the milk, slowly stir in the semolina and cook until thick. Leave to cool. Stir in egg and cooked onion and carrot. Season with rosemary, salt, pepper and nutmeg.

4 Place the semolina mixture on the 4 cabbage leaves and roll, tucking in the ends to form an envelope. Fasten with toothpicks. Bring the remaining stock to a boil, add cabbage rolls, reduce heat and simmer for 10 minutes.

5 Stir the sour cream into the cooked sliced cabbage and season with salt and pepper. Serve alongside the cabbage rolls, garnished with parsley.

East Indian Potato–Cauliflower Curry

Carbohydrates	●●●●	50 min.
Fat	●●	
Fiber	●●●	

Per serving: approx. 298 calories
13 g protein · 7 g fat · 46 g carbohydrates

FOR 2 SERVINGS:
2 firm potatoes
1 small cauliflower
1 tbsp (15 mL) oil
1 tomato
1 small green chili pepper
3 green (spring) onions
1 clove garlic
1 tbsp (15 mL) chopped fresh ginger
1 tbsp (15 mL) garam masala
⅓ cup (75 mL/75 g) low-fat yogurt
¼ tsp (1 mL) coarsely ground whole wheat flour
2 tbsp (30 mL) lemon juice
Salt and freshly ground pepper
2 tsp (10 mL) sesame seeds

1 Peel and dice the potatoes into ½-inch (2 cm) cubes. Separate the cauliflower florets and dice the stems.

2 Heat the oil in a wok or nonstick skillet (frying pan). Add potatoes and cauliflower and cook on medium heat, stirring constantly, for 20 minutes, adding a little hot water as needed.

3 Blanch the tomato in hot water, peel and dice finely. Set aside.

4 Cut the chili pepper lengthwise, core and slice finely. Slice the green onions into rings and set a little aside. Thinly slice the garlic. Combine the garlic, chili pepper and remaining green onions in another wok or skillet and brown lightly. Stir in ginger and garam masala. Mix in the yogurt and flour and stir until smooth. Stir in the tomato, then add to the potatoes and cauliflower. Cook on low heat for 10 minutes.

5 Season with lemon juice, salt and pepper. Garnish with sesame seeds and the reserved green onions, and serve.

VEGETABLES

East Indian Potato–Cauliflower Curry, right

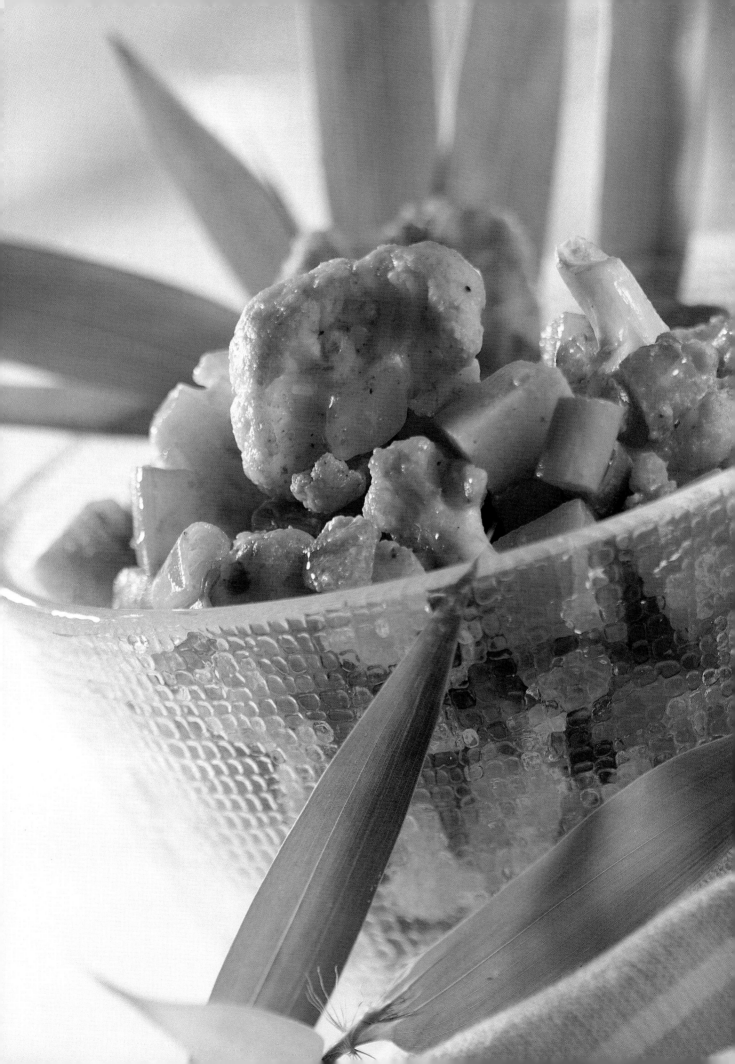

Broccoli–Red Pepper Vegetable Mix

Carbohydrates	●●●◖	40 min.
Fat	++	
Fiber	●●●	

Per serving: approx. 397 cal.
15 g protein · 23 g fat · 39 g carbohydrates

FOR 2 SERVINGS:
⅓ cup (75 mL/50 g) long-grain con-
    verted (parboiled) rice
¾ cup (175 mL) vegetable stock,
    divided
1 (1-lb/500 g) bunch broccoli
2 tbsp (30 mL) canola or vegetable
    oil
4 green (spring) onions
1 red pepper
1 to 2 tbsp (15 to 30 mL) chopped
    fresh ginger
2 tbsp (30 mL) lemon juice
Salt
Curry powder
¾ cup (175 ml/200 g) sour cream
2 tbsp (30 mL) chopped almonds

1 Combine the rice and ½ the vegetable stock and bring to a boil. Cook for 20 minutes on low heat.

2 Separate broccoli florets, peel the stems and slice finely. Slice the green onions and roughly chop the red pepper.

3 Heat the oil. Stir in the green onions and cook on low heat. Stir in the broccoli and red pepper and cook slightly. Pour in the remaining vegetable stock and cook the vegetables on low heat until crisp-tender, about 5 minutes.

4 Stir the ginger, lemon juice, salt and a little curry powder into sour cream. Combine with the vegetables and cook for another 5 minutes.

5 Toast the almonds in a non-stick skillet (frying pan) until golden. Sprinkle over the vegetables. Serve with the rice.

Spanish Potato–Fennel Omelet

Carbohydrates	●●●	1 hr.
Fat	●●●	(+ 10 min.
Fiber	●●●	baking)

Per serving: approx. 317 calories
16 g protein · 13 g fat · 33 g carbohydrates

FOR 2 SERVINGS:
3 small firm potatoes
1 tsp (5 mL) olive oil
1 onion
1 large fennel bulb
⅔ cup (150 mL) milk
2 eggs
Salt and freshly ground pepper
1 tomato

1 Cook potatoes in lightly salted water for 25 minutes. Drain, leave to steam dry, then dice finely. Finely slice the onion and fennel.

2 Heat the oil in a large skillet (frying pan) with an oven-proof handle. Stir in the onion and lightly sauté on low heat until translucent. Add the fennel and potatoes and cook slightly.

3 Preheat the oven to 375°C (190°C). Whisk together the milk and eggs and season with salt and pepper. Pour the egg mixture over the vegetables and leave to set on medium heat on the stove.

4 Thinly slice the tomato and lay the slices on top. Finish in the oven for 10 minutes, until golden.

 TIP: Boiled potatoes should be enjoyed with their skins on.

Hard-Cooked Eggs with Potatoes and Herb Sauce

Carbohydrates	●●◖	35 min.
Fat	+	
Fiber	●	

Per serving: approx. 358 calories
24 g protein · 18 g fat · 26 g carbohydrates

FOR 2 SERVINGS:
2 potatoes
Salt
2 eggs
1 bunch parsley
1 bunch chervil
1 bunch chives
⅔ cup (150 mL/150 g) low-fat quark
    or puréed cottage cheese
⅓ cup (75 mL/75 g) yogurt
1 tbsp (15 mL) hot mustard
1 tbsp (15 mL) white-wine vinegar
2 tbsp (30 mL) olive oil
Freshly ground pepper
Freshly grated nutmeg

1 Peel the potatoes and cook for 25 minutes in boiling salted water.

2 Pierce a hole in the eggshells and cook eggs in the boiling water for 8 minutes. Plunge into ice water immediately, then peel.

3 Finely chop the parsley, chervil and chives, and combine with quark, yogurt, mustard, vinegar and oil. Stir well and season with salt, pepper and a little nutmeg. Ladle the sauce onto plates. Cut the eggs in half and arrange on top of the sauce with the potatoes. Sprinkle with salt and pepper, garnish with additional herb sprigs and serve.

Broccoli–Red Pepper Vegetable Mix,
top
Spanish Potato–Fennel Omelet,
bottom left
Hard-Cooked Eggs with Potatoes
and Herb Sauce, bottom right

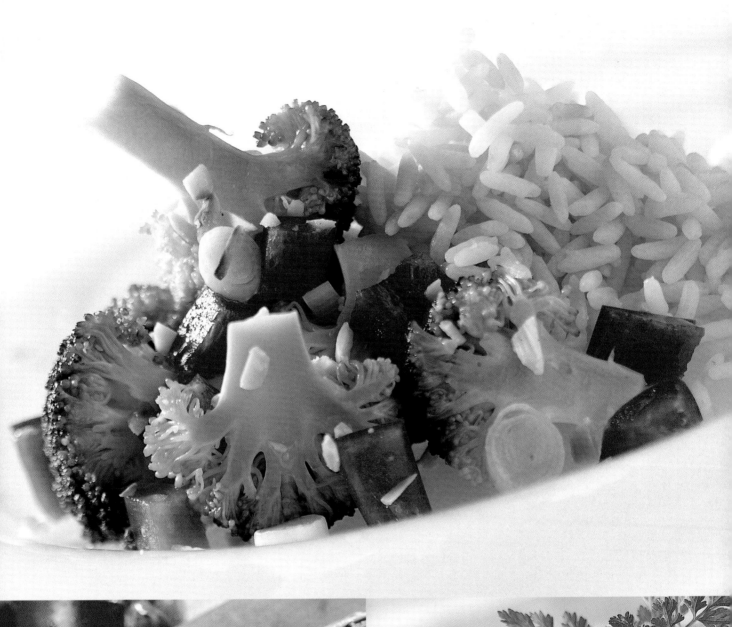

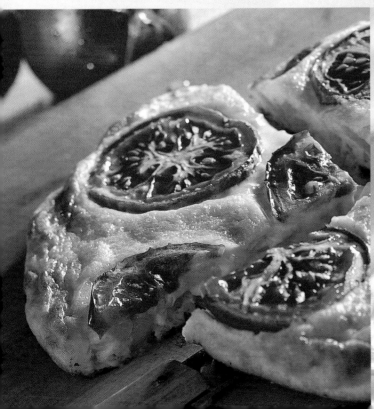

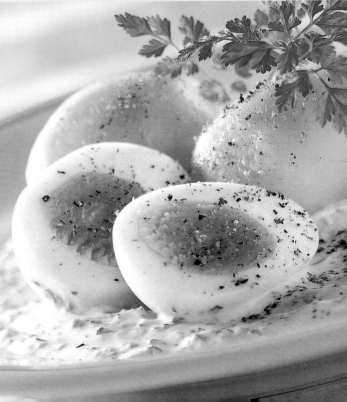

Potato Pancake with Sour Cream

Carbohydrates	●●●●●◖	1 hr. 15 min.
Fat	+	
Fiber	●●●	

Per serving: approx. 491 calories
24 g protein · 17 g fat · 63 g carbohydrates

FOR 2 SERVINGS:
5 firm potatoes
1 medium onion
Salt and freshly ground pepper
Freshly grated nutmeg
2 tsp (10 mL) crumbled dried rosemary
2 eggs
1 oz (30 g) smoked ham, rind removed
1 to 2 tbsp (15 to 30 mL) flour, if required
1 tsp (5 mL) oil
Flour
²/₃ cup (150 mL/150 g) sour cream
½ bunch chives

1 Peel and finely grate the potatoes and drain thoroughly in a fine sieve. Chop the onion and combine with the potatoes in a large mixing bowl. Season with 1 tsp (5 mL) salt, a little pepper, nutmeg and rosemary.

2 Using a fork, beat the eggs in a small bowl, then combine with the potatoes. Mix in the ham. If the dough is too moist, add flour as needed.

3 Preheat the oven to 425°F (220°C). Brush a medium-sized ovenproof dish with oil. Spoon the potato mixture into the dish, spreading until even, and cover with aluminum foil (shiny side down).

4 Bake the potato pancake for 30 minutes. Remove the foil and bake for another 15 minutes, until the top is light brown.

5 Meanwhile, chop the chives and mix with sour cream in a small bowl until smooth. Use dollops as garnish and serve what remains on the side.

Crêpes Stuffed with Sauerkraut

Carbohydrates	●●●●	20 min.
Fat	+	(+ 30 min. resting)
Fiber	●●	

Per serving: approx. 480 calories
35 g protein · 18 g fat · 45 g carbohydrates

FOR 2 SERVINGS:
¾ cup (175 mL) milk
2 eggs
Salt
¾ cup (175 mL/100 g) coarsely ground whole grain flour
1 cup (250 mL/200 g) sauerkraut
4 tsp (20 mL) canola or vegetable oil
¾ cup (175 mL/200 g) light spreadable cream cheese
¼ cup (50 mL/30 g) freshly grated Parmesan cheese
¼ cup (50 mL) chopped chives
Freshly ground pepper

1 Combine milk with eggs, salt and flour, and stir until smooth. Leave the batter to rest for 30 minutes. Separate the sauerkraut with a fork.

2 Make 8 crêpes. Heat about ½ tsp (2 mL) oil in an 8-inch (20 cm) nonstick skillet (frying pan). Ladle about 3 tbsp (45 mL) of batter into the skillet, tilt and swirl to cover the bottom. Cook on medium heat until lightly browned on the bottom and set. Flip the crêpe over and cook the other side until golden.

3 Immediately spread cream cheese on each crêpe, cover with sauerkraut, and sprinkle with Parmesan and chives. Season with pepper. Roll up the crêpes and keep warm.

!! **TIP:** Sauerkraut is an excellent source of vitamin C, its potassium has a purifying effect, and its high lactic acid content encourages the growth of beneficial intestinal flora.

Potato Pancake with Sour Cream, top
Crêpes Stuffed with Sauerkraut, bottom

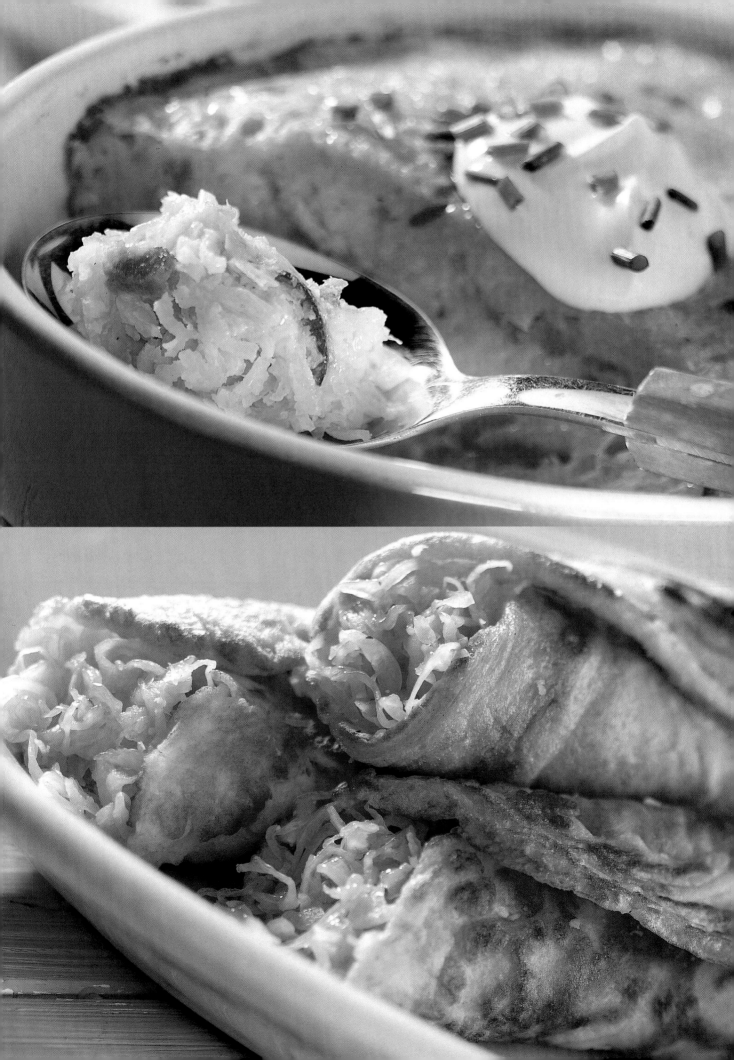

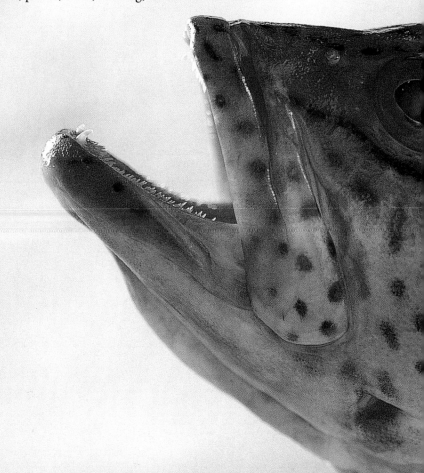

Fish and Seafood

Eating fish means filling up on energy!

If you include fish in your diet once or twice a week, you'll soon notice an increase in energy and fitness—fish is rich in easily digested protein and delivers valuable fatty acids and iodine for active metabolism.

Choose fish high in iodine, such as cod, salmon, halibut, salmon, red snapper, bream, ocean perch, plaice, tuna, herring, mackerel and shellfish.

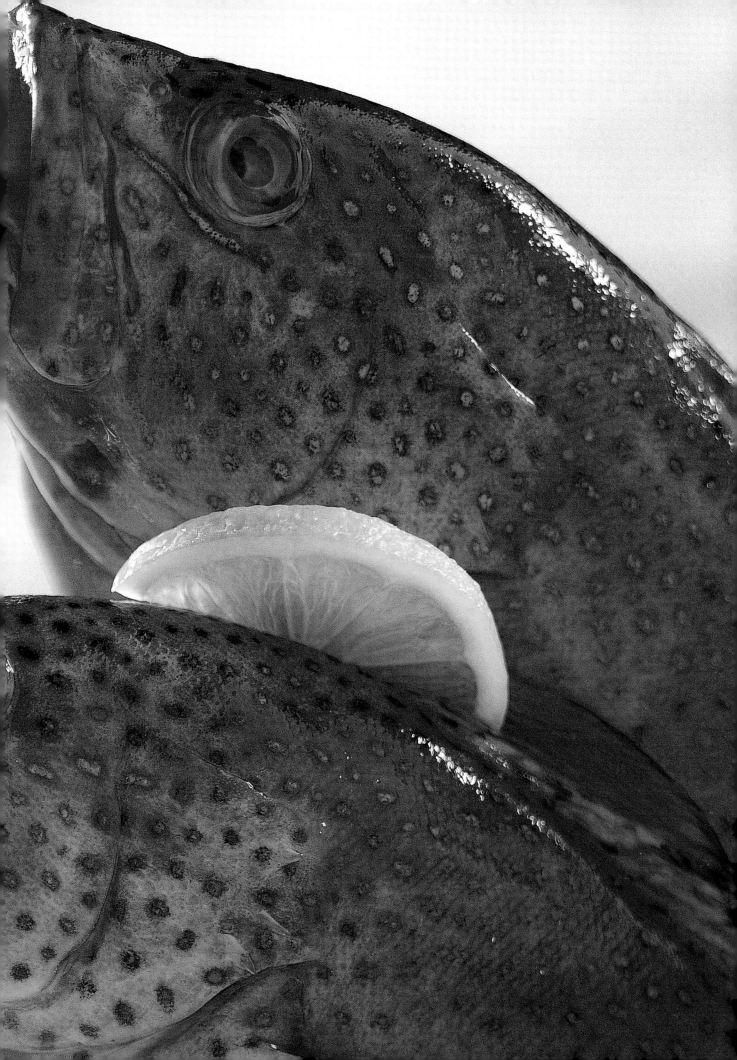

Smoked Trout Fillets with Warm Potato Salad

Carbohydrates	●●●◖	50 min.
Fat	–	
Fiber	●●	

Per serving: approx. 280 calories
17 g protein · 3 g fat · 38 g carbohydrates

FOR 2 SERVINGS:
Salt
2 large firm potatoes
3 tbsp (45 mL) hot vegetable stock
1 tbsp (15 mL) grated fresh horseradish
½ bunch fresh chives
½ bunch fresh dill
3½ oz (100 g) smoked trout fillets
2 radishes

1 Bring lightly salted water to a boil and cook the potatoes for 20 minutes. Drain, let steam slightly, peel while still hot and slice.

2 Combine vegetable stock and horseradish in a medium bowl. Season with a little salt. Finely chop the chives and dill and stir them in. Mix in the potatoes.

3 Slice the radishes. Arrange the trout and potatoes on two plates and garnish with radishes.

!! **TIP:** Like all types of fish, trout is rich in protein. The fat content of the delicate, sweet, nutty-tasting flesh varies according to type—but no need to worry about eating and enjoying it. Fish fat is generally rich in healthful omega-3 fatty acids, otherwise found primarily in such vegetable oils as canola and flaxseed.

Matjes Herring and Apple–Bean Salad

Carbohydrates	●●	25 min.
Fat	+++	(+ 1 hr. chilling)
Fiber	●●	

Per serving: approx. 590 calories
31 g protein · 42 g fat · 22 g carbohydrates

FOR 2 SERVINGS:
Salt
1¼ cups (300 mL/150 g) green beans
1 small onion
2 tart apples
1 small gherkin
1 bunch fresh chervil
Juice of 1 lemon
½ tsp (2 mL) hot mustard
⅓ cup (75 mL/75 g) sour cream
⅓ cup (75 mL/75 g) low-fat yogurt
4 Matjes (cured) herring fillets
Freshly ground pepper

1 In a small saucepan, bring salted water to a boil and cook the beans on medium heat for 10 minutes. Drain the beans and leave to cool, then cut into small pieces.

2 Finely chop the onion, apples, gherkin and chervil, and mix with the beans.

3 Combine lemon juice, mustard, sour cream and yogurt. Stir into the salad. Cut the herring into bite-size pieces and add to the salad. Season with salt and pepper and refrigerate for 1 hour before serving.

Smoked Trout Fillets with Warm Potato Salad, top
Herring and Apple–Bean Salad, bottom

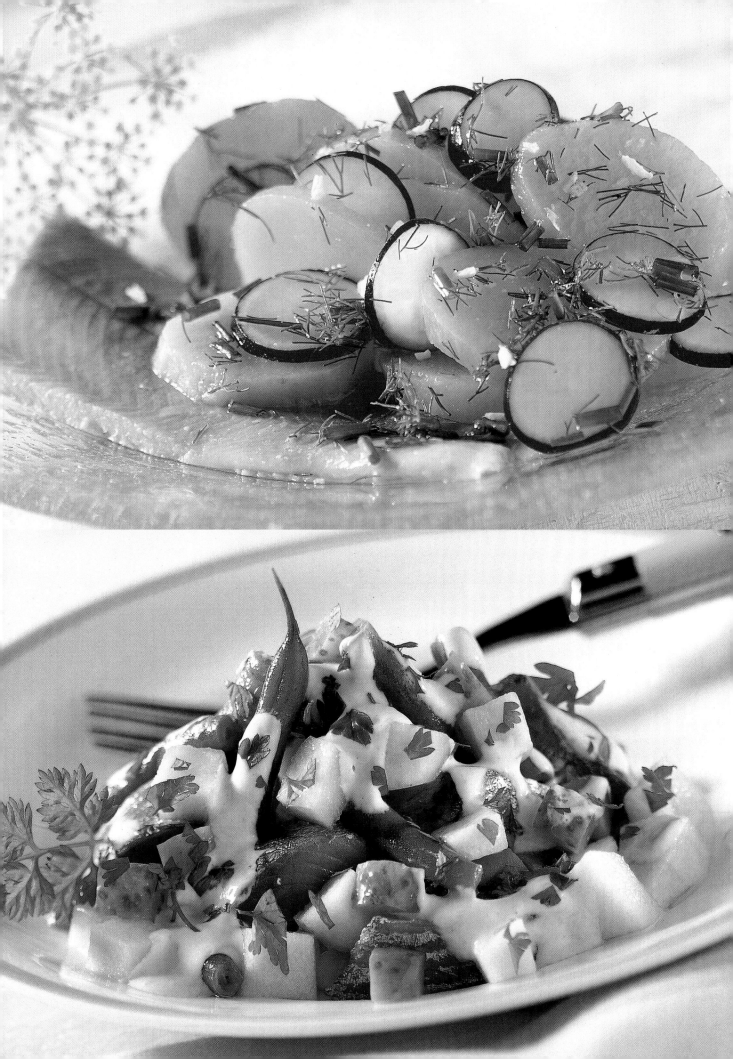

Cod with Summer Vegetables

Carbohydrates	●●●●	1 hr. 10 min.
Fat	+	
Fiber	●●●	

Per serving: approx. 517 calories
48 g protein · 15 g fat · 47 g carbohydrates

FOR 2 SERVINGS:
⅓ cup (75 mL/60 g) long-grain converted (parboiled) rice
½ cup (125 mL) salted boiling water
1 onion
1 green (spring) onion
1 leek
2 carrots
1 kohlrabi
2 tbsp (30 mL) canola or vegetable oil
2½ cups (625 mL) snow (mange-tout) peas
1¼ cups (300 mL) vegetable stock
2 small cod fillets
Salt and freshly ground pepper
Juice of 1 lemon
½ bunch fresh dill
¼ cup (50 mL/50 g) sour cream

1 Add the rice to the water. Cover and cook for 20 minutes on low heat.

2 Chop the onion. Finely slice the green onion and leek. Julienne the carrots and kohlrabi. Heat the oil. Stir in the onion, green onion and leek, and cook on medium heat until translucent. Stir in the carrots, kohlrabi and snow peas. Cook lightly, then pour in vegetable stock. Arrange the cod on top of the vegetables and cook, covered, on low heat for 20 minutes. Season with salt and pepper.

3 Finely chop the dill and combine it with the lemon juice and sour cream. Season with salt and pepper, and serve with the rice, fish and vegetables.

Plaice with Tomato Polenta

Carbohydrates	●●●●	1 hr. 30 min.
Fat	++	
Fiber	●●	

Per serving: approx. 527 calories
34 g protein · 22 g fat · 45 g carbohydrates

FOR 2 SERVINGS:
¾ cup (175 mL/100 g) cornmeal
2 cups (500 mL) vegetable stock
1 bunch fresh basil
3 eggs
3 tbsp (45 mL) tomato paste
2 tbsp (30 mL) olive oil, divided
Freshly ground pepper
2 tbsp (30 mL) milk
10 oz (300 g) plaice fillets
Salt
2 tbsp (30 mL) flour
2 tbsp (30 mL) chopped fresh parsley

1 Slowly pour the cornmeal into the vegetable stock, stirring constantly. Cook on low heat until thick, about 45 minutes.

2 Preheat the oven to 300°F (150°C). Chop the basil and combine it with 1 egg and the tomato paste. Stir into the cornmeal. Spread the mixture out on a baking sheet lined with parchment paper and bake in the preheated oven for 15 minutes. Leave to cool.

3 Cut the polenta into slices. Heat 1 tbsp (15 mL) of the olive oil and brown the polenta on both sides on medium heat. Season with pepper and keep warm.

4 Whisk milk with remaining 2 eggs. Season both sides of the fish with salt and pepper, coat with flour, then dip into eggs. Heat the remaining oil and brown the fish on both sides on medium heat, about 5 minutes a side. Arrange with the polenta on two plates, sprinkle with parsley and serve.

Salmon with Fettuccine

Carbohydrates	●●●●	45 min.
Fat	●●	
Fiber	●●	

Per serving: approx. 451 calories
46 g protein · 9 g fat · 46 g carbohydrates

FOR 2 SERVINGS:
Juice of 1 lemon
1 tsp (5 mL) walnut oil
2 tsp (10 mL) white-wine vinegar
1 shallot
Salt and freshly ground pepper
Ground coriander seeds
1 tbsp (15 mL) olive oil
2 carrots
1 small fennel bulb
1 zucchini (courgette)
2 small salmon fillets
2 sprigs fresh tarragon
3½ oz (100 g) fettuccine

1 Chop the shallot and combine with the lemon juice, walnut oil and vinegar. Season with salt, pepper and ground coriander. Set aside.

2 Slice the carrots, fennel and zucchini. Heat the olive oil, stir in the sliced vegetables and cook for 5 minutes.

3 Preheat the oven to 325°F (160°C). Cut two pieces of aluminum foil, about 8 x 12 inches (20 x 30 cm) each. Place ½ the vegetable mixture on each. Arrange salmon fillets and a sprig of tarragon on top and drizzle with the sauce. Wrap and seal tightly, and bake for 15 minutes.

4 Cook and drain the fettuccine. Arrange the fish and vegetables and the pasta on two plates and serve immediately.

**Cod with Summer Vegetables, top
Plaice with Tomato Polenta, bottom left
Salmon with Fettuccine, bottom right**

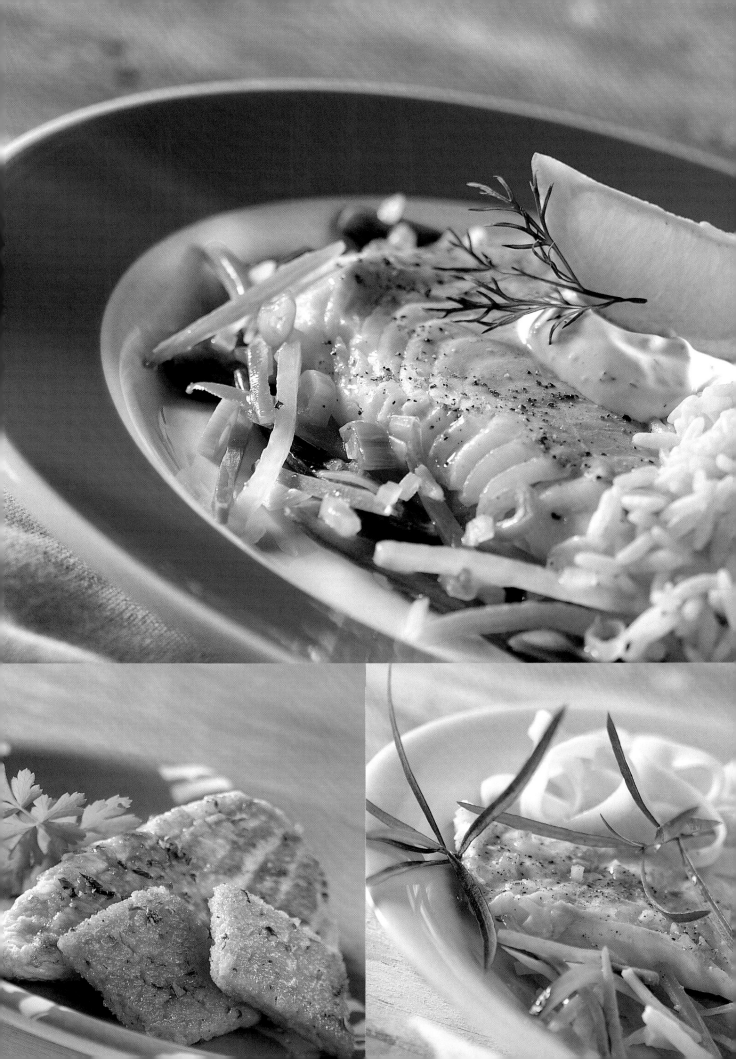

Grilled Red Bream or Red Snapper with Tarragon

Carbohydrates	–	20 min.
Fat	●●●	
Fiber	–	

Per serving: approx. 248 calories
33 g protein · 12 g fat · 1 g carbohydrates

FOR 2 SERVINGS:
2 small dressed red bream or red snappers, about 10 oz
   (300 g) each
Salt and freshly ground pepper
2 tbsp (30 mL) lime juice
Fresh tarragon or basil leaves
1 shallot
1 tbsp (15 mL) olive oil

1 Light or preheat a barbecue, indoor grill or oven broiler. Using a sharp knife, make 3 or 4 incisions at an angle on both sides of each fish. Season with salt and pepper and sprinkle with lime juice.

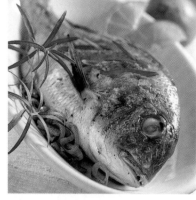

2 Slice the shallot and place ½ the slices and a little tarragon inside each fish.

3 Brush fish lightly with oil on both sides. Lightly oil the grill or a broiling pan. Cook on medium heat for 5 minutes on each side.

!! TIP: Baked potatoes and whole-grain bread go equally well with this dish. You can also serve a light vegetable salad for a well-balanced meal.

!! TIP: Red bream is ideal for barbecuing, but it shouldn't weigh more than 14 oz (400 g). You can substitute the slightly more expensive yellow bream, also sold as dorado.

Baked Salmon with Cucumber Salad

Carbohydrates	◖	50 min.
Fat	+	
Fiber	–	

Per serving: approx. 267 calories
23 g protein · 18 g fat · 4 g carbohydrates

FOR 2 SERVINGS:
½ onion
4 to 5 sprigs fresh dill
2 slices salmon, about 3½ oz (100 g) each
Salt
2 tsp (10 mL) oil, divided
2 tsp (10 mL) lemon juice
Finely grated zest of ½ lemon
1 tbsp (15 mL) fruit vinegar
½ tsp (2 mL) liquid honey
½ tsp (2 mL) medium mustard
Freshly ground pepper
Liquid sweetener
½ English cucumber

1 Preheat the oven to 350°F (180°C). Slice the onion and remove the stems of the dill. Brush the bottom of an ovenproof dish with 1 tsp (5 mL) of the oil. Spread the onion in the bottom and the dill stems over top.

2 Season salmon with salt on both sides, lay it on over the dill stems and sprinkle with lemon juice. Top with lemon zest. Cover dish with aluminum foil and bake for 15 minutes. Remove the foil, turn off the oven and leave the dish in the oven for 5 more minutes.

3 Finely slice the fronds of the dill and peel and dice the cucumber. Combine the vinegar, the remaining 1 tsp (5 mL) of oil, honey and mustard in a small bowl. Season with 2 pinches of salt, a little pepper and a dash of liquid sweetener. Toss with the dill and cucumber. Arrange salmon and cucumber salad on two plates, decorate with a twist of lemon peel, if desired, and serve with potatoes.

Baked Salmon with Cucumber Salad, right

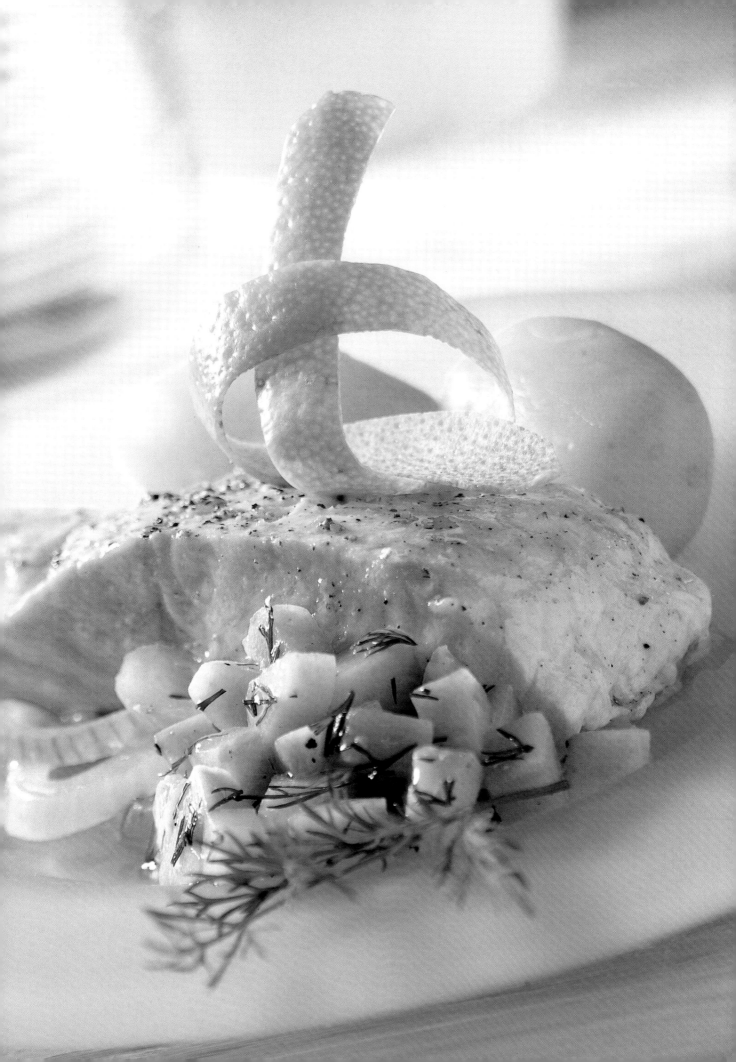

Exotic
Stir-Fry

Carbohydrates	●●●●	30 min.
Fat	●	
Fiber	●	

Per serving: approx. 336 calories
26 g protein · 6 g fat · 45 g carbohydrates

FOR 2 SERVINGS:
8 oz (250 g) fish fillets: salmon or cod
¼ cup (50 mL) fish or vegetable stock, divided
Freshly ground pepper
½ cup (125 mL/100 g) basmati rice, or a mixture of brown
    and wild rice
½ lime (organic preferred)
1 tbsp (15 mL) olive oil
1 green chili pepper
1 red pepper
1 cup (250 mL) unsweetened coconut milk
2 tbsp (30 mL) finely chopped coriander leaves
2½ tbsp (37 mL) peeled and finely sliced fresh ginger

1 Cut the fish into bite-size pieces. Combine with 2 tbsp (30 mL) of the stock and a pinch of pepper. Marinate in the refrigerator for 20 minutes.

2 Prepare the rice according to package directions.

3 Grate the lime zest and squeeze out the juice. Finely dice the chili and slice the red pepper. Heat the oil in a skillet (frying pan) and stir-fry the peppers on medium heat for 2 to 3 minutes, until tender-crisp. Stir in the coconut milk, ginger, lime zest and fresh coriander, and cook briefly to blend. Carefully stir in the fish and remaining stock, and cook for 3 to 4 minutes.

4 Pour the fish mixture into a bowl, remove the ginger and squeeze on 2 tbsp (30 mL) lime juice. Serve over the rice. If desired, garnish with rings of red chili, chopped fresh coriander and lime leaves.

Steamed
Trout

Carbohydrates	◀	40 min.
Fat	●●●	
Fiber	●	

Per serving: approx. 367 calories
55 g protein · 10 g fat · 8 g carbohydrates

FOR 2 SERVINGS:
2 small dressed trout, about 10 oz (300 g) each
2 tbsp (30 mL) lemon juice, divided
Salt and white pepper
3 or 4 fresh dill sprigs
1 cup (250 mL) fish or vegetable stock
3 to 4 cups (750 mL to 1 L) julienned or sliced vegetables:
    carrot, white turnip or daikon, leek, bok choy, Brussels
    sprout leaves, etc.
1 tbsp (15 mL) cornstarch or arrowroot
1 tbsp (15 mL) sour cream

1 Sprinkle fish with 1 tbsp (15 mL) of the lemon juice and season with salt and pepper. Place 1 sprig of dill inside each fish.

2 In a saucepan with a steamer insert, bring the stock to a boil. Arrange the trout in the insert. Stir the prepared vegetables into the stock, bring back to a boil, and place the insert on top. Cover and steam for 8 minutes.

3 Remove the trout and keep warm. Mix the cornstarch with the remaining 1 tbsp (15 ml) lemon juice and stir into the stock and vegetables. Cook until thickened, stir in the sour cream, and season with salt and pepper. Arrange the trout on two plates with the vegetables and garnish with the remaining dill.

 TIP: Potatoes, brown rice or a whole-grain baguette would be good with this dish.

Exotic Stir-Fry, top
Steamed Trout, bottom

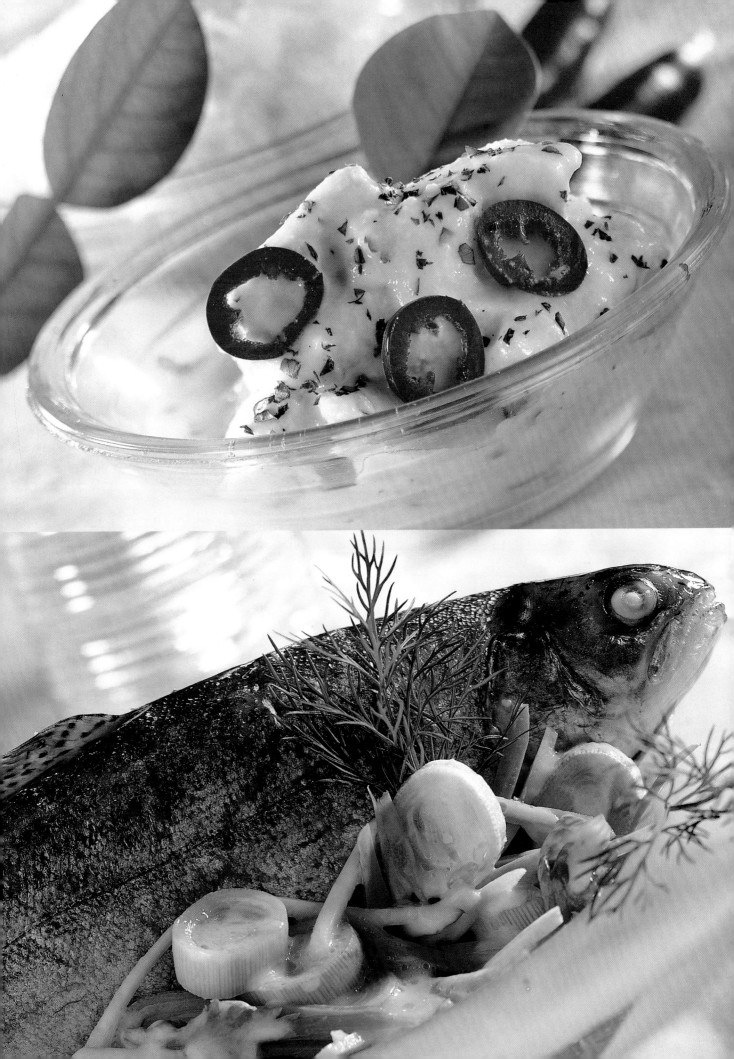

Bouillabaisse Provençale

Carbohydrates ●◖	1 hr. 30 min.
Fat ●●●	
Fiber ●	

Per serving: approx. 322 calories
133 g protein · 12 g fat · 17 g carbohydrates

FOR 2 SERVINGS:
2 firm medium potatoes
2 beefsteak tomatoes
½ onion
2 cloves garlic
½ bunch parsley
2 tbsp (30 mL) olive oil
2 bay leaves
Pinch ground saffron
Salt and freshly ground pepper
14-oz (400 g) monkfish fillet
2 cups (500 mL) boiling water

1 Slice the potatoes. Score, blanch, peel and dice the tomatoes. Chop the onion, garlic and parsley.

2 Heat the oil, stir in the onion and garlic, and lightly sauté on low heat until translucent. Add the potatoes and brown on medium heat. Stir in the tomatoes, parsley, bay leaves, saffron, salt and pepper. Cover and cook on low heat for 5 minutes.

3 Cut the fish into bite-size pieces. Combine with the vegetables and cook for 3 minutes. Pour in the water and simmer on medium heat for 15 to 20 minutes.

 TIP: A thinly sliced toasted baguette goes very well with this dish.

Oven-Baked Fillets with Vegetables

Carbohydrates ●●	30 min.
Fat ++	(+ 8 to 10 min. baking)
Fiber ●●●	

Per serving: approx. 167 calories
43 g protein · 23 g fat · 21 g carbohydrates

FOR 2 SERVINGS:
14 oz (400 g) rosefish, red snapper or ocean perch fillets
2 tbsp (30 mL) lemon juice
Salt and freshly ground pepper
2 tbsp (30 mL) flour
3 tbsp (45 mL) olive oil, divided
1 small eggplant (aubergine)
2 red peppers
1 small tomato
1 small zucchini (courgette)
3 sprigs fresh basil
3 sprigs fresh parsley
2 to 3 tbsp (30 to 45 mL) fresh bread crumbs
Fresh basil leaves

1 Sprinkle the fish with lemon juice, then season with salt and pepper. Dip in flour and shake off any excess.

2 Chop the eggplant and slice the red peppers, tomato and zucchini. Finely chop the basil and parsley. Heat 1 tbsp (15 mL) of the oil in a skillet (frying pan). Fry the fish on medium heat for 5 minutes on each side, then place in a medium-size ovenproof dish.

3 Rinse the skillet and heat another 1 tbsp (15 mL) oil. Cook the eggplant on medium heat for 5 to 6 minutes, turning occasionally. Stir in the red peppers, tomatoes and zucchini and steam for another 5 minutes. Season with salt and pepper.

4 Preheat the oven to 350°F (180°C). Spread the vegetables over the fish. Mix bread crumbs with the remaining 1 tbsp (15 mL) oil, chopped basil and parsley, and sprinkle on top. Bake in the preheated oven for 8 to 10 minutes. Garnish with additional basil leaves.

 TIP: Serve with a whole-grain baguette.

Bouillabaisse Provençale, top
Oven-Baked Fillets with Vegetables, bottom

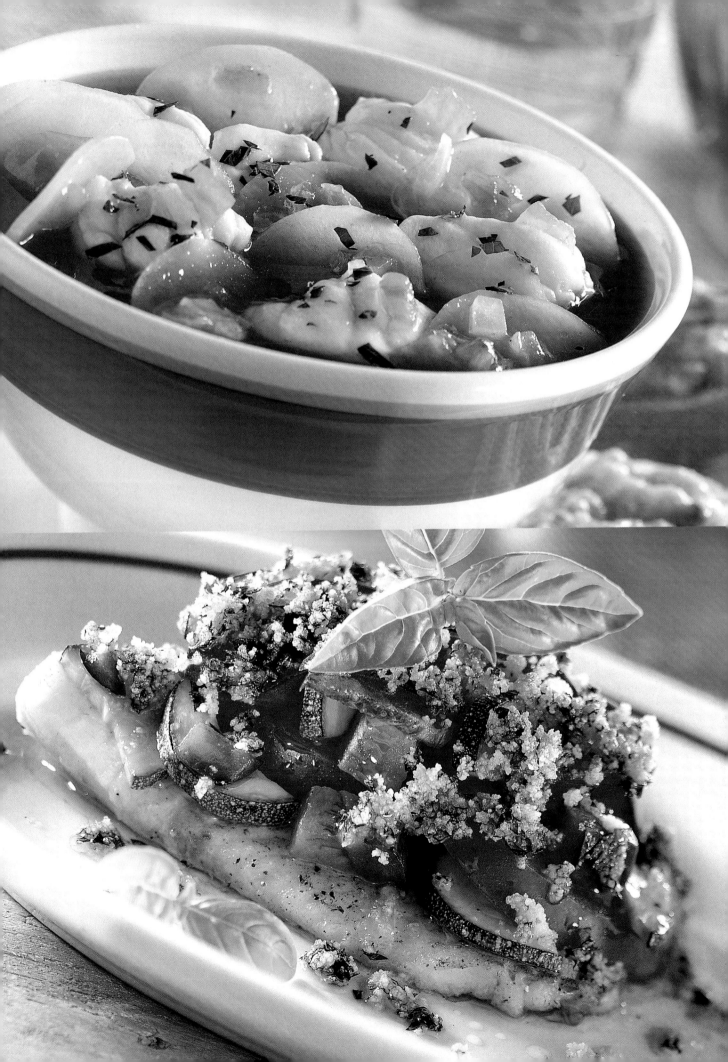

Plaice Pouches

Carbohydrates	●◖	30 min.
Fat	●●●	(+ 15 min. baking)
Fiber	●	

Per serving: approx. 280 calories
30 g protein · 12 g fat · 14 g carbohydrates

FOR 2 SERVINGS:
10 oz (300 g) spinach
2 green (spring) onions
10 oz (300 g) fresh or frozen plaice or sole fillets
Salt and freshly ground pepper
Lemon juice
2 tbsp (30 mL) butter
1 mealy (floury) potato
1 medium carrot
Pinch lemon zest
Pinch cayenne
1 tbsp (15 mL) chopped fresh parsley
1 tbsp (15 mL) chopped fresh dill
2 thin slices lemon

1 Slice the spinach. Cut the green onions in half lengthwise, then across. Thinly slice the potatoes and carrot.

2 Preheat the oven to 325°F (160°C). Cut 2 squares of aluminum foil, each 12 x 12 inches (30 x 30 cm), and grease with a little of the butter. Place ½ the spinach on each square, then cover with potatoes, carrot and onions. Season with salt and pepper. Place the fish on top of the vegetables, season with salt and pepper, and squeeze lemon juice over to taste.

3 Combine remaining butter with lemon zest, cayenne, parsley, dill and a little salt, and dot on the fish. Top with 1 lemon slice on each fillet.

4 Fold the foil to form a pouch, sealing tightly to ensure that no juice will leak out. Place the two pouches on a baking sheet and bake in the preheated oven for 20 minutes. Arrange the pouches on two plates, slice them open and peel back the tops.

!! **TIP:** You can prepare other fish fillets—salmon, cod, pike, perch, red snapper—the same way.

Swordfish–Zucchini (Courgette) Kebabs

Carbohydrates	◖	20 min.
Fat	+	
Fiber	●●	

Per serving: approx. 325 calories
33 g protein · 18 g fat · 8 g carbohydrates

FOR 2 SERVINGS:
10 oz (300 g) swordfish steaks, ¾ inch (2 cm) thick
2 tbsp (30 mL) olive oil, divided
1 tbsp (15 mL) lemon juice
1 tsp (5 mL) fresh thyme or ½ tsp (2 mL) dried
Salt and freshly ground pepper
4 shallots
4 yellow peppers
2 plum or other firm tomatoes
½ zucchini
½ bunch Italian (flat-leaf) parsley, stems removed

1 Dice the swordfish into ½-inch (1 cm) cubes. Combine 1 tbsp (15 mL) of the oil with the lemon juice, thyme, salt and pepper, and turn the fish in this mixture to coat the fish. Cover and marinate for 30 minutes.

2 Peel and halve the shallots. Halve the yellow peppers and cut into 1-inch (2.5 cm) pieces. Quarter the tomatoes. Slice the zucchini into ¾-inch (2 cm) rounds.

3 Preheat oven broiler or portable grill. Thread fish and vegetable pieces on 2 skewers, reserving the marinade. Brush the fish and vegetables with the remaining 1 tbsp (15 mL) oil and season lightly with salt and pepper. Broil or grill for 2 to 3 minutes per side, then drizzle with the marinade. Serve on a bed of parsley.

!! **TIP:** If you would rather fry the kebabs, use the remaining 1 tbsp (15 mL) oil to brush the skillet (frying pan) instead of the vegetables. Sauté on high heat for 2 to 3 minutes per side.

Plaice Pouches, top
Swordfish–Zucchini Kebabs, bottom

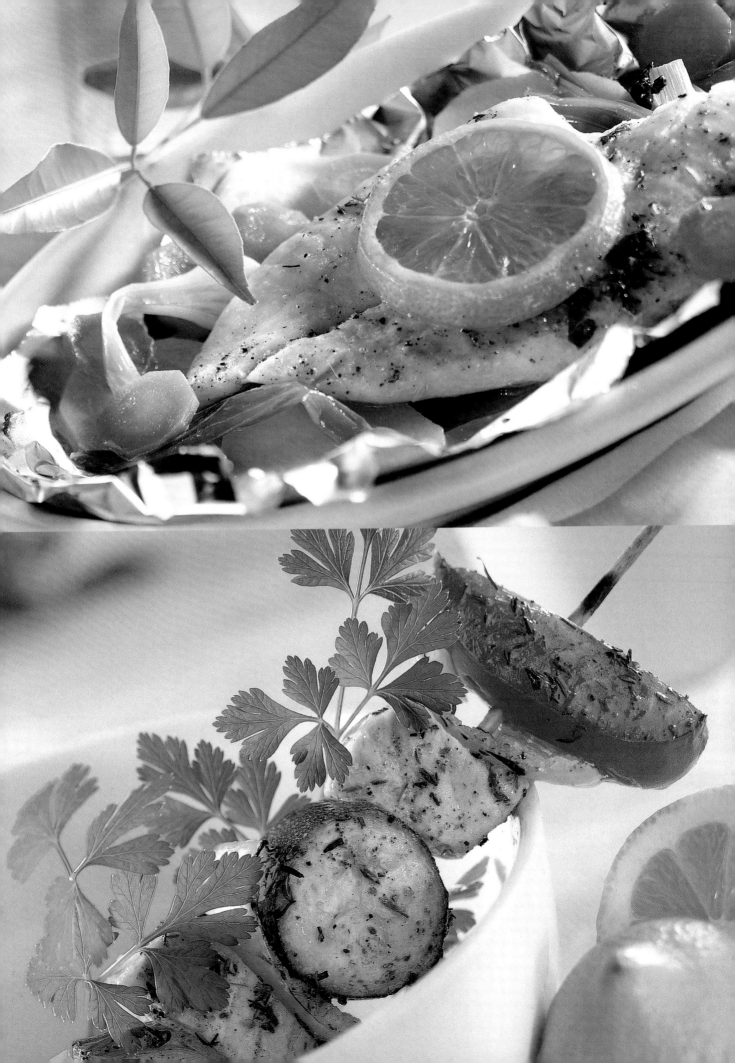

Fish Fillets with Zucchini (Courgette) and Tomatoes

Carbohydrates	●	1 hr.
Fat	●●	
Fiber	●	

Per serving: approx. 245 calories
31 g protein · 9 g fat · 11 g carbohydrates

FOR 2 SERVINGS:
8 oz (250 g) red snapper or salmon
　　fillets
2 tbsp (30 mL) lemon juice
Salt and white pepper
Ground coriander seeds
½ bunch basil
1½ zucchini
1 onion
4 tomatoes
2 tbsp (30 mL) freshly grated
　　Emmenthal cheese

1 Cut fish into pieces. Sprinkle with lemon juice and season with salt, pepper and ground coriander.

2 Chop the basil and coarsely grate the zucchini. Chop the onion and slice the tomatoes.

3 Preheat the oven to 325°F (160°C). Mix ½ the basil with the zucchini and place in a greased gratin dish. Season with salt and pepper. Arrange the fish, onion and tomatoes on top. Sprinkle with cheese and bake in the preheated oven for 30 minutes, or until fish is golden and cooked. Garnish with remaining basil and serve.

 TIP: A whole-grain baguette and tossed salad go well with this meal.

Grouper with Orange

Carbohydrates	●	25 min.
Fat	–	(+ 30 min.
Fiber	●●	marinating)

Per serving: approx. 195 calories
32 g protein · 3 g fat · 10 g carbohydrates

FOR 2 SERVINGS:
1 small orange (organic preferred)
1 onion
Salt
2 grouper or other firm fillets, about
　　5 oz (150 g) each
1 fennel bulb
1 green (spring) onion
2 tbsp (30 mL) sour cream
Freshly grated nutmeg
Freshly ground pepper

1 Grate a little zest off the orange and squeeze out the juice. Chop the onion and combine with the orange zest and juice and ½ tsp (2 mL) salt. Coat both sides of the fish in this mixture, cover and marinate for 30 minutes.

2 Halve the fennel and slice finely. Slice the green onion in half lengthwise and julienne. Blanch both in boiling water for 1 to 2 minutes, then plunge into ice water and drain.

3 Preheat the oven to 350°F (180°C). Layer the blanched vegetables in a greased gratin dish. Combine the sour cream and 2 to 3 tbsp (30 to 45 mL) of the marinade and spread over the vegetables. Lay the fish on top and season lightly with nutmeg and pepper. Bake in the preheated oven for 15 minutes, drizzling occasionally with orange marinade. Serve immediately with the cooked vegetables on top of the fillets.

Catfish with Tomatoes

Carbohydrates	◖	25 min.
Fat	+	
Fiber	●	

Per serving: approx. 290 calories
21 g protein · 18 g fat · 6 g carbohydrates

FOR 2 SERVINGS:
2 sprigs fresh rosemary
Zest and juice of ½ lemon
Salt and white pepper
Pinch dried chili flakes
8 oz (250 g) catfish or salmon fillets
2 tbsp (30 mL) olive oil. divided
1 onion
1 clove garlic
6 plum tomatoes

1 Chop the rosemary leaves and combine with the lemon zest and juice, salt, pepper and chili flakes. Cut the fish to make 2 servings and coat with the seasoning mixture.

2 Chop the onion and garlic. Score, blanch, peel and dice the tomatoes. Heat 1 tbsp (15 mL) of the oil, stir in the onion and garlic, and lightly sauté on low heat until translucent. Stir in the tomatoes, season with salt and pepper, and simmer for 10 minutes.

3 Heat the remaining 1 tbsp (15 mL) oil. Brown the fish for 2 to 3 minutes on each side on low heat. Serve with the tomatoes. Garnish with wedges of lemon and additional rosemary sprigs, if desired.

Fish Fillets with Zucchini and
Tomatoes, top
Grouper with Orange, bottom left
Catfish with Tomatoes, bottom right

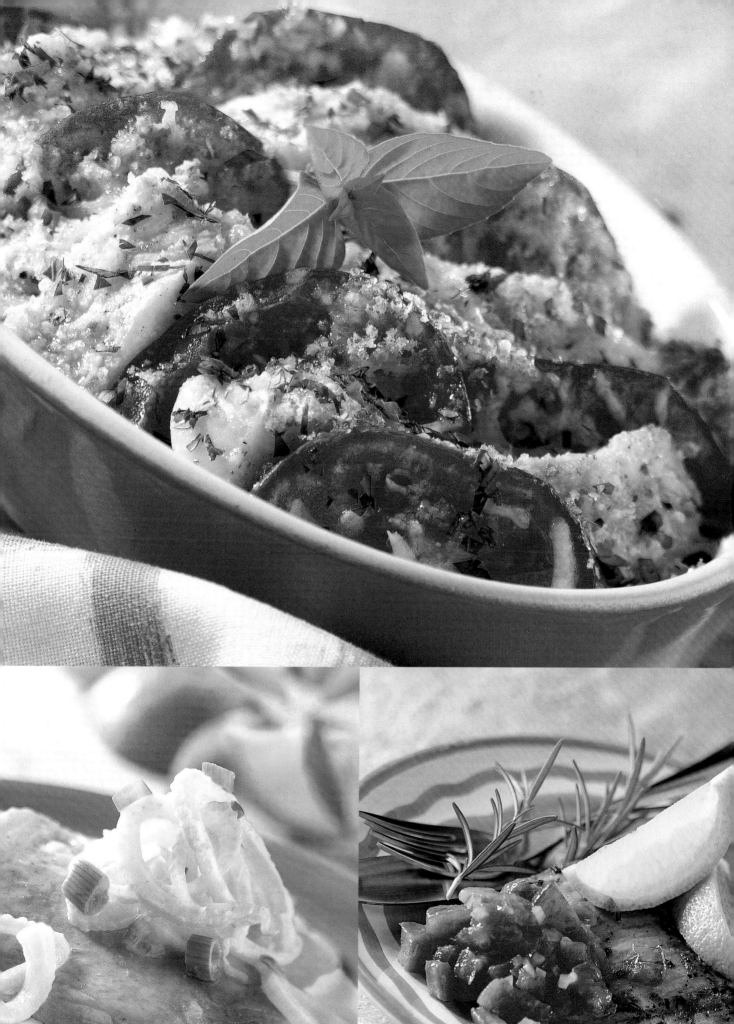

Shrimp Curry with Rice

Carbohydrates	●●●●	30 min.
Fat	+	
Fiber	●	

Per serving: approx. 427 calories
24 g protein · 17 g fat · 44 g carbohydrates

FOR 2 SERVINGS:
²/₃ cup (150 mL) chicken stock
½ cup (125 mL/75 g) basmati rice
2 tbsp (30 mL) sesame oil
1 large onion
1 banana
¾ cup (175 mL) tomato sauce or puréed tomatoes
7 oz (200 g) cooked frozen shrimp
Salt and freshly ground pepper
Curry powder
1 bunch parsley

1 Bring the chicken stock to a boil. Stir in the rice and cook, covered, on low heat for 20 minutes, stirring occasionally.

2 Dice the onion. Heat the oil in a skillet (frying pan). Stir in the onion and curry powder to taste and gently sauté on low heat until translucent and fragrant. Peel the banana, cut into pieces and add to the onion. Mix in the tomato sauce, turn the heat up to medium and cook for 3 minutes. Add shrimp and cook for another 2 minutes. Season with salt and pepper.

3 Chop the parsley. Combine the shrimp curry and cooked rice, arrange on two plates and sprinkle with parsley.

TIPS: Basmati rice is one of the most interesting types of rice because of its unique aroma. You can also use a more economical long-grain rice in this dish. If you're concerned about nutrition, choose converted (parboiled) long-grain rice instead of white—it offers a greater variety of important vitamins and minerals.

Stir-Fried Shrimp

Carbohydrates	◖	45 min.
Fat	●●●	
Fiber	–	

Per serving: approx. 207 calories
17 g protein · 14 g fat · 5 g carbohydrates

FOR 2 SERVINGS:
1 clove garlic
2 tbsp (30 mL) light soy sauce
1 tsp (5 mL) sunflower or vegetable oil
Pinch grated galangal (optional)
Pinch ground coriander seeds
10 medium shrimp, peeled and deveined
1 green (spring) onion
1 tbsp (15 mL) lime juice
1 tsp (5 mL) chopped fresh ginger
Pinch sugar
Salt and freshly ground pepper
1 tsp (5 mL) fresh coriander leaves
1 tsp (5 mL) sesame oil
2 tbsp (30 mL) peanut or vegetable oil
1 zucchini (courgette)
1 or 2 mild or hot chili peppers

1 Chop the the garlic and combine with the soy sauce, sunflower oil, galangal, if using, ground coriander and 1 tbsp (15 mL) water. Stir shrimp in this mixture to coat, and marinate for 20 minutes.

2 Finely chop the green onion and fresh coriander. Mix with the lime juice, ginger, sugar, salt, pepper and sesame oil. Stir in 1 to 2 tbsp (15 to 30 mL) water.

3 Slice the zucchini and cut the peppers into 1-inch (2.5 cm) pieces. Heat the peanut oil in a wok. Stir-fry individual servings of the shrimp, zucchini and peppers for 2 minutes, adding marinade as needed. Serve with the lime sauce and rice.

TIP: Galangal (pronounced guh-LANG-gul), also known as Laos ginger, Siamese ginger and Thai ginger, is a rhizome often used in Southeast Asian cuisine. It is related to ginger, but it has a spicy, pungent flavor all its own.

Shrimp Curry with Rice, top
Stir-Fried Shrimp, bottom

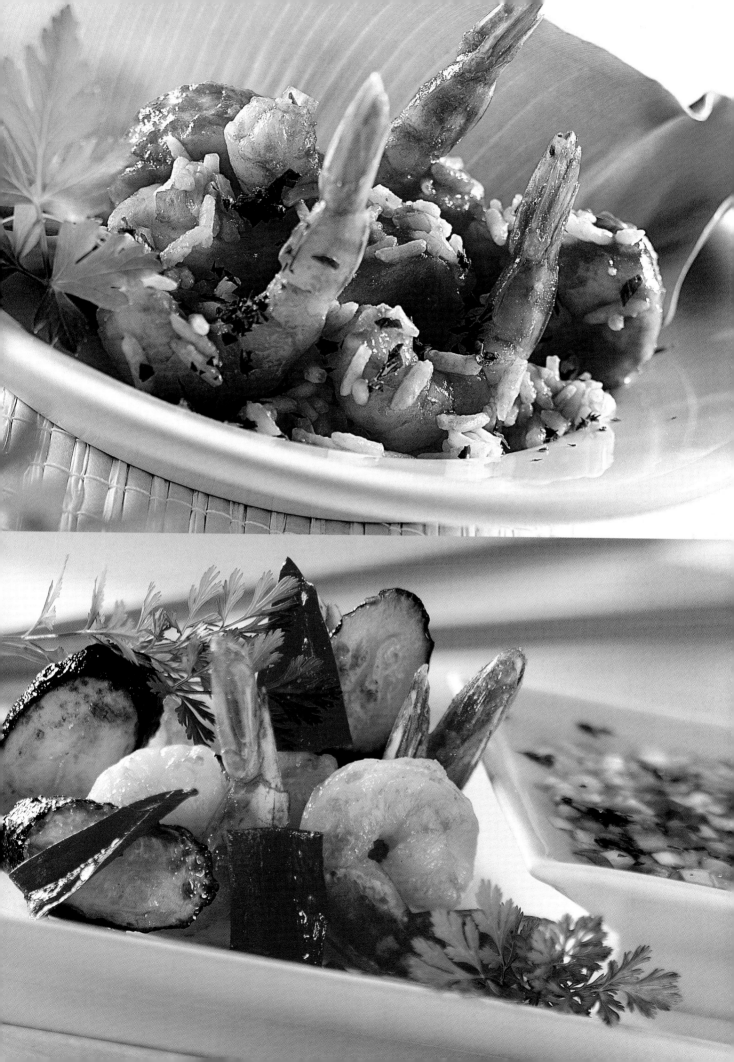

Meat and Poultry

Less is more...

Meat is an excellent source of protein and important nutrients, such as iron, vitamin B_{12} and zinc, that occur only in small quantities in vegetables. Depending on the type, however, meat also contains high levels of saturated fats, cholesterol and purine—dietary elements that can have a negative impact on your health.

So enjoy meat and meat products less often—2 to 3 servings a week make sense in a health-conscious diet—and choose better-quality cuts, preferably organically produced.

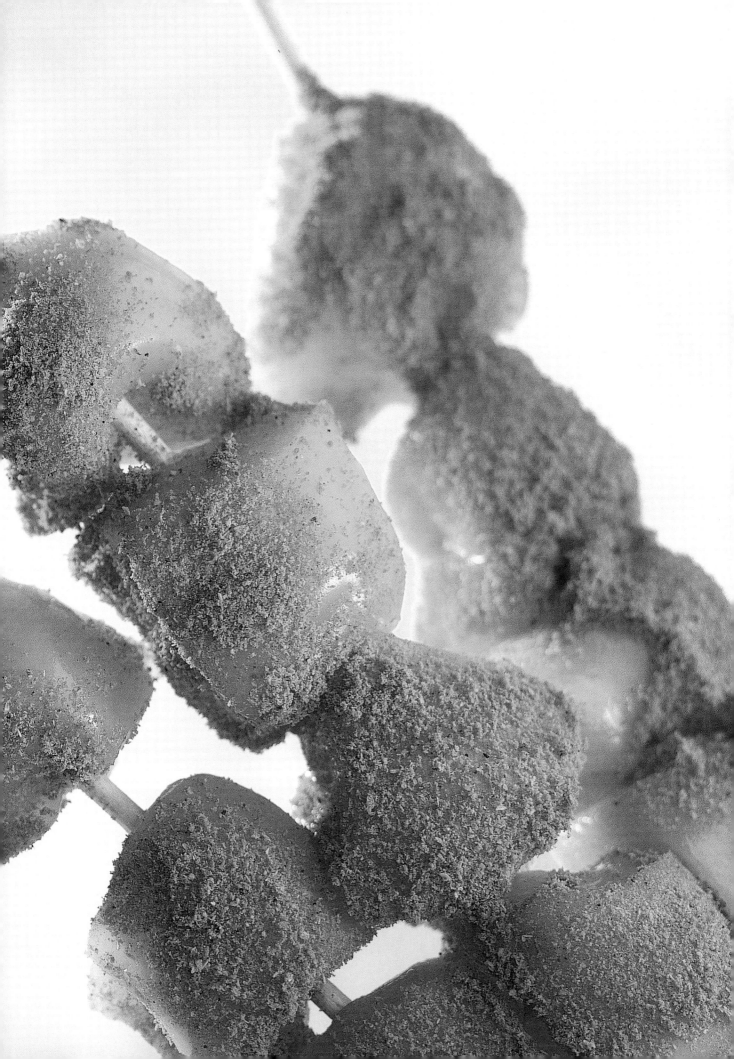

Pork Cutlets with Vegetables

Carbohydrates	●●●●◖	50 min.
Fat	●●●	
Fiber	●●	

Per serving: approx. 399 calories
25 g protein · 12 g fat · 43 g carbohydrates

FOR 2 SERVINGS:
1 tbsp (15 mL) olive oil
1 onion
1 small clove garlic
½ cup (125 mL/100 g) long-grain
   brown rice
3 tbsp (45 mL) dry white wine
1 cup (250 mL) water
Salt
1 carrot
½ fennel bulb
⅓ cup (75 mL/75 g) low-fat yogurt
2 tsp (10 mL) lemon juice
1 tbsp (15 mL) chopped parsley
5½ oz (160 g) pork cutlet
Sweet paprika
Crumbled dried rosemary
1 tbsp (15 mL) oil

1 Chop the onion and garlic. Heat the oil, stir in the onion and garlic, and lightly sauté. Stir in the rice and cook briefly. Add wine and water, and season lightly with salt. Cook, covered, on low heat for 40 minutes.

2 Slice the carrot and fennel and arrange on two plates. Combine the yogurt with lemon juice, parsley and a pinch of salt. Drizzle over the vegetables.

3 Flatten the pork with a meat tenderizer and season with salt, paprika and rosemary. Cut into 6 small pieces and brown in hot oil for 3 minutes each side. Serve with the vegetables and rice.

Beef Patties with Herbs and Red Pepper

Carbohydrates	●◖	35 min.
Fat	++	
Fiber	●●●	

Per serving: approx. 217 calories
16 g protein · 10 g fat · 15 g carbohydrates

FOR 2 SERVINGS:
1 slice whole-grain bread
2 tbsp (30 mL) low-fat milk
3½ oz (100 g) lean ground beef
1 onion
1 red pepper
½ bunch parsley
5 sprigs fresh thyme or ½ tsp (2 mL)
   dried
1 small carrot
1 to 2 tbsp (15 to 30 mL) low-fat
   quark or puréed cottage cheese
1 tbsp (15 mL) flour
Salt and freshly ground pepper
1 tsp (5 mL) canola or vegetable oil

1 Remove the crust, dice the bread finely and soak in the milk.

2 Finely chop the onion, red pepper, parsley and thyme. Finely grate the carrot. Combine ground beef, onion, pepper, carrot, quark, soaked bread, parsley and thyme, adding flour as needed to bind. Season with salt and pepper.

3 Form 4 patties. Heat the oil in a nonstick skillet (frying pan) and cook the patties for 5 to 6 minutes on each side on medium heat, until brown.

Pork and Peppers

Carbohydrates	◖	30 min.
Fat	●●	
Fiber	●	

Per serving: approx. 188 calories
27 g protein · 7 g fat · 8 g carbohydrates

FOR 2 SERVINGS:
1 yellow and 1 green pepper
1 red onion
7 oz (200 g) pork tenderloin
1 clove garlic
6 sage leaves
6 sprigs fresh thyme or ¾ tsp
   (4 mL) dried
2 tsp (10 mL) olive oil, divided
1½ tsp (7 mL) coarsely ground
   whole wheat flour
⅔ cup (150 mL) vegetable stock
Salt and freshly ground pepper

1 Slice the peppers into thin strips. Cut the onion into wedges. Slice pork into thin strips. Finely slice the garlic, shred the sage leaves and chop the thyme leaves.

2 Heat 1 tsp (5 mL) of the oil in a skillet (frying pan) or wok. Brown the meat on medium heat and set aside.

3 Heat the remaining oil and lightly fry the peppers, onion and garlic. Mix in the sage and thyme, dust with flour, then stir in the stock. Season with salt and pepper. Cook for 5 minutes. Stir pork in and reheat.

Pork Cutlets with Vegetables, top
Beef Patties with Herbs and Red
Pepper, bottom left
Pork and Peppers, bottom right

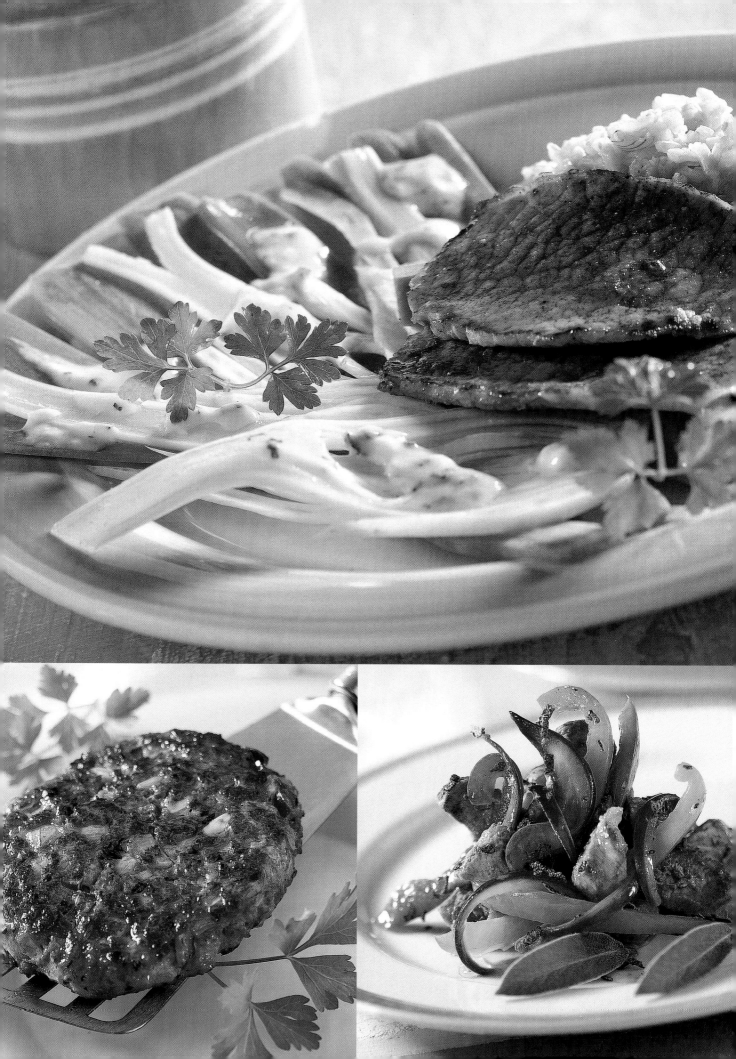

Pork with Lentils

Carbohydrates	●●●◖	1 hr.
Fat	+	
Fiber	●●●	

Per serving: approx. 520 calories
46 g protein · 19 g fat · 40 g carbohydrates

FOR 2 SERVINGS:
1 onion
1 carrot
2 ribs celery
1 tbsp (15 mL) olive oil
½ cup (125 mL/100 g) red lentils
1¼ cups (300 mL) meat stock, divided
2 tbsp (30 mL) white-wine vinegar
Cayenne
Salt and freshly ground pepper
10 oz (300 g) pork tenderloin
1 tbsp (15 mL) canola or vegetable oil
½ tsp (2 mL) curry powder
5 tbsp (75 mL) grape juice
¼ cup (50 mL/50 g) sour cream

1 Chop the onion and carrot and slice the celery crosswise. Heat the olive oil in a medium saucepan. Stir in the onion, carrot and celery, and cook, covered, on medium heat for 10 minutes.

2 Stir in the the lentils and pour in ¾ cup (175 mL) of the stock. Season with the vinegar, a little cayenne, salt and pepper. Cook, covered, on low heat for 40 minutes.

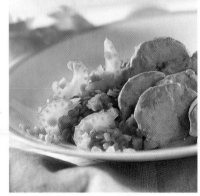

3 Slice the pork into thin medallions. Heat the canola oil and cook the pork on medium heat until brown. Season with salt, pepper and curry powder. Remove, set aside and keep warm.

4 Deglaze the pan with the grape juice, add the remaining ½ cup (125 mL) of stock, and cook on high heat until reduced. Stir in the sour cream and reheat the pork in the sauce. Serve with the lentils.

Pork with a Savory Topping

Carbohydrates	●●	50 min.
Fat	+++	
Fiber	●●●	

Per serving: approx. 588 calories
44 g protein · 33 g fat · 20 g carbohydrates

FOR 2 SERVINGS:
1 small Savoy cabbage
10 oz (300 g) pork tenderloin
Salt and freshly ground pepper
4 tsp (20 mL) clarified butter, divided
½ cup (125 mL) dry white wine
2 oz (60 g) ham
1 medium white onion
2 cloves garlic
2 medium tomatoes
3 tbsp (45 mL/20 g) raisins
1 small sprig fresh thyme
1 small sprig fresh marjoram
1 tbsp (15 mL) blanched chopped almonds
1 tbsp (15 mL) pine nuts

1 Remove the tender leaves from the cabbage and blanch in boiling water for 3 minutes. Remove, plunge into ice water and drain.

2 Season the meat with salt and pepper. Heat 2 tsp (10 ml) butter, add the meat and brown lightly on all sides. Slice the meat thickly and place in an ovenproof dish. Deglaze the pan with ½ the wine and pour over the meat. Arrange the cabbage leaves on top.

3 Preheat oven to 350°F (180°C). Dice the ham, chop the onion and garlic, and score, blanch, peel and dice the tomatoes. Brown the ham, onion, garlic, tomatoes and raisins in the remaining 2 tsp (10 mL) butter. Pour in the remaining wine. Place this mixture on the cabbage leaves. Top with thyme and marjoram. Bake for 20 minutes.

5 Toast the almonds in a dry nonstick skillet (frying pan), crush slightly, and sprinkle over top along with the pine nuts. Bake for another 10 minutes.

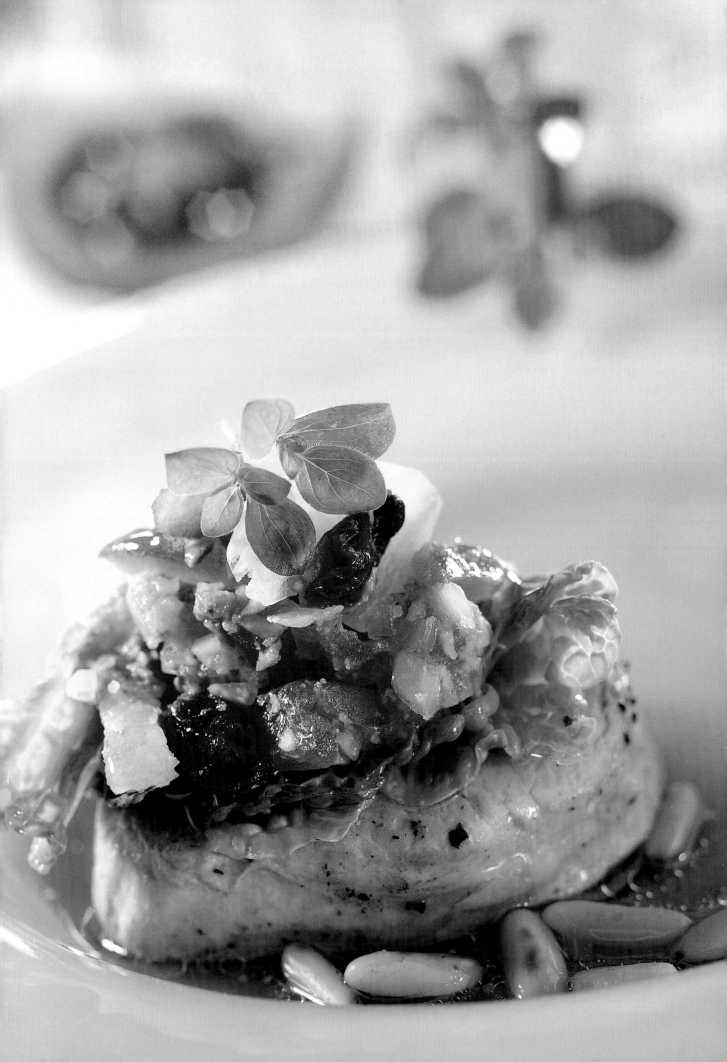

Veal Rouladen with Ham and Cheese

Carbohydrates ◖	30 min.
Fat +++	
Fiber –	

Per serving: approx. 643 calories
58 g protein · 43 g fat · 5 g carbohydrates

FOR 2 SERVINGS:
2 thin 6-oz (175 g) veal cutlets
4 paper- thin slices prosciutto
4 small slices pecorino cheese
1 clove garlic
2 tbsp (30 mL) chopped fresh parsley
2 tbsp (30 mL) vegetable oil, divided
Salt and freshly ground pepper
12 fresh basil leaves
¼ cup (50 mL) dry white wine
¼ cup (50 mL) vegetable stock
2 tbsp (30 mL/30 g) crème fraîche or sour cream

1 Using a meat hammer, tenderize and flatten the veal. Cut the pieces in two. Cover each piece with a slice of prosciutto and a slice of pecorino.

2 Chop the garlic and pound with the parsley and 1 tbsp (15 mL) of the oil in a mortar to form a thick paste. Lightly season with salt and pepper.

3 Spread the paste over the cheese, then place 2 basil leaves on top. Roll and fasten with toothpicks.

4 Heat the remaining 1 tbsp (15 mL) of oil in a skillet (frying pan) and fry the rouladen on medium heat until golden. Pour in wine and stock. Cook, covered, on low heat for 10 minutes. Stir in the crème fraîche and season with salt and pepper. Arrange the rouladen and sauce on warm plates. Garnish with remaining basil and serve.

 TIP: Brown rice goes well with this dish.

 TIP: Instead of using veal, you can prepare the rouladen with turkey.

Veal with Swiss Chard and Potatoes

Carbohydrates ●●	45 min.
Fat +	
Fiber ●●	

Per serving: approx. 409 calories
44 g protein · 16 g fat · 22 g carbohydrates

FOR 2 SERVINGS:
10 oz (300 g) veal (shoulder)
1 medium onion
1 clove garlic
1 cup (500 mL) water
2 tbsp (30 mL) olive oil
Juice of ½ lemon
Salt and freshly ground pepper
2 firm potatoes
10 oz (300 g) Swiss chard, beet greens or spinach
¼ cup (50 mL/30 g) freshly grated Parmesan cheese

1 Cut the veal into bite-size pieces. Finely chop the onion and garlic. Heat the oil in a heavy saucepan and brown the meat on all sides on medium heat. Stir in the onion and garlic and sauté until translucent. Add the water and lemon juice. Season with salt and pepper. Cook, covered, on medium heat for 15 minutes.

2 Peel and cut the potatoes in quarters or wedges and coarsely chop the Swiss chard. Mix the potatoes into the meat mixture and simmer for 15 minutes, or until potatoes are tender. Stir in Swiss chard and cook, covered, for another 3 minutes. Season with salt and pepper. Arrange on two plates, sprinkle with Parmesan and serve.

TIP: When served with potatoes, pasta or rice and a large serving of vegetables, meat is a healthful choice. The recommended amount is 3 to 5 oz (85 to 140 g) per person per meal, no more than 3 times a week.

Veal Rouladen with Ham and Cheese, top
Veal with Swiss Chard and Potatoes, bottom

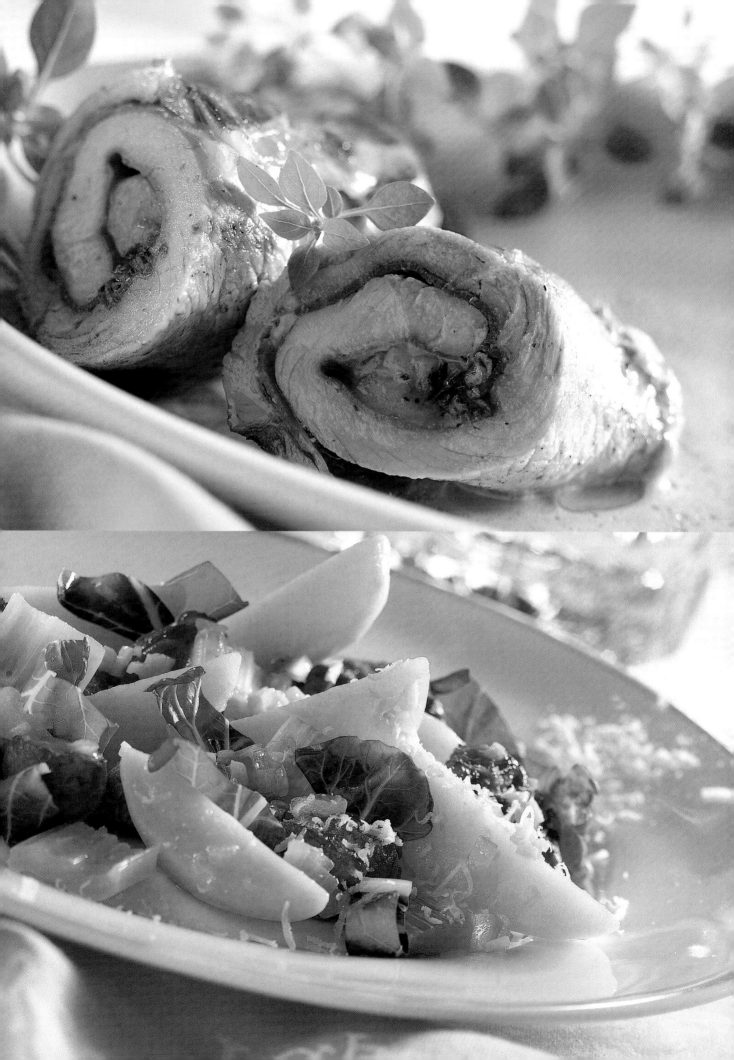

Lamb Curry with Tomatoes and Zucchini (Courgette)

Carbohydrates	●●●●●◖	2 hrs.
Fat	+++	(+ 4 hrs. marinating)
Fiber	●●●	

Per serving: approx. 625 calories
30 g protein · 25 g fat · 68 g carbohydrates

FOR 2 SERVINGS:
7 oz (200 g) lean lamb (leg)
Salt
2 tsp (10 mL) Madras curry powder, divided
1 small clove garlic
1 tbsp (15 mL) olive oil
1 onion
3 beefsteak tomatoes
2 bay leaves
1 small red pepper
1 carrot
1 small zucchini
½ handful fresh coriander
⅔ cup (150 mL/120 g) basmati rice

1 Remove any fat and sinews from the lamb and dice. Finely chop the garlic. Combine meat with ½ tsp (2 mL) salt, 1 tsp (5 mL) of the curry powder and the garlic. Stir to coat, and refrigerate, covered, for at least 4 hours.

2 Finely chop the onion and purée the tomatoes. Heat the oil and stir-fry the lamb and onion, seasoning with the remaining 1 tsp (5 mL) curry powder and 1 tsp (5 mL) salt. Stir in the tomatoes and bay leaves and bring to a boil. Cook, covered, on low heat for 1 hour.

3 Coarsely chop the red pepper and zucchini, slice the carrot, and finely chop the fresh coriander. Stir the red pepper, carrot and zucchini into the meat mixture, bring to a boil and simmer, covered, for 30 to 40 minutes. Stir in the coriander just before serving.

4 Meanwhile, cook the rice in lightly salted water according to package directions and serve on the side.

‼ **TIP:** Instead of using fresh coriander, you can season with a mixture of 4 crushed coriander seeds and 1 tbsp (15 mL) chopped fresh parsley leaves.

Lamb with Beans and Red Peppers

Carbohydrates	●●●●	50 min.
Fat	+	
Fiber	●●●	

Per serving: approx. 450 calories
27 g protein · 18 g fat · 44 g carbohydrates

FOR 2 SERVINGS:
½ cup (125 mL/75 g) long-grain converted (parboiled) rice
1 cup (250 g) boiling salted water
7 oz (200 g) boned lamb chops
1 tbsp (15 mL) olive oil
1 large onion
2½ cups (625 mL) beef broth
Salt and freshly ground pepper
2½ cups (625 mL/300 g) green beans
2 red peppers
2 cloves garlic
Dried thyme
Dried chili flakes

1 Add rice to water. Cover and cook for 20 minutes on low heat, stirring occasionally.

2 Dice the lamb and finely chop the onion. Heat the oil in a medium saucepan and brown the meat on all sides. Stir in onion and sauté until translucent. Pour in the broth and season with salt and pepper. Simmer on medium heat for 10 to 15 minutes.

3 Meanwhile, cut the beans into bite-size pieces, coarsely dice the red peppers and chop the garlic. Stir the beans, peppers, garlic and thyme into the meat and cook for a further 10 minutes. Season with salt and chili flakes and serve with the rice.

‼ **TIP:** Red peppers enhance a meal not only with their bright red color, but also with their high vitamin C content, which is higher than that of green peppers.

Lamb Curry with Tomatoes and Zucchini, top
Lamb with Beans and Red Peppers, bottom

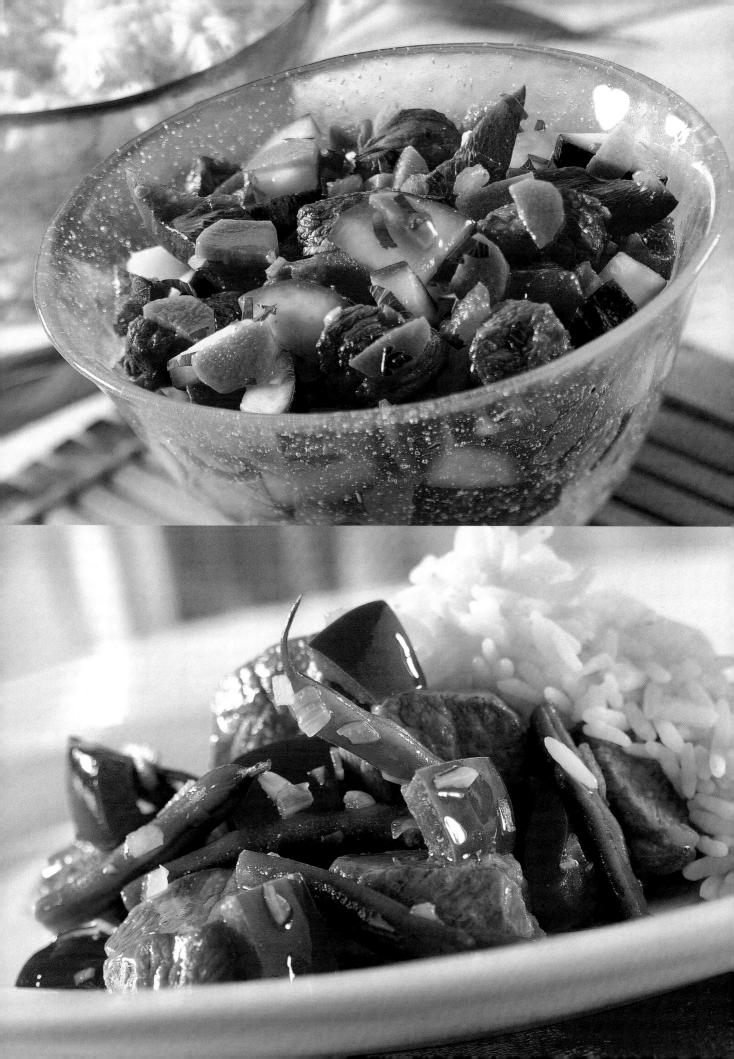

Rosemary Beef Stew

Carbohydrates	●●●	1 hr. 40 min.
Fat	+	
Fiber	●●●	

Per serving: approx. 433 calories
39 g protein · 15 g fat · 35 g carbohydrates

FOR 2 SERVINGS:
10 oz (300 g) stewing beef
1 onion
1 clove garlic
2 tbsp (30 mL) olive oil
4 tomatoes
2 carrots
2 potatoes
1 bay leaf
¾ cup (175 mL) beef broth
4 sprigs fresh rosemary
Salt and freshly ground pepper

1 Cut the beef into bite-size pieces and chop the onion and garlic. Heat the oil in a large, heavy saucepan or Dutch oven and sauté the onion and garlic. Stir in the meat and brown on all sides.

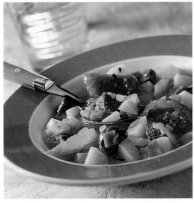

2 Score, blanch, peel and quarter the tomatoes. Peel and chop the carrots and potatoes. Stir these in with the bay leaf. Pour in the broth and simmer, covered, for 1 hour, or until meat is tender.

3 Chop the rosemary leaves and use them to season the stew just before serving, along with salt and pepper to taste.

Beef à la Ficelle

Carbohydrates	●●	1 hr.
Fat	●●	
Fiber	●●●	

Per serving: approx. 312 calories
36 g protein · 8 g fat · 24 g carbohydrates

FOR 2 SERVINGS:
6 cups (1.5 L) vegetable stock
1½ cups (375 mL) peeled, diced potatoes
10 oz (300 g) lean beef, such as round steak
2 large carrots
3 green (spring) onions
3 ribs celery
1 tbsp (15 mL) light thickener
Salt and freshly ground pepper

1 Bring the stock to a boil in a large saucepan. Add the potatoes and cook, covered, for 5 minutes.

2 Wind kitchen twine around the meat and make a loop at each end. Insert a long cooking spoon through the loops and pull tight.

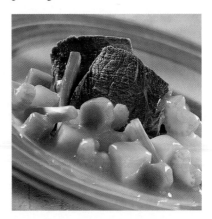

3 Peel and dice the carrots, slice the green onions and celery crosswise, and stir into the saucepan. Place the cooking spoon across the top of the pot so the meat hangs in the stock. Simmer, covered, for 30 minutes. Remove the meat, thicken the stock, and add salt and pepper. Slice the meat and serve with the vegetables and sauce.

Beef Stew with Tomatoes and Olives

Carbohydrates		30 min.
Fat		(+1 hr. braising)
Fiber		

Per serving: approx. 458 calories
33 g protein · 30 g fat · 6 g carbohydrates

FOR 2 SERVINGS:
10 oz (300 g) stewing beef
1 slice (rasher) lean bacon
1 tsp (5 mL) olive oil
2 onions
2 cloves garlic
½ cup (125 mL) meat or vegetable stock
½ cup (125 mL) dry red wine
2 tomatoes
Salt and freshly ground pepper
1 small sprig fresh rosemary
1 small sprig fresh thyme
3 tbsp (45 mL) pitted green olives
3 sprigs Italian (flat-leaf) parsley

1 Dice the beef and bacon and finely chop the onions and garlic. Heat the oil in a medium saucepan or Dutch oven and brown the bacon on medium heat. Stir in and brown the beef, then the onions and garlic.

2 Meanwhile, dice the tomatoes. Pour the stock and wine into the saucepan and bring to a boil. Stir in the tomatoes, and season with salt and pepper. Place the rosemary and thyme on top, cover and braise gently on low heat for 1 hour.

3 Slice and stir in the olives 15 minutes before the end of the cooking time. Chop and stir in the parsley just before serving. Garnish with additional herbs, if desired.

Beef Stew with Tomatoes and Olives, right

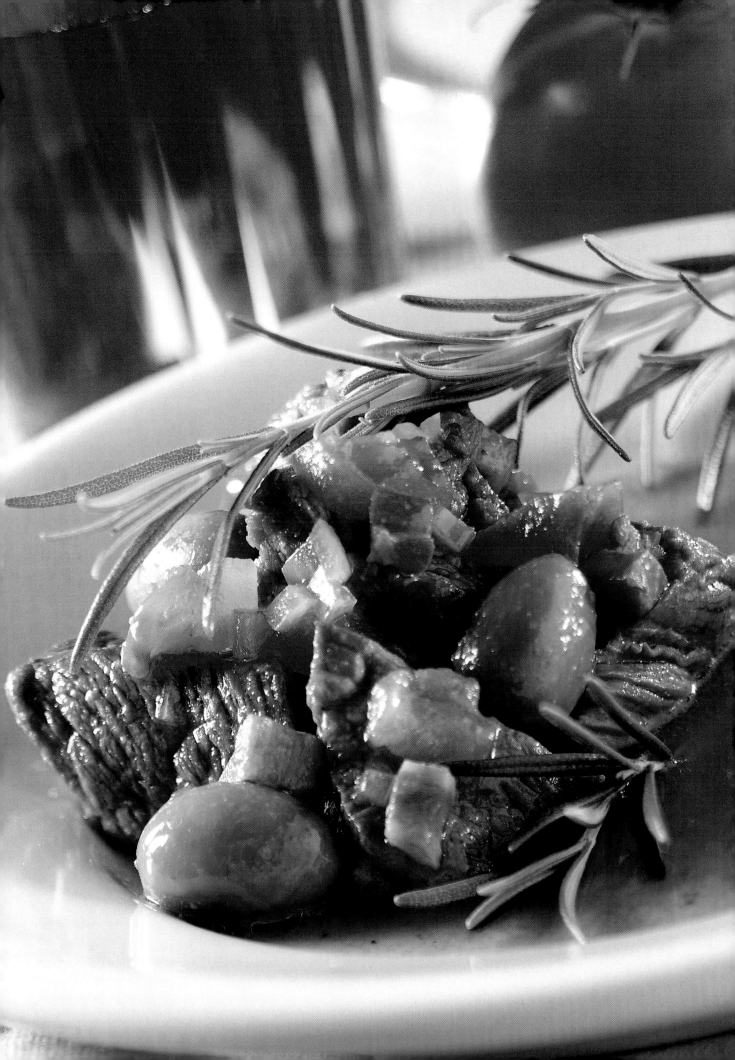

Braised Chicken Legs with Roasted Potatoes and Cabbage Salad

Carbohydrates	●●●	1 hr. 45 min.
Fat	++	
Fiber	●●●	

Per serving: approx. 458 calories
30 g protein · 22 g fat · 34 g carbohydrates

FOR 2 SERVINGS:
3 beefsteak tomatoes
2 dried apricots
2 small onions
2 tbsp (30 mL) tomato paste
1 tsp (5 mL) + 2 tbsp (30 ml) fruit vinegar
Salt
Liquid sweetener
Hot pepper sauce
2 (4-oz/125 g) skinless chicken legs
Sweet paprika
2 baking potatoes
1 tsp (5 mL) olive oil
Dried rosemary
2 cups (500 mL/150 g) shredded tender green cabbage
1 tbsp (15 mL) chopped Italian (flat-leaf) parsley
3 tbsp (45 mL) water
1 tbsp (15 mL) sunflower oil
1/2 tsp (2 mL) medium-hot mustard

1 Quarter the tomatoes. Purée 2 and dice the third. Combine in a large saucepan or Dutch oven. Chop the apricots and stir in. Finely dice the onions and add 1/2 to the saucepan. Stir in the tomato paste, the 1 tsp (5 mL) vinegar and 2 pinches salt. Bring to a boil and simmer, uncovered, for 2 minutes. Splash in sweetener and hot pepper sauce to taste.

2 Preheat the oven to 425°F (220°C). Peel the potatoes, if desired, and cut into wedges or "fingers." Place on a baking sheet, brush lightly with oil, and season with salt, rosemary and a little paprika. Roast on the bottom rack of the preheated oven for 5 to 10 minutes.

3 Rub the chicken with salt and paprika and arrange in a greased baking dish. Pour tomato sauce over and cover with aluminum foil. Place on the middle rack of the oven and bake for 35 to 40 minutes (turn the potatoes at least once in this time). Remove the foil from the chicken and bake for another 10 minutes, until the chicken is done and the potatoes lightly browned and cooked through.

4 Meanwhile, make the salad. Combine cabbage with parsley and remaining diced onion in a small saucepan. Add the water, the 2 tbsp (30 mL) vinegar, oil and mustard. Cover and cook for 4 minutes. Season with salt and sweetener and toss.

Chicken Breasts with Rice and Peas

Carbohydrates	●●●●●	30 min.
Fat	++	
Fiber	●●	

Per serving: approx. 675 calories
15 g protein · 22 g fat · 57 g carbohydrates

FOR 2 SERVINGS:
3 oz (85 g) cooked ham
1 onion
4 tbsp (60 mL) olive oil, divided
1 2/3 cups (400 mL) chicken stock, divided
1 cup (250 mL/75 g) thawed frozen peas
2/3 cup (150 mL/100 g) long-grain rice
10 oz (300 g) skinless boneless chicken breasts
Salt and freshly ground pepper
1/4 cup (50 mL/30 g) freshly grated Parmesan cheese
1 bunch parsley
2 tbsp (30 mL/30 g) sour cream

1 Cut the ham into strips and dice the onion. Heat 2 tbsp (30 mL) of the oil in a medium saucepan, stir in onion and gently sauté on low heat until translucent. Add ham and brown lightly.

2 Bring 1 1/4 cups (300 mL) of the stock to a boil. Stir the peas and rice into the onion–ham mixture, stir to coat, then pour in a little hot stock. Gradually add all the stock and cook, covered, on low heat for 15 minutes.

3 Heat the remaining oil and brown the chicken on all sides. Stir in remaining stock and cook on low heat for 10 minutes.

4 Meanwhile, chop most of the parsley. Season the rice mixture with salt and pepper. Fold in Parmesan and parsley. Remove chicken from the pan and slice. Stir the sour cream into the pan juices, cook briefly, and serve with the chicken and rice. Garnish with the remaining parsley leaves.

Braised Chicken Legs with Roasted Potatoes and Cabbage Salad, top
Chicken Breasts with Rice and Peas, bottom

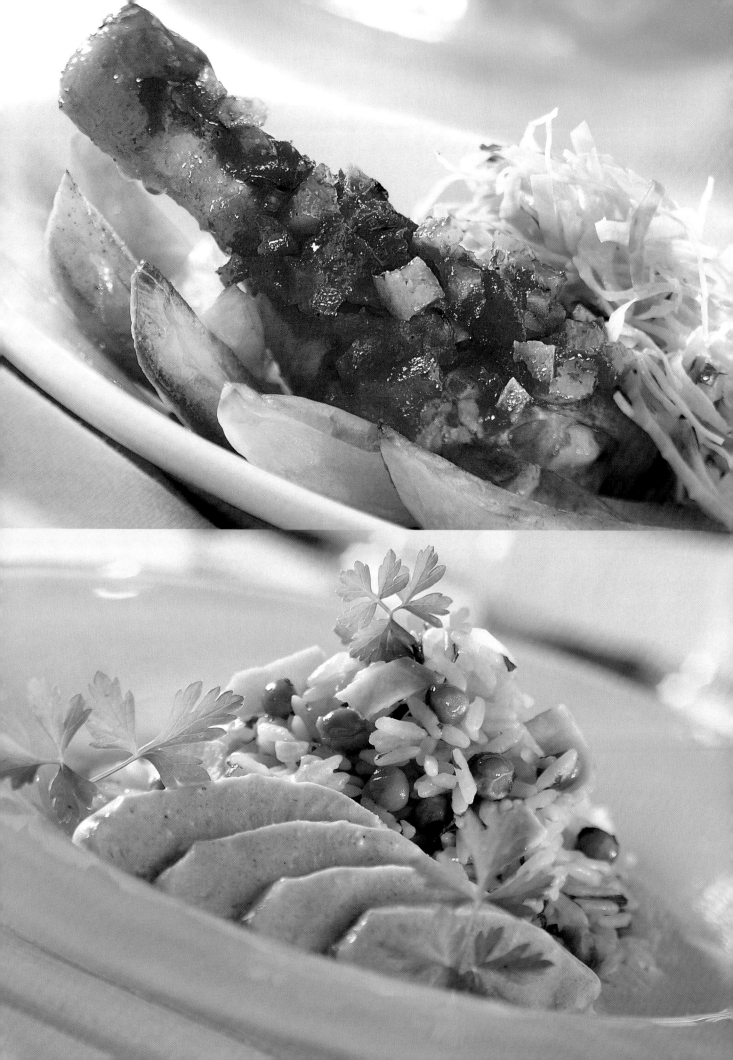

Chicken Breasts in Curry Sauce with Basmati Rice

Carbohydrates ●●●		40 min.
Fat +		
Fiber ●		

Per serving: approx. 423 calories
36 g protein · 17 g fat · 33 g carbohydrates

FOR 2 SERVINGS:
½ cup (125 mL/75 g) basmati rice
1 cup (250 mL) boiling salted water
½ cup (125 mL) unsweetened coconut milk
½ cup (125 mL) chicken or vegetable stock
Juice of 1 lime
4 sprigs fresh coriander
Curry powder
Sambal oelek or other hot chili-based sauce
Salt and freshly ground pepper
8 oz (250 g) skinless boneless chicken breasts
2 tbsp (30 mL) sesame oil
1 small red pepper

1 Add rice to water and cook, covered, on low heat for 20 minutes, stirring occasionally.

2 Chop the fresh coriander. Combine coconut milk and stock and bring to a boil. Add lime juice, coriander, curry powder, sambal oelek, salt and pepper to taste.

3 Cut the chicken and red pepper into fine strips. Heat the oil in a skillet (frying pan) or wok. Brown the chicken and pepper strips on medium heat. Stir in the coconut-milk mixture and simmer on medium heat for 10 minutes. Serve with rice on the side.

 TIP: Large shrimp, shelled and deveined, and fish stock are tasty substitutes for the chicken and stock in this recipe.

Chicken Tonnato with Vegetables

Carbohydrates ●		50 min.
Fat +		
Fiber ●●●		

Per serving: approx. 461 calories
56 g protein · 21 g fat · 11 g carbohydrates

FOR 2 SERVINGS:
1 lb (500 g) mixed chicken parts, or ½ a small chicken
Freshly ground pepper
2 medium carrots
3 ribs celery
1 onion
4 cups (I L) water
Juice of 1 lemon, divided
Salt
½ (6 oz/170 g) can water-packed tuna, drained
1 tbsp (15 mL) capers
2 tbsp (30 mL) olive oil, divided
1 egg yolk
2 tbsp (30 mL) chopped Italian (flat-leaf) parsley
2 tbsp (30 mL) chopped fresh basil
Fresh basil leaves

1 Rub chicken with pepper. Cut carrots and celery into large pieces. Quarter the onion. In a soup pot, combine water with ½ the lemon juice and 1 tsp (5 mL) salt. Add carrots, celery and onion, and bring to a boil. Add the chicken and cook on low heat for 40 minutes. Remove 2 tbsp (30 mL) of the stock and leave to cool.

2 In a small saucepan, combine tuna with capers and 1 tsp (5 mL) oil. Mash with a potato masher. Whisk egg yolk, a pinch of salt and 1 tbsp (15 mL) of the lemon juice until smooth. Stir in another 1 tsp (5 mL) oil. Stir in the parsley, chopped basil and the 2 tbsp (30 mL) cooled stock, and cook until thick. Season with salt, pepper and the remaining lemon juice.

4 Lift chicken from the stock, remove skin and bones, and arrange on two plates. Drizzle the tuna sauce over the chicken. Spoon the vegetables onto the plates and garnish with lemon wedges and basil leaves.

Chicken Breasts in Curry Sauce with Basmati Rice, top
Chicken Tonnato with Vegetables, bottom

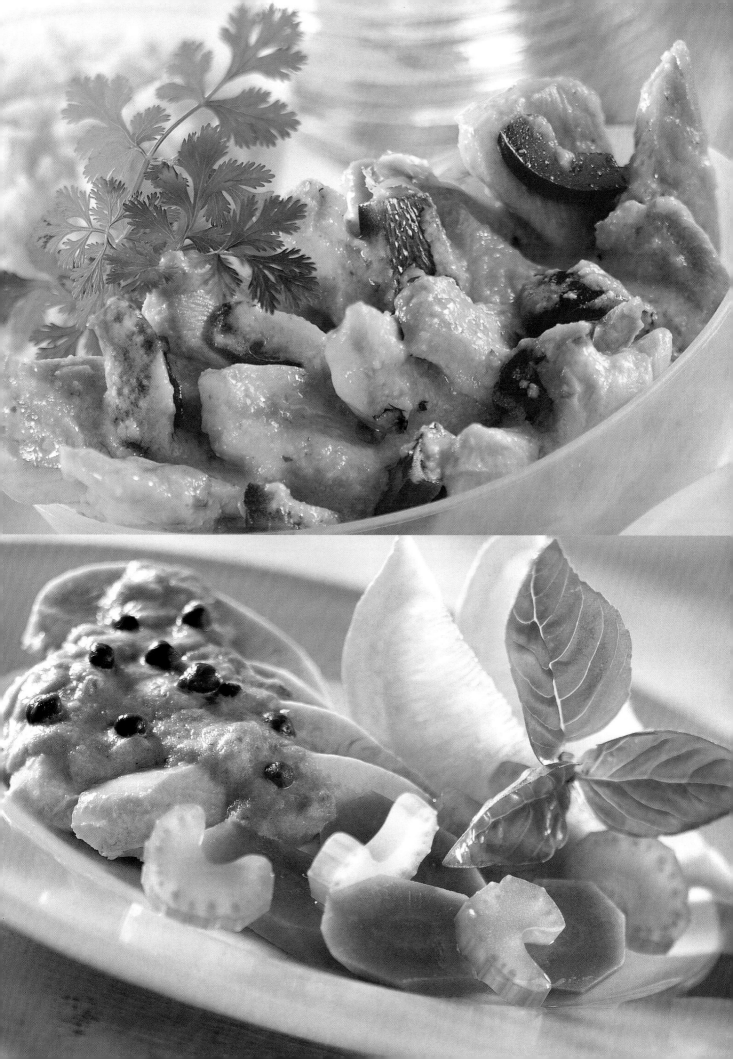

Chicken Skewers with Lentil Sauce

Carbohydrates ●●	35 min.
Fat —	
Fiber ●●	

Per serving: approx. 267 calories
33 g protein · 3 g fat · 24 g carbohydrates

FOR 2 SERVINGS:
7 oz (200 g) skinless boneless chicken breasts
2 tbsp (30 mL) soy sauce
1 tsp (5 mL) sambal oelek or other hot chili-based sauce
1 cup (250 mL) vegetable stock
3 shallots
1 tsp (5 mL) curry powder
½ cup (125 mL/75 g) red lentils
½ bunch chives

1 Cut the chicken into ½-inch (1 cm) cubes. Combine soy sauce with sambal oelek in a small bowl and add chicken. Stir to coat, and refrigerate for 15 minutes.

2 Meanwhile, finely chop the shallots and mix into the stock in a medium saucepan. Stir in the curry powder. Bring to a boil, stir in the lentils and cook, covered, on low heat for 6 to 8 minutes.

3 Preheat a table grill or oven broiler. Slide chicken pieces onto 6 skewers and grill for 6 minutes on all sides, until golden.

4 Remove a little of the lentil mixture from the saucepan and set aside. Mash the remainder with a potato masher. Bring back to a boil, adding water as needed.

5 Arrange skewers on plates with the lentil sauce. Snip the chives and sprinkle on top of the sauce with the reserved lentils.

!! TIP: Without the skin, chicken and turkey are very low fat, but they dry out quickly. Brown them only briefly or brush with a marinade containing vegetable oil.

Turkey Cutlet with Lentils

Carbohydrates ●●●●	50 min.
Fat ●●●	(+ 15 min. marinating)
Fiber ●●	

Per serving: approx. 447 calories
48 g protein · 11 g fat · 44 g carbohydrates

FOR 2 SERVINGS:
10 oz (300 g) skinless boneless turkey breast
Juice of 1 orange
2 tbsp (30 mL) soy sauce
⅓ cup (75 mL/50 g) long-grain converted (parboiled) rice
⅔ cup (150 mL) boiling salted water
¾ cup (175 mL) chicken stock
⅓ cup (75 mL/50 g) green lentils
1 leek
1 tbsp (15 mL) walnut oil
1 tbsp (15 mL) cider vinegar
Salt and freshly ground pepper
Cayenne
1 tbsp (15 mL) canola or vegetable oil

1 Flatten the turkey slightly with a meat tenderizer. Combine orange juice and soy sauce in a flat bowl. Add turkey, turn to coat, and marinate for 15 minutes.

2 Add rice to water and cook, covered, on low heat for 20 minutes, stirring occasionally.

3 Bring the stock to a boil. Stir in the lentils and cook on medium heat for 40 minutes.

4 Meanwhile, cut the leek lengthwise, wash thoroughly, and slice the white and light green parts into fine strips. Stir into the lentils 15 minutes before the end of the cooking time. Remove from the heat and leave to cool slightly. Stir in walnut oil, vinegar, salt, pepper and cayenne.

5 Remove turkey from the marinade and pat dry with a paper towel. Heat the canola oil in a skillet (frying pan) and brown the turkey on medium heat on each side for 4 minutes. Arrange on top of the warm lentils. Serve with rice, and half-moons of sliced orange, if desired.

Chicken Skewers with Lentil Sauce, top
Turkey Cutlet with Lentils, bottom

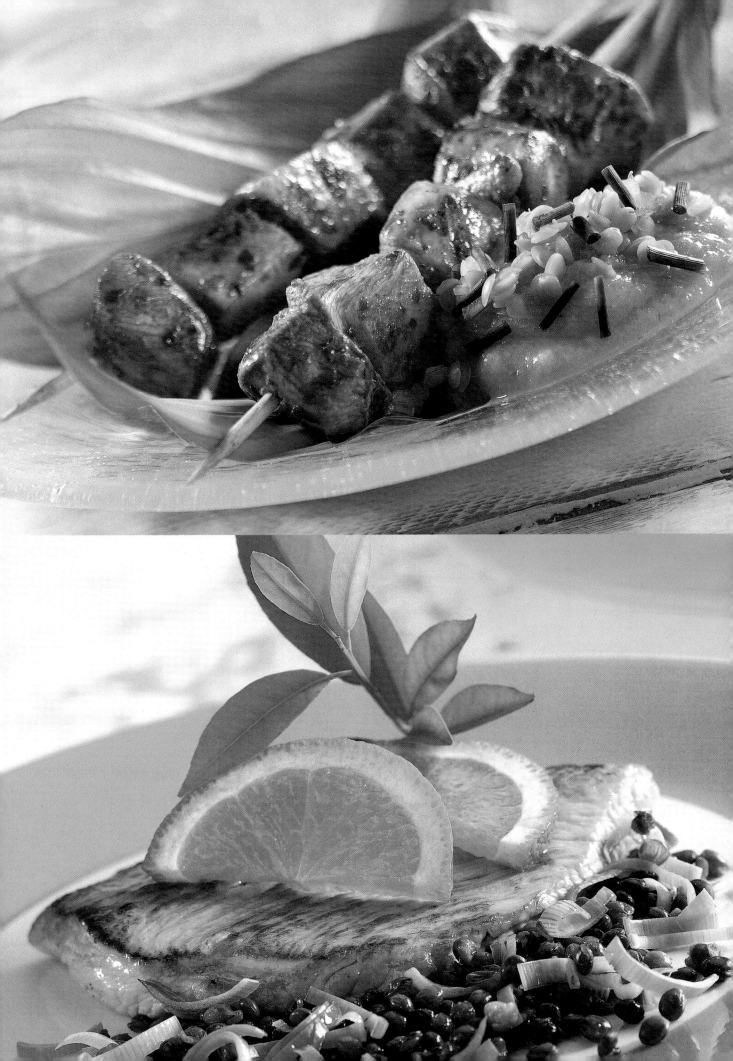

Turkey–Cucumber Clay Pot Casserole

Carbohydrates	◖	1 hr. 25 min.
Fat	●	
Fiber	●	

Per serving: approx. 217 calories
38 g protein · 4 g fat · 7 g carbohydrates

FOR 2 SERVINGS:
10 oz (300 g) skinless boneless turkey breast
Salt and freshly ground pepper
Ground coriander seeds
1 English cucumber
1 bunch green (spring) onions
3 to 4 sprigs fresh lovage, or celery tops with leaves
1 cup (250 mL) vegetable stock
1 tbsp (15 mL) lemon juice
Sweet paprika

1 Cut turkey into bite-size pieces. Season with salt, pepper and ground coriander, and refrigerate, covered, for 15 minutes.

2 Soak the bottom and lid of a clay roasting pot for 15 minutes. Halve and slice the cucumber and chop the green onions and lovage. Remove the bottom of the clay pot from the water, but leave it wet. Put in the vegetables and stock, and season with salt and pepper.

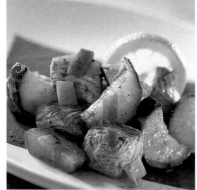

3 Cover the clay pot with its lid and place in the middle of a cold oven. Turn the oven on to 350°F (180°C) for about 30 minutes.

4 Remove the clay pot from the oven and stir in the turkey. Cook for a further 30 minutes. Season with salt, pepper and lemon juice. Sprinkle with paprika just before serving.

Turkey with Brown Rice Risotto

Carbohydrates	●●●●	2 hr.
Fat	●●●	(+4 hrs. soaking)
Fiber	●●●	

Per serving: approx. 506 calories
49 g protein · 13 g fat · 48 g carbohydrates

FOR 2 SERVINGS:
1/8 oz (4 g) dried porcini (cèpes) mushrooms
1 tbsp (15 mL) spelt
1 thin leek
3 carrots
1½ cups (375 mL) peeled, finely chopped celery root
Salt
1 clove garlic
1 small sprig fresh rosemary
14 oz (400 g) turkey thigh
Sweet paprika
1 small onion
1 tbsp (15 mL) sunflower oil
½ cup (125 mL/100 g) long-grain brown rice
1 bay leaf
1⅔ cups (400 mL) cold water
1 tbsp (15 mL) chopped fresh parsley

1 Soak the mushrooms and spelt in separate bowls of water for at least 4 hours. Soak the bottom and lid of a clay pot for 15 minutes. Slice the leek lengthwise, wash thoroughly and cut into strips. Chop the carrot, celery root, garlic and rosemary leaves. Put the vegetables in the clay pot and season with salt, rosemary and garlic.

2 Rub turkey with salt and paprika. Brown, fatty side down, in a hot skillet (frying pan) for 4 minutes. Lay the turkey on top of the vegetables, browned side up. Put the oven rack in the second slot from the bottom and slide the pot in. Turn the heat on to 350°F (180°C) and bake for 1 hour. Turn off the heat and leave the pot in the oven for ½ hour.

3 Meanwhile, drain mushrooms and spelt, reserving the mushroom soaking water. Slice mushrooms finely, chop onion, and brown both in hot oil. Combine the rice with the spelt and add ¼ cup (50 mL) of the mushroom water. Stir in the bay leaf, cold water and 2 pinches of salt. Bring to a boil and cook, uncovered, for 40 to 45 minutes.

4 Slice the turkey and arrange on a plate with the vegetables. Sprinkle the risotto with parsley and serve with the turkey.

Turkey with Brown Rice Risotto, right

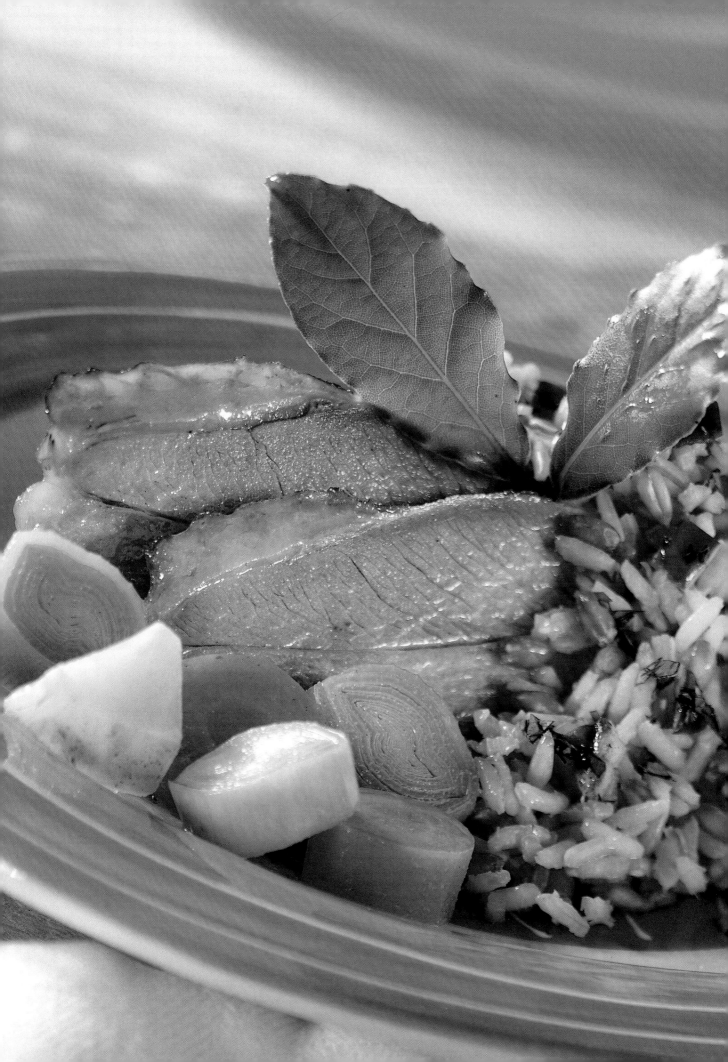

Chinese Fondue

Carbohydrates	◖	45 min.
Fat	●	
Fiber	●	

Per serving: approx. 474 calories
49 g protein · 9 g fat · 48 g carbohydrates

FOR 2 SERVINGS:
2 tsp (10 mL) sunflower oil, divided
1 small red onion
1 clove garlic
½ English cucumber
1 tsp (5 mL) sugar
Pinch curry powder
1 tbsp (15 mL) rice vinegar
Salt and freshly ground pepper
1 red and 1 green chili pepper
1 cooking onion
8 to 12 cups (2 to 3 L) vegetable stock
2 tbsp (30 mL) soy sauce
½ cup (125 mL/75 g) rice noodles
10 oz (300 g) skinless boneless chicken breasts
1 small Chinese (Napa) cabbage
2 carrots
2½ tbsp (37 mL/20 g) fresh ginger

1 Chop the red onion and grate the cucumber. Heat 1 tsp (5 mL) of the oil and stir in the red onion. Peel and press or grate garlic and mix it in. Stir in cucumber. Stir in sugar, curry powder, vinegar, salt and pepper. Simmer, covered, for 15 minutes. Leave to cool.

2 Finely slice the chili peppers and chop the cooking onion. Stir-fry briefly in the remaining oil. Pour in the stock and season with soy sauce. Simmer, covered, for 15 minutes.

3 Pour warm water over the noodles and let stand until softened, then drain. Slice the chicken, cabbage and carrots. Arrange on a plate with the noodles.

4 Bring the stock to a boil. Fill a fondue pot ½ full with stock and light the burner. Peel ginger, add to stock and simmer. People can then cook their chosen ingredients in the stock, in a small sieve. Serve cucumber sauce on the side.

Chicken Stir-Fry

Carbohydrates	●●●●	40 min.
Fat	●●●	(+ 1 hr. marinating)
Fiber	●●●	

Per serving: approx. 356 calories
29 g protein · 20 g fat · 15 g carbohydrates

FOR 2 SERVINGS:
7 oz (200 g) skinless boneless chicken breasts
1 clove garlic
4 tsp (20 mL/10 g) fresh ginger
2 tbsp (30 mL) soy sauce
½ tsp (2 mL) sambal oelek or other hot chili-based sauce
½ bunch green (spring) onions
2 tbsp (30 mL) sunflower oil
Pinch ground coriander seeds
Pinch fresh lemon grass
Pinch fresh galangal (optional)
3 cups (750 mL/200 g) chopped bok choy
⅔ cup (150 mL/100 g) diced fresh or canned pineapple
¼ cup (50 mL) chicken stock
Juice of ½ lime
Salt
1 tbsp (15 mL) toasted flaked almonds

1 Slice the chicken into strips. Use a garlic press or micrograter to crush the garlic and ginger into a bowl. Stir in soy sauce and sambal oelek. Add chicken, stir to coat, and marinate in the refrigerator for 1 hour.

2 Chop the green onions and set aside 1 tsp (5 mL). In a wok or deep skillet (frying pan), heat the oil and stir-fry the chicken until brown. Stir in ground coriander, lemon grass, galangal, green onions, bok choy and pineapple, and stir-fry for 5 minutes. Stir in stock and lime juice. Cover and cook on medium heat for 5 minutes. Season with salt.

3 Garnish with the reserved green onion and the flaked almond and serve.

!! **TIP:** Instead of bok choy—an Asian green in the cabbage family—you could use Savoy cabbage, Chinese (Napa) cabbage or broccoli.

Chinese Fondue, top
Chicken Stir-Fry, bottom

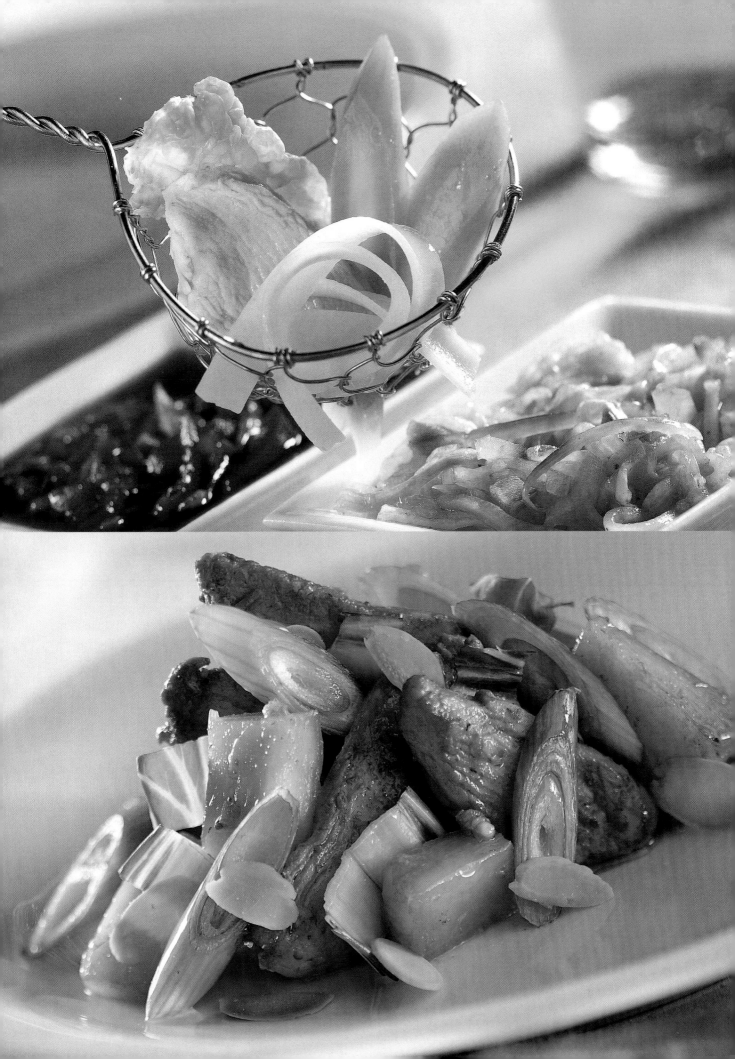

Couscous with Rabbit

Carbohydrates	●●●●◖	1 hr. 10 min.
Fat	++	
Fiber	●●●	

Per serving: approx. 559 calories
70 g protein · 27 g fat · 53 g carbohydrates

FOR 2 SERVINGS:
5 tbsp (75 mL) water
½ cup (125 mL/75 g) couscous
1 cup (250 mL) venison or other meat stock, divided
2 rabbit fillets
1 tbsp (15 mL) canola or vegetable oil
Salt and freshly ground pepper
1 tbsp (15 mL) port
2 tbsp (30 mL/30 g) crème fraîche or sour cream
12 oz (375 g) snow (mange-tout) peas
2 carrots

1 Pour water over the couscous, fluff with a fork and transfer to a large sieve. Set on top of a saucepan containing ¾ cup (175 mL) hot stock. Cover with a tea towel and the lid of the saucepan, and steam on low heat for 30 minutes. (Or pour the hot stock over instant couscous, cover and leave for 5 to 10 minutes.)

2 Preheat the oven to 200°F (100°C). Remove the skin and sinews from the rabbit. Heat the oil in a skillet (frying pan) and brown the meat on all sides on medium heat. Season with salt and pepper. Finish in the preheated slow oven for 30 minutes.

3 Combine the remaining stock with the port and bring to a boil. Stir in the crème fraîche and reduce by ½ on low heat.

4 Slice the carrots and cook for 5 minutes in a little salted water. Add the snow peas and cook for another 5 minutes. Season with salt and pepper.

5 Cut up the rabbit and serve with the couscous, port sauce and vegetables.

!! **TIP:** You can buy the traditional couscous in Middle Eastern, health-food and some grocery stores, but the much faster precooked kind is almost everywhere now.

Sweet and Sour Duck

Carbohydrates	●●◖	50 min.
Fat	++++	
Fiber	●	

Per serving: approx. 674 calories
44 g protein · 42 g fat · 29 g carbohydrates

FOR 2 SERVINGS:
2 small duck breasts
White pepper
2 tbsp (30 mL) rice wine
1 tbsp (15 mL) ketchup
2 tbsp (30 mL) rice vinegar
5 tbsp (75 mL) water
1 tsp (5 mL) sugar
2 tsp (10 mL) cornstarch
2 tsp (10 mL) sunflower oil
2 tbsp (30 mL) light soy sauce
1 onion
1 clove garlic
4 ribs celery
2 slices fresh or canned pineapple
5 oz (150 g) fresh or ¾ cup (175 mL) canned lychees
Hot chili sauce or hot pepper sauce

1 Remove the skin and fat from the duck and cut the meat into bite-size cubes. Rub with pepper and sprinkle with wine. Marinate for 10 minutes.

2 Combine ketchup, vinegar, water, sugar and cornstarch.

3 Heat the oil in a large skillet (frying pan) or wok. Brown the duck over high heat, remove and sprinkle with soy sauce.

4 Chop the onion, garlic and celery, and stir-fry for 1 minute. Give the ketchup mixture a stir and pour into the wok with the vegetables. Bring to a boil.

5 Chop the pineapple, hull and pit the lychees, and stir them in. Gently mix in the duck. Continue to stir for 1 to 2 minutes, until warm. Season with chili sauce or hot pepper sauce to taste.

Couscous with Rabbit, top
Sweet and Sour Duck, bottom

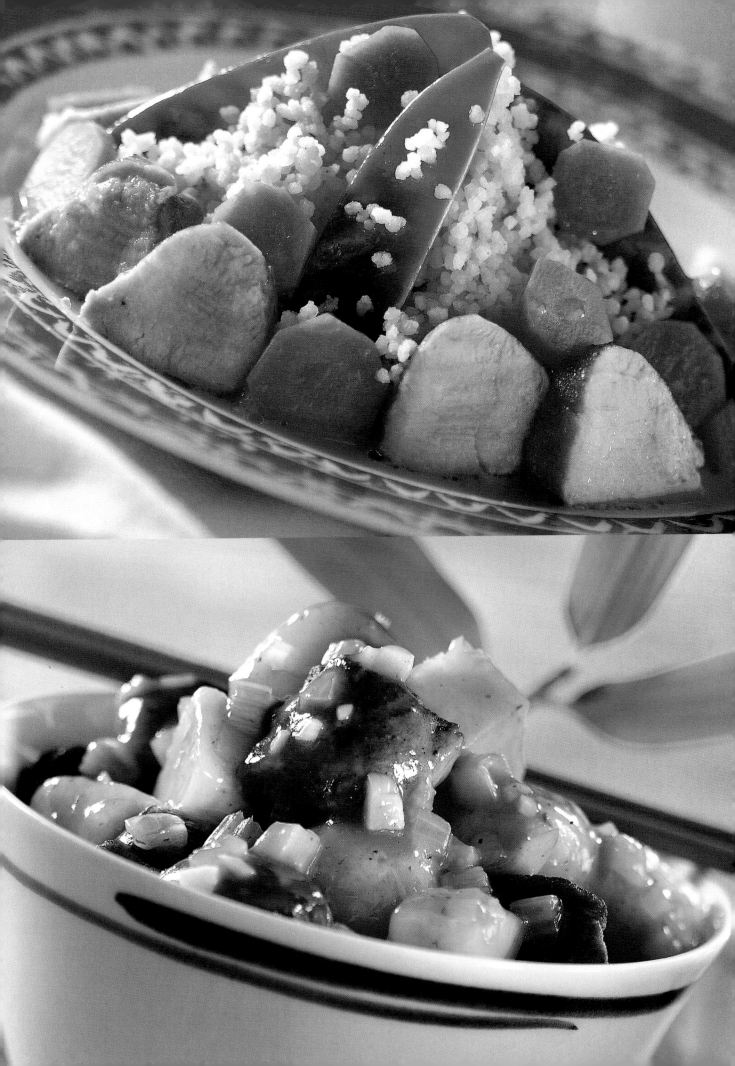

Venison Medallions with Chanterelles, Onions and Pears

Carbohydrates	●◀	
Fat	●●	
Fiber	●●●	

45 min.

Per serving: approx. 312 calories
31 g protein · 8 g fat · 19 g carbohydrates

FOR 2 SERVINGS:
¼ tsp (1 mL) black peppercorns
½ tsp (2 mL) dried juniper berries
½ tsp (2 mL) dried rosemary
Salt and freshly ground pepper
8 oz (250 g) venison steak
1 red onion
2 small pears
2 tbsp (30 mL) lemon juice
1 tsp (5 mL) sunflower oil
7 oz (200 g) chanterelle mushrooms
1 tsp (5 mL) coarsely ground whole wheat flour
½ cup (125 mL) dry rosé wine
1 handful fresh chervil

1 Combine peppercorns, juniper berries, rosemary, salt and pepper in a mortar and crush. Cut the meat into 1½-inch (4 cm) medallions and rub with the crushed seasonings.

2 Cut the onion into small wedges. Peel, quarter, core and slice the pears crosswise; sprinkle immediately with lemon juice.

3 Heat the oil in a nonstick skillet (frying pan) and brown the meat quickly on both sides on medium heat. Finish cooking each side on low heat for 3 minutes. Remove and keep warm.

4 Fry the onion wedges in the skillet, then brown the chanterelles quickly on medium heat.

5 Sprinkle flour into the skillet, brown slightly and moisten with wine. Add pears and cook for 1 or 2 minutes. Season with salt and pepper.

6 Arrange medallions, onions, mushrooms and pears on two plates, sprinkle with chervil and serve.

Venison Medallions with Chanterelles, Onion and Pears, top
Saddle of Venison with Cranberry Sauce and Lamb's Lettuce, bottom

Saddle of Venison with Cranberry Sauce and Lamb's Lettuce

Carbohydrates	●●●◀	
Fat	++	
Fiber	●●	

1 hr. 20 min.

Per serving: approx. 584 calories
62 g protein · 22 g fat · 37 g carbohydrates

FOR 2 SERVINGS:
1-lb (500 g) saddle of venison (shoulder or blade)
Salt; sweet paprika
1 small carrot
⅓ cup (75 mL) diced celery root
1 small onion
1 sprig fresh thyme; 1 bay leaf; 3 dried juniper berries
2 potatoes
2 oz (60 g) lamb's lettuce (corn salad, mâche), watercress or arugula (rocket)
4 oz (120 g) radicchio
Juice of ½ orange, divided
1 tsp (5 mL) balsamic vinegar
1 tbsp (15 mL) olive oil
½ tsp (2 mL) Dijon mustard
½ tsp (2 mL) orange marmalade
Freshly ground pepper
1 small shallot
1 tsp (5 mL) margarine
2 tsp (10 mL) whole-berry cranberry sauce
2 tbsp (30 mL/30 g) sour cream

1 Preheat the oven to 350°F (180°C). Season venison with salt and paprika. Peel and dice the carrots, celery root and onion. Place a 20-inch (50 cm) roasting bag on a shallow pan and put in the carrots, celery root, onion, thyme, bay leaf and juniper berries. Lay the saddle on top, meat side up. Add 2 tbsp (30 mL) water and seal. Pierce the top. Roast for 45 minutes.

2 Peel and cut the potatoes into quarters or eighths. Boil in salted water for 20 minutes.

3 Tear the lamb's lettuce and radicchio into bite-size pieces. Combine 1 tsp (5 mL) orange juice with the vinegar, oil, mustard, marmalade, salt and pepper and toss ½ with the lettuces.

4 Chop and gently sauté the shallot in hot margarine. Cut open the roasting bag. Wrap the meat in aluminum foil and reserve the roasting juices. Stir ⅓ cup (75 mL) of the meat juices in with the shallot along with the cranberry sauce, the remaining orange juice and dressing and the sour cream. Simmer briefly and season with salt. Slice the meat and serve with the potatoes, cranberry sauce, lettuces and slices of orange.

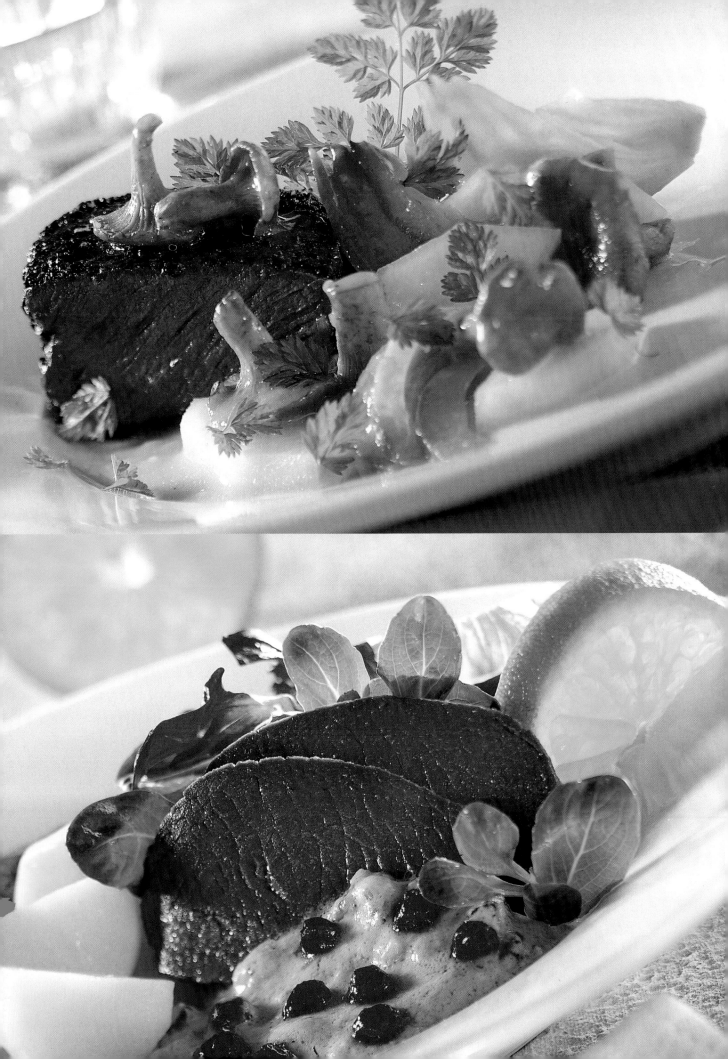

Pasta, Rice and Company

Potatoes and pasta, rice, whole grains and legumes — anywhere, anytime!

In scientific circles, it has long been established that diabetics don't have to avoid these fundamentally nutritious, carbohydrate-rich foods. With their abundance of vitamins, minerals and energy, whole-grain products offer the best value. What's more, their fiber slows the transfer of carbs to the bloodstream and ensures that hunger doesn't set in too quickly.

Legumes such as lentils, peas and beans contain a high level of quality protein and are becoming increasingly popular. Today, these important foods go far beyond the traditional casseroles to form the base for sophisticated salads, sides and main dishes.

Vegetarian Lasagna

Carbohydrates	●●●●	30 min.
Fat	+	(+ 35 to 40 min. baking)
Fiber	●●●	

Per serving: approx. 466 calories
29 g protein · 19 g fat · 43 g carbohydrates

FOR 2 SERVINGS:
5 tomatoes
7 oz (200 g) spinach
2 tbsp (30 mL) canola or vegetable oil
2 onions
1 kohlrabi
1½ cups sliced mushrooms
Freshly grated nutmeg
Salt and freshly ground pepper
6 oven-ready or fresh lasagna noodles
3½ oz (100 g) mozzarella cheese
¼ cup (50 mL/30 g) freshly grated Parmesan cheese

1 Cut the tomatoes into eighths. Wash the spinach, remove large stems and drain. Chop the onions; peel and dice the kohlrabi.

2 Heat the oil and lightly sauté the onions on low heat until translucent. Stir in the kohlrabi and brown lightly. Stir in the spinach and tomatoes. Cook, covered, for 10 minutes. Mix in the mushrooms and cook slightly. Season with nutmeg, salt and pepper.

3 Preheat the oven to 350°F (180°C). Dice or grate the mozzarella. Grease a 9- x 9-inch (23 x 23 cm) ovenproof dish and place 2 uncooked lasagna noodles in the bottom. Cover with ⅓ each of the vegetables, mozzarella and Parmesan. Repeat for 2 more layers, ending with cheese.

4 Bake for 35 to 40 minutes, or until the noodles are cooked and the top is golden.

Tomato Lasagna

Carbohydrates	●●●	1 hr.
Fat	●●●	(+ 35 to 40 min. baking)
Fiber	●	

Per serving: approx. 319 calories
20 g protein · 11 g fat · 34 g carbohydrates

FOR 2 SERVINGS:
1 tbsp (15 mL) olive oil
1 large onion
2 beefsteak tomatoes
Salt
½ tsp (2 mL) dried herbes de Provence
½ handful fresh basil leaves
½ cup (125 mL) low-fat quark or puréed cottage cheese
1 tbsp (15 mL) ketchup or tomato paste
1 extra-large egg
6 oven-ready or fresh lasagna noodles
2 tbsp (30 mL/15 g) freshly grated Parmesan cheese

1 Coarsely chop the onion and quarter the tomatoes. Heat the oil and sauté the onion on low heat until translucent. Stir in the tomatoes, ½ tsp (2 mL) salt and the herbes de Provence. Cook, covered, on low heat for 15 minutes. Using a hand-held blender or potato masher, purée the mixture in the saucepan.

2 Chop the basil and combine with the quark, ketchup, egg and a pinch of salt.

3 Preheat the oven to 350°F (180°C). Spread a thin layer of the tomato mixture in the bottom of a 9- x 9-inch (23 x 23 cm) ovenproof dish. Cover with 2 uncooked lasagna noodles. Spread on another layer of tomato and 2 more lasagna noodles. Cover with ½ the quark mixture, then the remaining tomato mixture. Cover with the last 2 lasagna noodles and spread the rest of the quark on top. Sprinkle with Parmesan.

4 Bake for 35 to 40 minutes, or until the noodles are cooked and the top is golden.

Vegetarian Lasagna, top
Tomato Lasagna, bottom

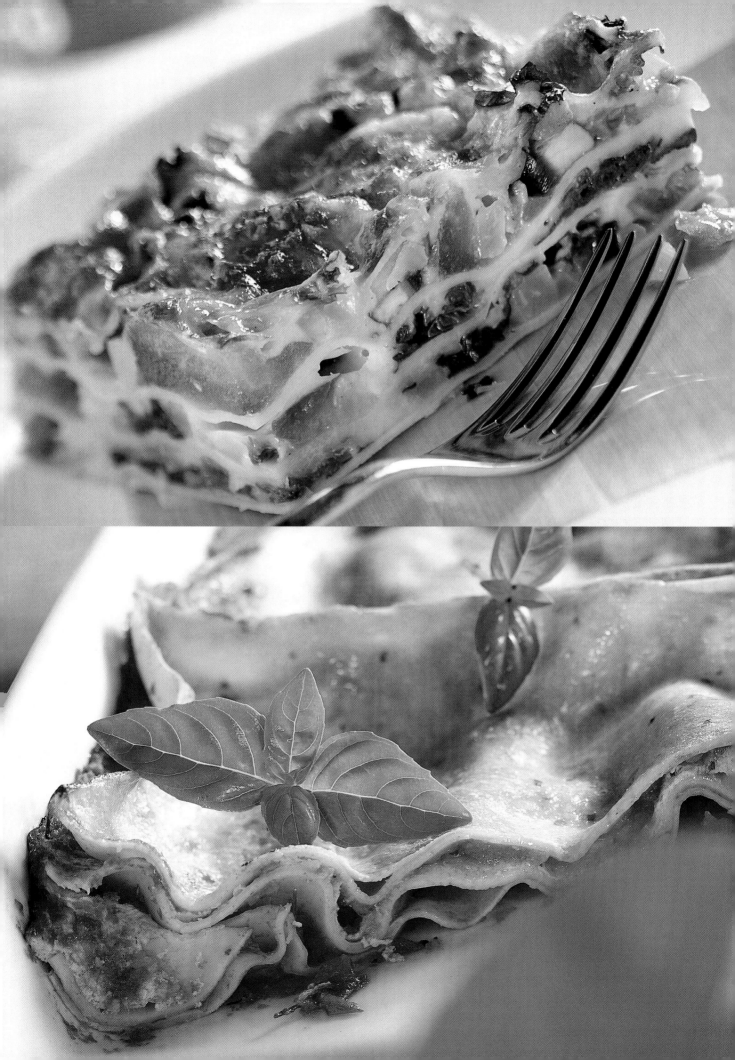

Pesto Spaetzle

Carbohydrates	●●●◖	40 min.
Fat	●●●	(+ 30 min.
Fiber	●	resting)

Per serving: approx. 318 calories
12 g protein · 11 g fat · 42 g carbohydrates

FOR 2 SERVINGS:
1 tbsp (15 mL) olive oil
1 onion
5 tomatoes
1 tbsp (15 mL) pine nuts
2 bunches basil
1 clove garlic
1 cup (250 mL/100 g) pastry flour
1 extra-large egg
Salt

1 Chop the onion and score, blanch, peel and dice the tomatoes. Heat the oil, stir in the onion and tomatoes, and simmer on low heat for 10 minutes.

2 Toast the pine nuts in a dry nonstick skillet (frying pan). Make a paste of the pine nuts, basil leaves and garlic in a blender or food processor.

3 Combine flour, egg, a little salt and 3 tbsp (45 mL) water to form a smooth batter. Stir in the basil mixture and beat until the batter thickens, adding water as needed. Leave to rest for 30 minutes.

4 Bring a large pot of salted water to a boil. Drop in the batter by pressing it through a colander, ricer or spaetzle cutter, or by cutting lengths from a wet board with a bench knife. Cook for 4 minutes, or until the noodles float to the surface. Drain and serve on two plates with the tomato sauce on the side.

Pasta with Cabbage

Carbohydrates	●●●●	45 min.
Fat	●	
Fiber	●●	

Per serving: approx. 257 calories
9 g protein · 4 g fat · 46 g carbohydrates

FOR 2 SERVINGS:
1 tsp (5 mL) canola or vegetable oil
1 onion
5 cups (1.25 L) shredded green cabbage
2 tsp (10 mL) white-wine vinegar
⅔ cup (150 mL) vegetable stock
Salt and freshly ground pepper
Caraway seeds
3½ oz (100 g) small pasta squares or large bow ties

1 Chop the onion. Heat the oil, stir in the onion and gently sauté on low heat until translucent. Stir in the cabbage and cook for 1 to 2 minutes. Add vinegar and vegetable stock, season with salt, pepper and caraway, and simmer for 20 minutes.

2 Bring a large pot of salted water to a boil. Stir in the pasta squares (or wide noodles broken into rough squares) or bow ties. Cook on medium heat for 10 minutes. Drain and combine with the cabbage.

!! **TIP:** If you have difficulty digesting cabbage, remove the core and the middle ribs of the leaves—these parts contain elements that cause flatulence. Coarsely ground caraway seeds also help minimize gas.

Spelt Spaetzle

Carbohydrates	●●●◖	35 min.
Fat	●●●	
Fiber	●●	

Per serving: approx. 310 calories
16 g protein · 11 g fat · 37 g carbohydrates

FOR 2 SERVINGS:
¾ cup (175 mL/100 g) whole-grain spelt flour
Salt
Freshly ground nutmeg
1 extra-large egg
1 tsp (5 mL) sunflower oil
1 small onion
2 oz (60 g) cooked ham
⅔ cup (150 mL/140 g) white-wine sauerkraut
1 tbsp (15 mL) chopped fresh parsley
Freshly ground pepper
Thin wedges of apple

1 Combine the spelt, 2 pinches salt and a little nutmeg. Make a well in the center and crack the egg into it. Starting in the center, knead to form a soft dough, gradually adding ⅓ cup (75 mL) cold water, as needed.

2 Bring a large pot of salted water to a boil. Drop in the batter by pressing it through a colander, ricer or spaetzle cutter. Cook for 4 minutes, or until the noodles float. Remove, rinse with cold water and drain.

3 Chop the onion and ham. Heat the oil, stir in onion and sauté until translucent. Stir in the ham and brown for 1 or 2 minutes. Stir in the spaetzle and brown for 1 minute.

4 Combine sauerkraut, parsley, salt and pepper, and mix with the spaetzle. Arrange on two plates and garnish with thin slices of apple (raw or lightly sautéed) and additional parsley leaves.

Pesto Spaetzle, top
Pasta with Cabbage, bottom left
Spelt Spaetzle, bottom right

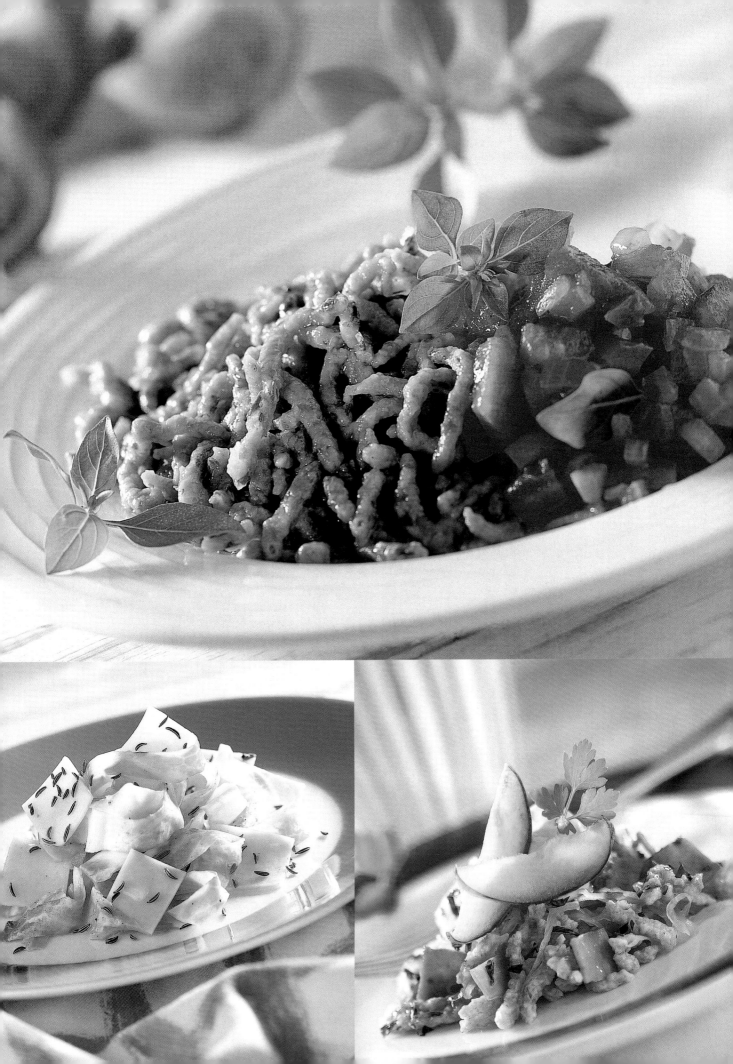

Risotto with Artichokes

Carbohydrates	●●●●●	
Fat	●●●	45 min.
Fiber	●●●	

Per serving: approx. 425 calories
14 g protein · 10 g fat · 60 g carbohydrates

FOR 2 SERVINGS:
4 small artichokes
Juice of 1 lemon
1½ cups (375 mL) low-sodium vegetable stock
2 tsp (10 mL) olive oil
1 shallot
½ cup (125 mL/120 g) arborio rice
¼ cup (50 mL) dry white wine
2 tbsp (30 mL/30 g) cream
Salt and freshly ground pepper
Freshly grated nutmeg
¼ cup (50 mL/30 g) freshly grated Parmesan cheese

1 Wash the artichokes. Remove the outside leaves and trim the inside ones. Peel the bottoms and stems. Scoop out chokes with a teaspoon. Cut into eighths and place in water with lemon juice.

2 Heat the stock.

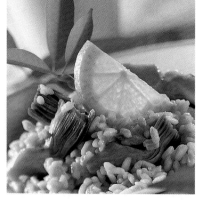

3 Finely chop the shallot. Heat the oil, stir in the shallot and sauté on low heat until translucent. Drain the artichokes, mix in and brown for 3 minutes, stirring. Stir in the rice and cook until translucent.

4 Add wine and stir. When the wine is absorbed, start gradually adding hot stock until it is absorbed, stirring often so the rice doesn't stick. Cook for 20 minutes in all, or just until al dente.

5 Stir in cream, salt, pepper, a pinch of nutmeg and ½ the Parmesan. Garnish with remaining Parmesan and some half-moons of lemon.

Rice with Squid and Vegetables

Carbohydrates	●●●●◖	
Fat	+	40 min.
Fiber	●●●	

Per serving: approx. 479 calories
25 g protein · 17 g fat · 52 g carbohydrates

FOR 2 SERVINGS:
2 small artichokes
Juice of ½ lemon
7 oz (200 g) dressed squid
1 clove garlic
3 tbsp (45 mL) olive oil, divided
⅔ cup (150 mL/100 g) small peas
2 tomatoes
½ cup (125 mL) water
5 threads saffron
½ cup (125 mL/100 g) short-grain rice
1 cup (250 mL) fish or vegetable stock
1 small fennel frond
3 sprigs Italian (flat-leaf) parsley
Pinch cayenne
Pinch dried chili flakes
Salt and freshly ground pepper

1 Wash the artichokes, remove the hard outer leaves and trim the tips of the others right to the fleshy stems. Scoop out the choke and peel the bottoms. Cut into quarters and place in a little water with lemon juice.

2 Cut the squid into quarters. Finely chop the garlic; peel and dice the tomatoes. Heat 2 tbsp (30 mL) of the oil. Stir in the squid and sauté for 2 minutes; remove and set aside. Drain the artichokes and sauté in the oil remaining in the pan. Stir in the peas, tomatoes and garlic, and brown lightly. Stir in the squid. Pour in the ½ cup (125 mL) water and heat.

3 Soak the saffron in 2 tbsp (30 mL) water. Rinse and drain the rice. Heat the remaining 1 tbsp (15 ml) oil and stir-fry the rice until translucent. Stir in squid mixture. Add a little stock and the saffron and water, and cook on low heat. Finely chop and stir in the fennel and parsley. Season with cayenne, chili flakes, salt and pepper. Gradually add remaining stock until all the liquid is absorbed, stirring constantly. Cook the rice for 20 minutes, just until al dente.

Rice with Squid and Vegetables, right

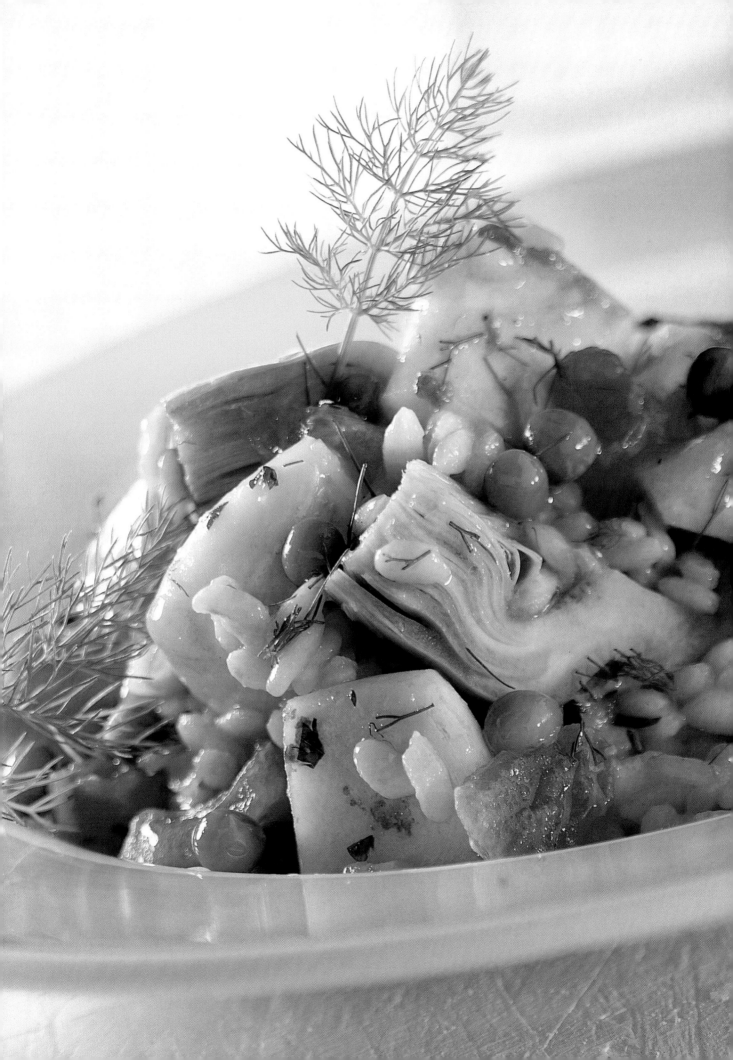

Brown Rice with Carrots

Carbohydrates ●●●●●   45 min.
Fat ●●●
Fiber ●●●

Per serving: approx. 365 calories
10 g protein · 12 g fat · 57 g carbohydrates

FOR 2 SERVINGS:
²⁄₃ cup (150 mL/120 g) long-grain brown rice
2 cups (500 mL) lightly salted boiling water
1 tbsp (15 mL) sunflower seeds
5 medium carrots
4 green (spring) onions
2 tsp (10 mL) olive oil
Salt
Sugar
½ handful fresh coriander
⅓ cup (75 mL/75 g) sour cream
½ tsp (2 mL) lemon juice

1 Add rice to the water and cook, covered, on low heat for 40 minutes. Toast the sunflower seeds in a dry skillet (frying pan) until golden and leave to cool.

2 Finely grate the carrots and chop the green onions. Heat the oil. Stir in carrots and onions and sauté on medium heat for about 2 minutes. Season with 2 pinches of salt and a little sugar. Cover and cook on low heat for 5 minutes.

3 Chop the coriander and mix with the sour cream, lemon juice and a little salt.

4 Drain the rice and top with the vegetables. Sprinkle with sunflower seeds. Serve the coriander sauce on the side.

Brown Rice Jambalaya

Carbohydrates ●●●●◖   50 min.
Fat ●
Fiber ●●●

Per serving: approx. 319 calories
8 g protein · 6 g fat · 53 g carbohydrates

FOR 2 SERVINGS:
1¼ cups (300 mL) vegetable stock
½ cup (125 mL/100 g) short-grain brown rice
1 tbsp (15 mL) oil
1 large onion
1 clove garlic
1 chili pepper
1 small rib celery
1 red pepper
14-oz (398 ml) can tomatoes
1 tbsp (15 mL) tomato paste
½ bunch Italian (flat-leaf) parsley
Pinch ground cloves
Salt and freshly ground pepper
Hot pepper sauce

1 Bring the stock to a boil. Stir in the rice and cook, covered, on low heat for 30 to 40 minutes.

2 Chop the onion, garlic and parsley. Slice the chili pepper, celery and red pepper. Heat the oil, stir in the onion and garlic, and sauté until translucent. Stir in the chili pepper, celery and red pepper. Cook for 3 to 4 minutes, stirring.

3 Stir in the tomatoes and juice, crushing the tomatoes. Stir in tomato paste and ½ the parsley. Season with cloves, salt, pepper and hot pepper sauce. Simmer, uncovered, for 10 minutes.

4 Drain the rice, stir into the vegetables and heat quickly. Season with salt and pepper, sprinkle with the remaining parsley and serve.

Rice with Cucumbers and Capers

Carbohydrates ●●●●   35 min.
Fat +
Fiber ●●

Per serving: approx. 364 calories
15 g protein · 16 g fat · 46 g carbohydrates

FOR 2 SERVINGS:
1²⁄₃ cups (400 mL) vegetable stock, divided
½ cup (125 mL/100 g) short-grain converted (parboiled) rice
1 tbsp (15 mL) canola or vegetable oil
¾ cucumber
3 tbsp (45 mL/45 g) crème fraîche or sour cream
½ tsp (2 mL) hot mustard
1 tbsp (15 mL) capers
Salt and freshly ground pepper
½ bunch parsley

1 Bring 1 cup (250 mL) of the vegetable stock to a boil, stir in rice and cook, covered, on low heat for 20 minutes, stirring occasionally.

2 Peel, halve, seed and slice the cucumber. Heat the oil and lightly braise cucumber for 5 minutes. Add remaining ²⁄₃ cup (150 mL) stock. Stir in the crème fraîche and mustard. Cook, covered, on low heat for 15 minutes.

3 Stir the cooked rice into the cucumber mixture. Add capers and season with salt and pepper. Stir in ½ the parsley and sprinkle the rest on top. Serve immediately.

Brown Rice with Carrots, top
Brown Rice Jambalaya, bottom left
Rice with Cucumbers and Capers,
bottom right

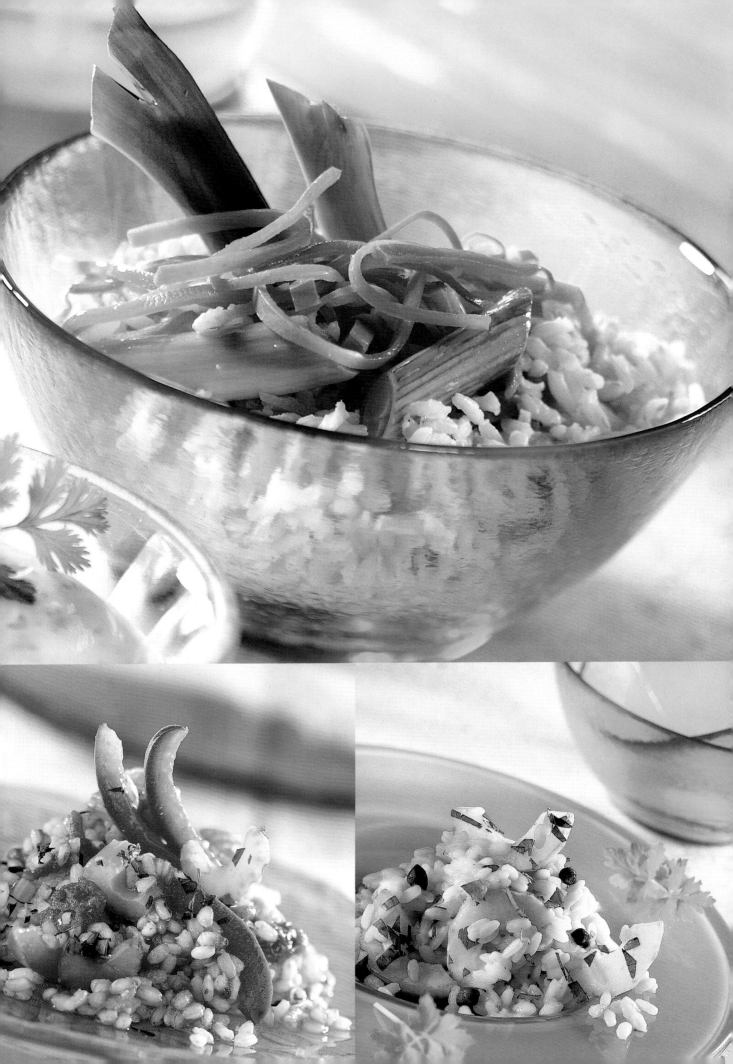

Millet Soufflé with Peas

Carbohydrates	●●●		40 min.
Fat	●●●		(+ 25 min. baking)
Fiber	●		

Per serving: approx. 321 calories
18 g protein · 11 g fat · 36 g carbohydrates

FOR 2 SERVINGS:
¼ cup (50 mL/50 g) millet
¾ cup (175 mL) vegetable stock
1⅓ cups (325 mL/200 g) frozen peas
3 eggs
Salt and freshly ground pepper
⅔ cup (150 mL) carrot juice
1 tbsp (15 mL) cornstarch
½ bunch parsley
Curry powder

1 Stir millet into vegetable stock and cook, covered, on low heat for 20 minutes, stirring occasionally. After the first 10 minutes, stir in the peas.

2 Preheat the oven to 350°F (180°C). Separate the eggs. Beat the yolks lightly and fold into the millet. With clean beaters, beat the whites until stiff and fold in. Season with salt and pepper. Grease two small ramekins. Spoon ½ the millet mixture into each and bake for 25 minutes.

3 Bring the carrot juice to a boil. Mix the cornstarch with a little cold water, stir it in and cook until thickened. Leave to cool. Chop and stir in the parsley, and season with salt, pepper and curry powder. Serve with the soufflés.

!! **TIP:** Millet is an important staple in many countries. If you find the mineral-packed small yellow grains tasty, you can serve them combined with vegetables or rice anytime. For 2 servings, add 1 cup (250 mL) millet to 3 cups (750 mL) boiling water and cook, covered, on low heat for 15 to 20 minutes.

Millet Risotto with Fennel

Carbohydrates	●●●●◖		55 min.
Fat	●●●		
Fiber	●●●		

Per serving: approx. 393 calories
20 g protein · 14 g fat · 51 g carbohydrates

FOR 2 SERVINGS:
1 large beefsteak tomato
1¼ cups (300 mL) chicken stock
1 large fennel bulb
1 large onion
1 clove garlic
1 tbsp (15 mL) olive oil
½ cup (125 mL/120 g) millet
⅓ cup (75 mL/40 g) freshly grated Parmesan cheese
Salt and freshly ground pepper

1 Score the tomatoes crosswise, blanch, peel, quarter and purée. Combine the tomatoes and stock. Bring to a boil and cook on low heat for a few minutes.

2 Slice the fennel finely. Set the leaves aside. Finely chop the onion and garlic. Heat the oil, stir in the onion and garlic, and gently sauté on low heat until translucent. Stir in the fennel and millet and cook briefly. Gradually add the tomato mixture, making sure that the millet is covered with liquid and stirring often. Cook for about 20 minutes.

3 Stir in the Parmesan and season with salt and pepper. Chop the fennel leaves and sprinkle on top, if desired.

!! **TIP:** Fennel isn't everyone's favorite. In this recipe, you can substitute diced peppers, carrots, celery, eggplant (aubergine), mushrooms or asparagus. Asparagus and mushrooms cook faster and shouldn't be added until the last 10 minutes of cooking time.

Millet Soufflé with Peas, top
Millet Risotto with Fennel, bottom

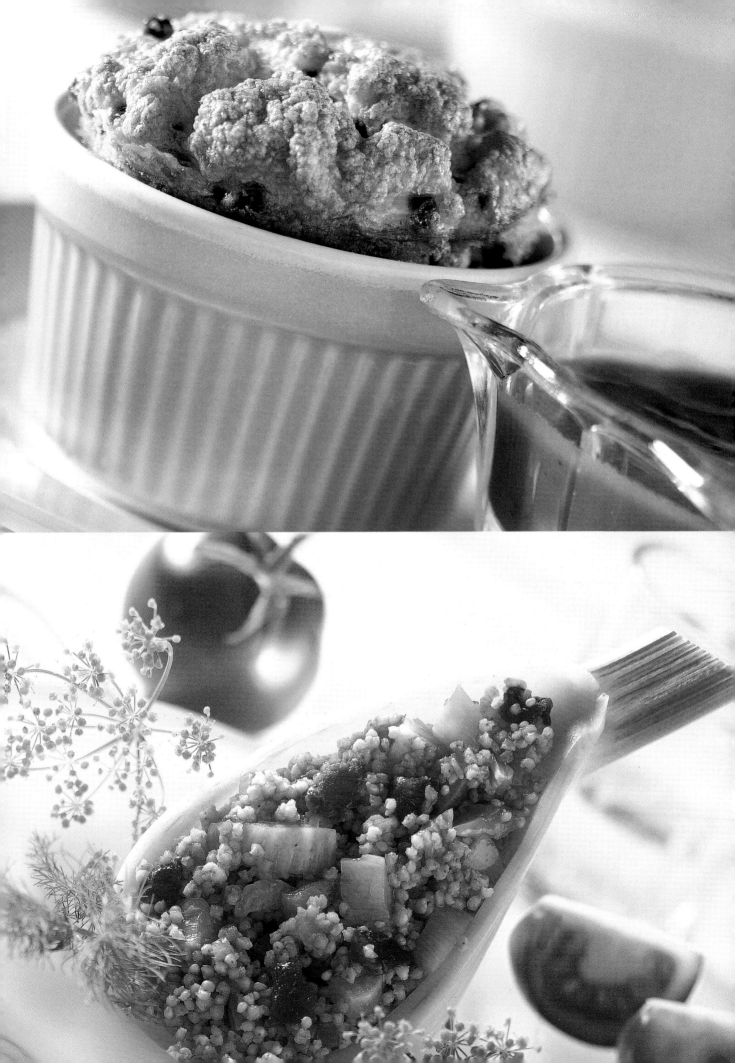

Quinoa with Carrots and Leeks

Carbohydrates ●●●◖
Fat ●●
Fiber ●●●

40 min.

Per serving: approx. 265 calories
10 g protein · 7 g fat · 39 g carbohydrates

FOR 2 SERVINGS:
1⅓ cups (325 mL) salted water
⅔ cup (150 mL/100 g) quinoa
2 small leeks
1 clove garlic
2 large carrots
1 tbsp (15 mL) canola or vegetable oil
½ cup (125 mL) vegetable stock
½ tsp (2 mL) mild mustard
Turmeric
Salt
½ bunch parsley

1 Bring the water to a boil. Stir in the quinoa and cook, covered, on low heat for 20 minutes.

2 Cut the white and light green parts of the leek into rounds. Finely slice the garlic, dice the carrots and chop the parsley.

3 Heat the oil. Stir in the garlic, carrots and leek, and sauté on medium heat for 1 to 2 minutes. Pour in the stock and simmer on medium heat for 15 minutes.

4 Stir in the cooked quinoa and season with mustard, turmeric, salt and ½ the parsley. Sprinkle remaining parsley on top and serve.

!! **TIP:** You can buy quinoa (pronounced KEEN-wah) at health-food stores. In fact not a grain but the seed of a plant in the goosefoot family, this ancient and protein-rich food can be used in the same way as rice or millet. Follow the package directions—it's easy to overcook.

Bulgur with Tomatoes and Peppers

Carbohydrates ●●●●◖
Fat ●●●
Fiber ●●●

55 min.

Per serving: approx. 328 calories
11 g protein · 10 g fat · 52 g carbohydrates

FOR 2 SERVINGS:
¾ cup (175 mL/120 g) bulgur
1 medium onion
4 yellow peppers
2 tomatoes
1 tbsp (15 mL) butter
¾ cup (175 mL) vegetable or chicken stock
Salt and freshly ground pepper
1 tbsp (15 mL) chopped walnuts
3 tbsp (45 mL) chopped fresh parsley

1 Rinse the bulgur in cold water and drain. Chop the onion and peppers; score, blanch, peel and dice the tomatoes.

2 Heat the butter in a medium saucepan. Stir in the onion, peppers and tomatoes, and cook for 2 minutes on medium heat, stirring constantly. Pour in the stock, bring to a boil, and season with salt and pepper. Stir in the bulgur and cook, covered, on low heat until the liquid is absorbed. Remove from the heat.

3 Toast the walnuts in a dry nonstick skillet (frying pan) until golden and stir into the bulgur. Stir in the parsley. Put a clean tea towel over the saucepan, cover, and leave the bulgur to swell for another 30 minutes.

!! **TIP:** You can find bulgur—a type of cracked wheat—in health-food or Middle Eastern grocery stores. It can be served on its own, with roasted or barbecued chicken, or with fried meatballs and salad.

Quinoa with Carrots and Leeks, top
Bulgur with Tomatoes and Peppers, bottom

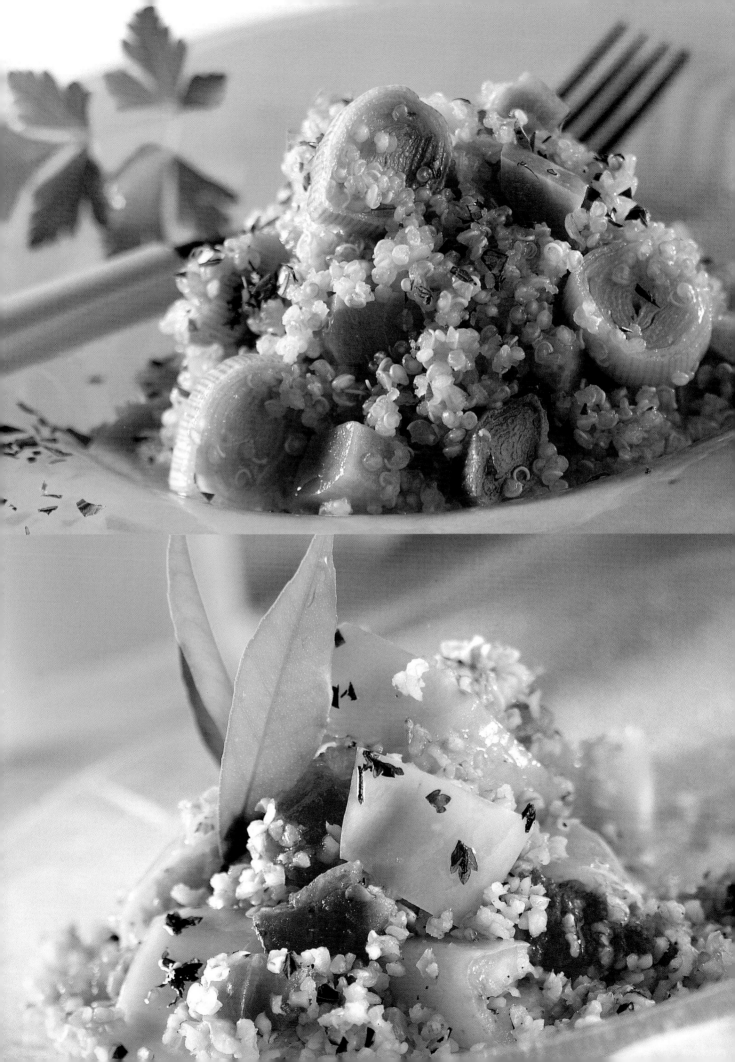

Spelt Gnocchi with Cheese Sauce

Carbohydrates ●●●
Fat ●●●
Fiber ●●

45 min.

Per serving: approx. 337 calories
17 g protein · 13 g fat · 36 g carbohydrates

FOR 2 SERVINGS:
3 oz (85 g) coarsely ground green spelt
1¾ cup (425 mL) vegetable stock, divided
½ cup (125 mL/100 g) low-fat quark or puréed cottage cheese
1 extra-large egg
3 tbsp (15 mL) chopped fresh parsley, divided
1 tsp (5 mL) herbed salt
Whole wheat flour
1 tsp (5 mL) oil
1 small onion
½ oz (15 g) low-fat herbed hard Swiss cheese
4 tbsp (60 mL/60 g) sour cream

1 Toast the spelt in a dry skillet (frying pan) on medium heat until fragrant. Bring ¾ cup (175 mL) of the stock to a boil. Stir in spelt and cook, covered, on low heat for 15 minutes. Leave to cool slightly.

2 Combine quark, egg, 1 tbsp (15 mL) of the parsley and herbed salt. Stir in the spelt, then 1 tbsp (15 mL) flour.

3 Finely chop the onion. Heat the oil, stir in the onion and sauté lightly. Sprinkle with 1 heaping tsp (7 mL) flour, cover and brown quickly. Pour in the remaining 1 cup (250 mL) stock and bring to a boil. Grate in the cheese and stir in the sour cream and remaining 2 tbsp (30 mL) parsley. Simmer on low heat.

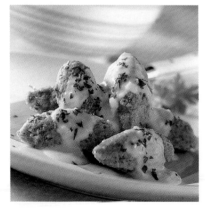

4 Form 12 gnocchi from the spelt mixture and cook in a large pot of boiling salted water until they float. Remove and drizzle with cheese sauce.

Barley with Beets

Carbohydrates ●●●●
Fat ●●●
Fiber ●●

1 hr. 25 min.

Per serving: approx. 358 calories
13 g protein · 14 g fat · 44 g carbohydrates

FOR 2 SERVINGS:
½ cup (125 mL/100 g) barley
1⅔ cups (400 mL) vegetable stock
2 red beets
1 bunch green (spring) onions
1 tbsp (15 mL) canola or vegetable oil
¼ cup (50 mL/30 g) freshly grated Parmesan cheese
½ bunch parsley
Salt and freshly ground pepper

1 Combine barley with vegetable stock and bring to a boil. Place beets on top of the barley and cook, covered, on low heat for 1 hour.

2 Remove the beets, peel and dice finely. Thinly slice the white and light green parts of the green onions. Chop most of the parsley. Heat the oil, stir in the onions and sauté on medium heat.

3 Add the barley, cooking water and beets, and cook for 10 minutes. Stir in the chopped parsley and ½ the Parmesan. Season with salt and pepper. Serve topped with the remaining Parmesan and parsley leaves.

!! TIP: Red beets are related to sugar beets, but 3½ oz (100 g) contain only about 7.5 g carbohydrates when cooked. Beets have a fine earthy, agreeable taste and match well with herring and horseradish. They are also delicious served raw in a salad.

PASTA, RICE AND COMPANY

Barley with Beets, right

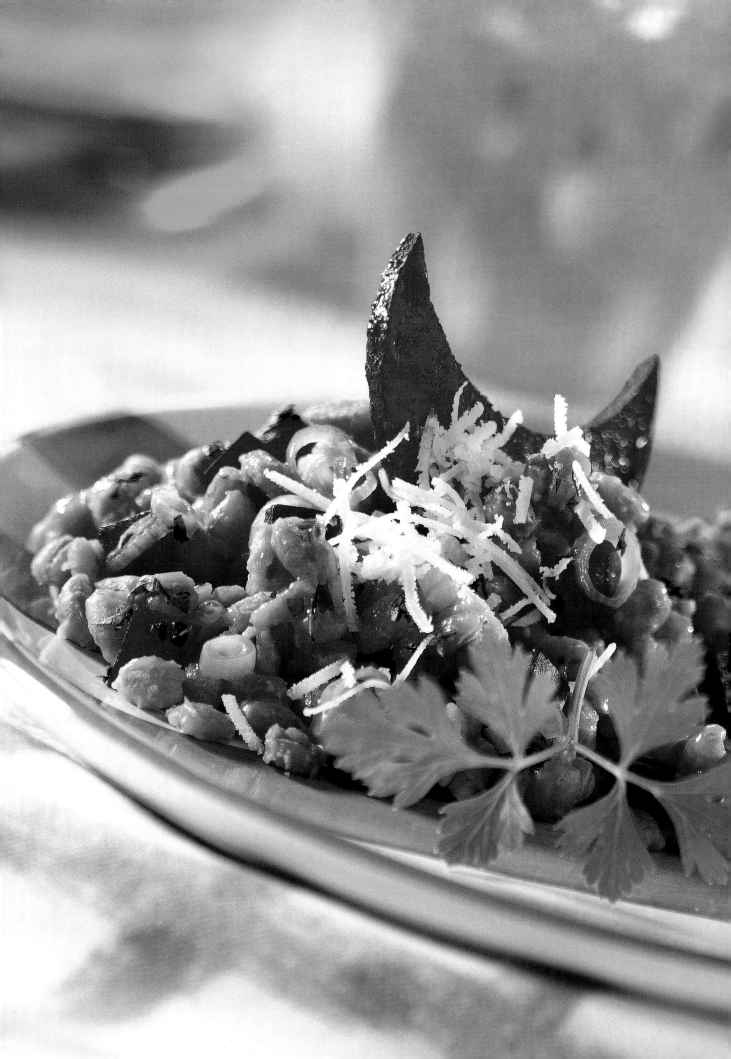

Vegetable Skewers with Red-Pepper Chutney

Carbohydrates	●◀	1 hr.
Fat	+	
Fiber	●●●	

Per serving: approx. 257 calories
5 g protein · 19 g fat · 17 g carbohydrates

FOR 2 SERVINGS:
2 onions
2 small red peppers
1 small piece ginger
3 tbsp (45 mL) olive oil, divided
Curry powder
¼ cup (50 mL) cider vinegar
1 tsp (5 mL) lemon juice
1 tsp (5 mL) sugar
Salt and freshly ground pepper
1 small ear corn
¾ cup (175 mL) vegetable stock
1 small eggplant (aubergine)
1 small zucchini (courgette)
6 to 10 cherry tomatoes
1 clove garlic

1 Chop the onions, red peppers and ginger. Heat 2 tbsp (30 mL) of the oil, stir in onions and sauté. Stir in red peppers and brown. Stir in ginger, curry powder to taste, vinegar, lemon juice and sugar. Cook on low heat for 30 minutes. Season with salt and pepper, and set aside.

2 Cook the corn in boiling water for 4 to 5 minutes. Slice the eggplant and zucchini. Heat the stock and stir in the eggplant and zucchini. Cook for 10 minutes. Remove and drain on a paper towel.

3 Cut the corn into rounds about as thick as the eggplant and zucchini. Starting and ending with cherry tomatoes, alternate the vegetables on 2 or 3 skewers.

4 Chop the garlic and heat the remaining 1 tbsp (15 ml) oil in a large skillet (frying pan). Sauté the garlic on medium heat. Lay in the vegetable skewers and brown on all sides. Arrange on two plates with the red-pepper chutney.

Eggplant (Aubergine) with Chickpeas

Carbohydrates	●●◀	1 hr.
Fat	●●	(+ 12 hrs. soaking)
Fiber	●●●	

Per serving: approx. 254 calories
14 g protein · 9 g fat · 30 g carbohydrates

FOR 2 SERVINGS:
½ cup (125 mL/100 g) dried chickpeas
1 onion
1 eggplant
3 tomatoes
1 tbsp (15 mL) olive oil
1 clove garlic
½ bunch fresh rosemary
1 tbsp (15 mL) white-wine vinegar
Salt and freshly ground pepper

1 Soak chickpeas in water to cover for 8 to 12 hours, or overnight.

2 Dice the onion and eggplant. Score, blanch, peel and coarsely dice the tomatoes. Heat the oil, stir in the onion and sauté on medium heat until translucent. Stir in the eggplant and sauté until light gold in color.

3 Finely chop or grate the garlic. Drain the chickpeas, stir into the eggplant along with the garlic and tomatoes, and simmer on low heat for at least 30 minutes. Chop the rosemary leaves and stir in with the vinegar, salt and pepper.

!! **TIP:** If you prefer softer chickpeas, simmer for 45 minutes. The important nutrients in tomatoes aren't affected by long cooking times—in fact, cooking tomatoes makes these nutrients more easily accessible.

Vegetable Skewers with Red-Pepper Chutney, top
Eggplant with Chickpeas, bottom

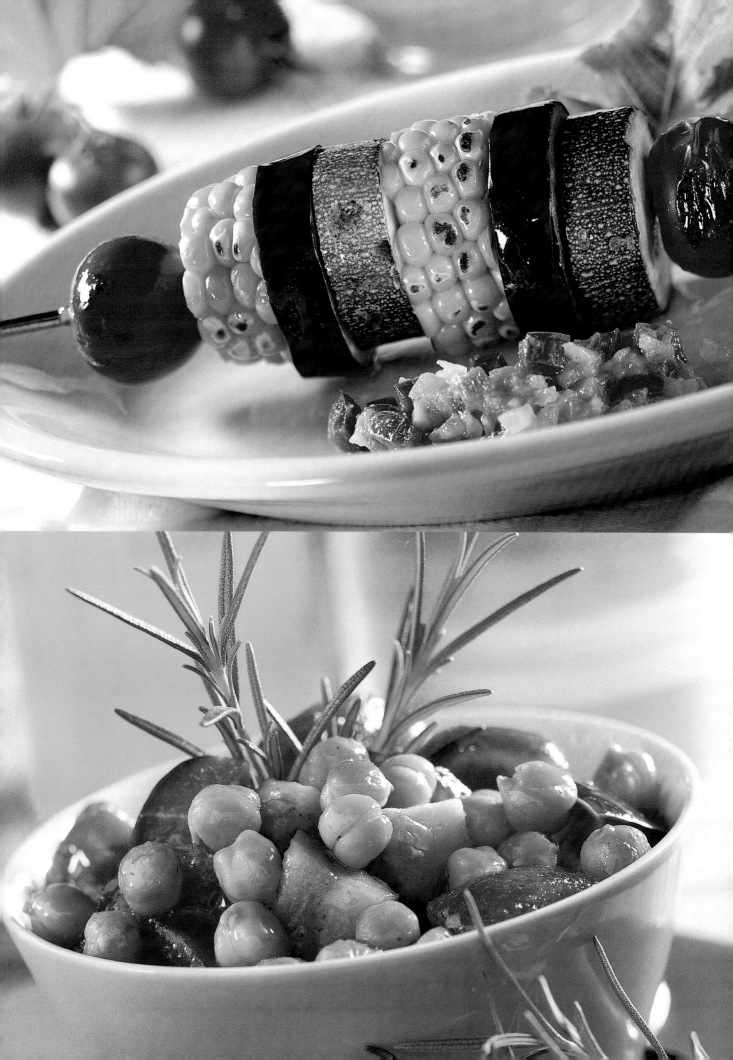

Spicy Chili Con Carne

Carbohydrates	●●●●	
Fat	++	
Fiber	●●●	

1 hr.

Per serving: approx. 533 calories
45 g protein · 20 g fat · 43 g carbohydrates

FOR 2 SERVINGS:
1 onion
1 clove garlic
1 tbsp (15 mL) canola or vegetable oil
7 oz (200 g) ground beef
19-oz (540 mL) can red kidney beans
2 green jalapeno or serrano peppers
5 tomatoes
1 tsp (5 mL) dried oregano
Salt and freshly ground pepper
Sugar

1 Chop the onion and garlic. Heat the oil in a large skillet. Stir in the onion and garlic, and sauté on medium heat until translucent. Stir in the ground beef and brown for 10 minutes.

2 Seed and finely chop the jalapenos. Thinly slice the tomatoes. Drain the beans and stir into the ground beef along with the peppers, tomatoes and oregano. Simmer on low heat for 20 minutes. Season with salt, pepper and a little sugar.

!! **TIP:** You can also make a meatless chili. Broil (grill) 1 large red pepper in the oven or over the flame of a gas burner. Sprinkle with salt and cover with a damp towel. After 5 minutes, slip off the skin and chop coarsely. Sauté the onion and garlic as described above, stir in the red pepper, hot peppers and tomatoes, and simmer for 20 minutes. Thicken with tomato paste and season with cayenne and basil.

Lentil Curry with Rice

Carbohydrates	●●●●● ◖	
Fat	●●	
Fiber	●●●	

55 min.

Per serving: approx. 407 calories
18 g protein · 9 g fat · 63 g carbohydrates

FOR 2 SERVINGS:
½ cup (125 mL/75 g) brown rice
1 cup lightly salted boiling water
1 bunch green (spring) onions
1 clove garlic
1 kohlrabi
1 tsp (5 mL) olive oil
1⅔ cups (400 mL) vegetable stock, divided
½ cup (125 mL/100 g) red lentils
4 tbsp (60 mL/60 g) sour cream
Curry powder
Ground coriander seeds
Salt and freshly ground pepper

1 Add the rice to the water and cook, covered, on low heat for 40 minutes, stirring occasionally.

2 Thinly slice the white and light green parts of the green onions. Chop the garlic and peel and dice the kohlrabi. Heat the oil, stir in the garlic and sauté on medium heat until translucent. Stir in the kohlrabi and green onions and brown slightly. Pour in ½ the stock and cook, covered, on low heat for 20 minutes.

3 Stir lentils into the remaining stock and bring to a boil. Cook, covered, on low heat for 8 to 10 minutes. Stir into the kohlrabi mixture and cook until lentils are soft but not mushy. Cool slightly, stir in the sour cream, and season with curry powder, ground coriander, salt and pepper to taste. Serve with the rice.

Spicy Chili Con Carne, top
Lentil Curry with Rice, bottom

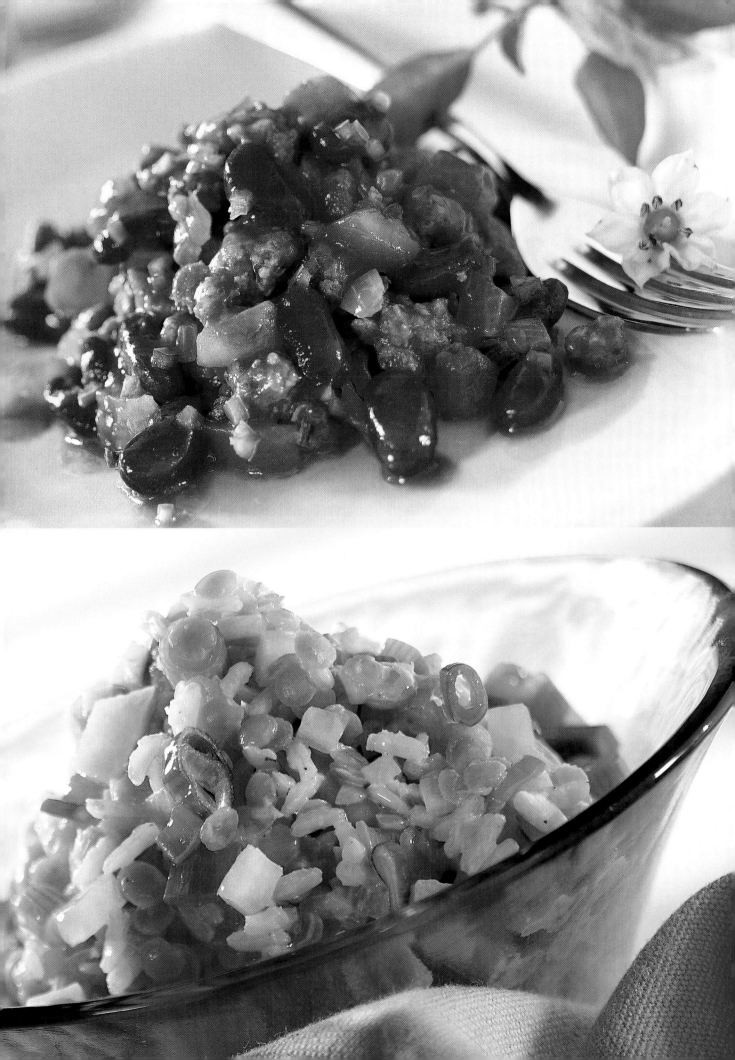

Sweets and Desserts

Not always, but more often

Fresh fruits, yogurt and cottage cheese or quark are frequently featured in refreshing desserts to please everyone, not just those with a sweet tooth. After a light, low-calorie meal—and only then—can dessert be a bit more extravagant.

Fruit desserts are relatively high in fructose. If the main dish of a meal is high in carbohydrates, prepare only half the amount of dessert and serve it with quark, cottage cheese or yogurt.

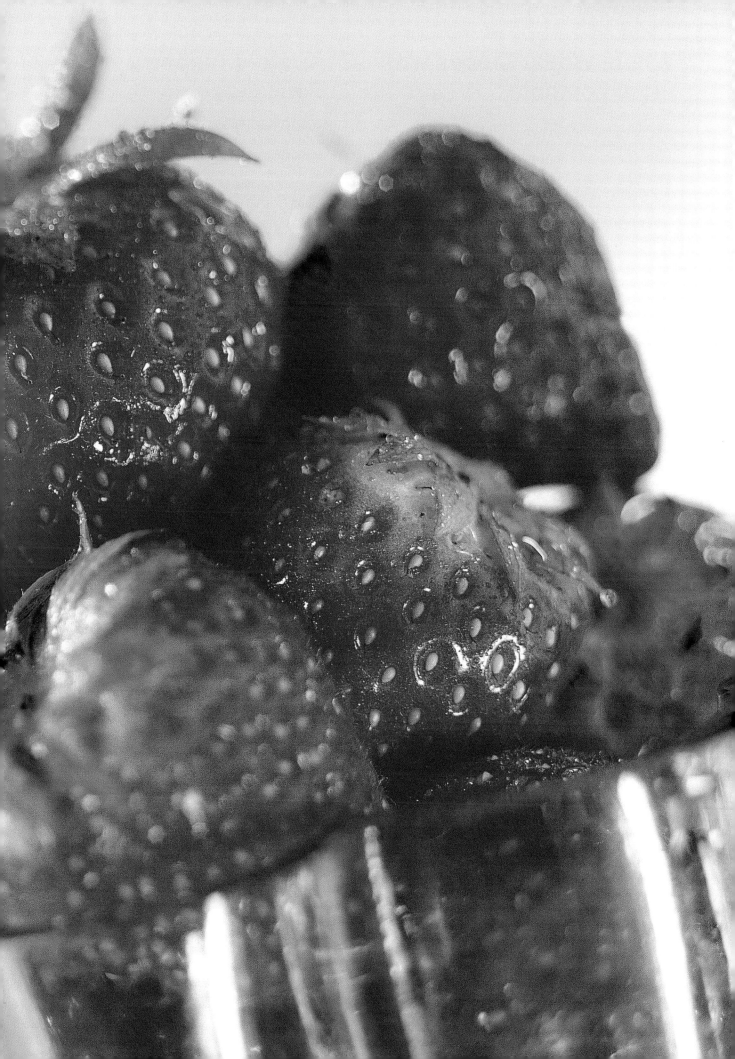

Whole Wheat Crêpes with Plum Compote

Carbohydrates	●●●●●	40 min.
Fat	+	(+ 15 minutes resting)
Fiber	●●●	

Per serving: approx. 455 calories
13 g protein · 16 g fat · 61 g carbohydrates

FOR 2 SERVINGS:
4 plums
4 tsp (20 mL/10 g) fresh ginger
Lemon zest
¼ cup (50 mL) dry red wine
Liquid sweetener
1 egg
1 cup (250 mL) low-fat milk
¾ cup (175 mL/100 g) coarsely ground whole wheat flour
½ vanilla bean
Salt
4 tsp (20 mL/20 g) clarified butter, divided
½ tsp (2 mL) ground cinnamon
1 tsp (5 mL) brown sugar

1 Pit and quarter the plums and grate the ginger. Combine with a small piece of lemon zest and the wine, and simmer on low heat for 15 minutes. Stir in a few drops of sweetener and leave to cool.

2 Separate the egg and whisk the yolk with the milk. Gradually sift in flour, stirring. Slice the vanilla bean lengthwise. Scrape out the seeds and add with a bit of grated lemon zest to the batter. Let stand for 15 minutes. Stir in a little sweetener. Beat the egg white and 1 pinch of salt until stiff and fold into the batter.

3 Heat 1 tsp (5 mL) of the butter in a nonstick skillet (frying pan). Pour in ¼ of the batter, enough to coat the bottom, and cook until golden. Flip and cook until golden on the other side.

4 Make 3 more crêpes and arrange on two plates. Sprinkle with cinnamon and brown sugar and serve with the plum compote.

 TIP: You can also use prunes in this recipe. Soak in the wine overnight, then cook for 10 minutes as described above.

Apple–Blueberry Pancakes

Carbohydrates	●●●	30 min.
Fat	++	(+ 10 min. resting)
Fiber	●●●	

Per serving: approx. 410 calories
12 g protein · 23 g fat · 32 g carbohydrates

FOR 2 SERVINGS:
2 eggs
½ cup (125 mL) low-fat milk
½ tsp (2 mL) vanilla sugar
2⅓ tbsp (35 mL/20 g) sugar
½ cup (125 mL/60 g) coarsely ground whole wheat flour
Pinch salt
1 tart apple
Liquid sweetener
2 tbsp (30 mL/30 g) clarified butter
⅔ cup (150 mL/100 g) blueberries

1 Separate the eggs and whisk the yolks with the milk, vanilla sugar and sugar. Gradually sift in the flour, stirring. Let stand for 10 minutes.

2 Combine egg whites and salt and beat until stiff. Fold into the batter. Peel, core and thinly slice the apple and fold in. Add sweetener to taste.

3 Heat a little of the butter in a nonstick skillet (frying pan). Pour in ¼ of the batter and sprinkle ¼ of the blueberries on top. Cook on one side until golden, then slide onto a plate. Brush a little more butter on the skillet and heat; return pancake to the pan and cook the other side.

4 Prepare 3 more pancakes. Serve warm.

 TIP: If you use frozen berries, first thaw them and drain. Save the juice to use as a fruit sauce.

TIP: To make vanilla sugar, add 1 or 2 vanilla beans—or even the scraped pods—to about 2 cups (500 mL/400 g) granulated sugar and store in a covered container.

Whole Wheat Crêpes with Plum Compote, top
Apple–Blueberry Pancakes, bottom

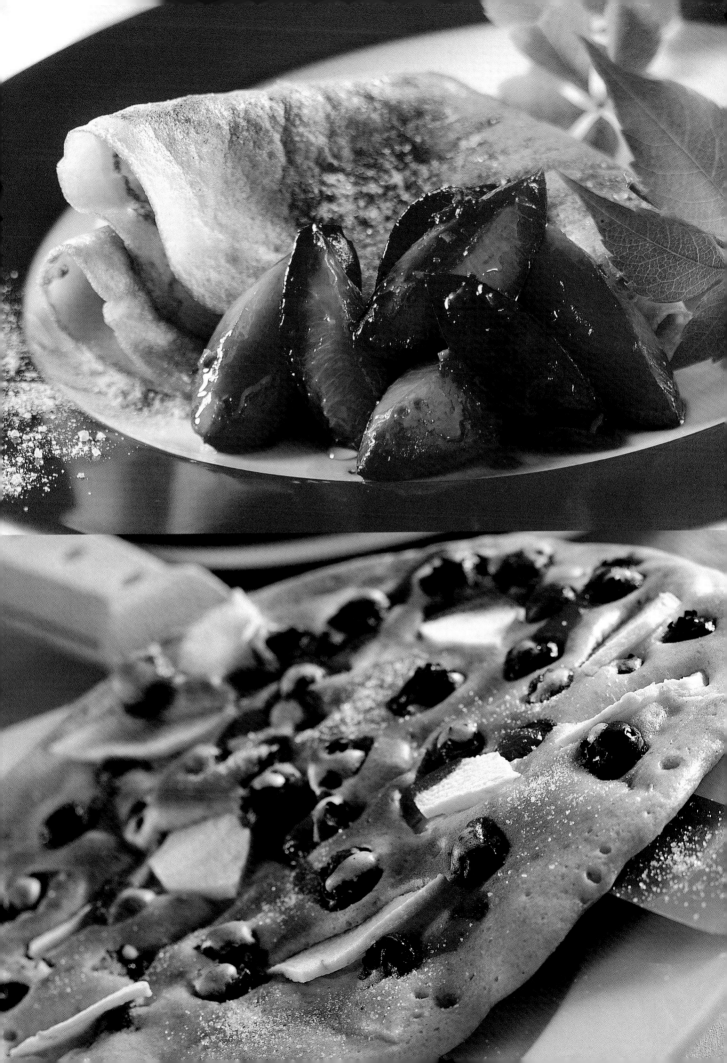

Ricotta Cream with Kiwi–Gooseberry Purée

Carbohydrates	●◖	20 min.
Fat	●	
Fiber	●	

Per serving: approx. 126 calories
8 g protein · 4 g fat · 13 g carbohydrates

FOR 2 SERVINGS:
1 ripe kiwi fruit
½ lemon (organic preferred)
1 cup (250 mL/150 g) gooseberries
Liquid sweetener
¼ cup (50 mL/60 g) ricotta
¼ cup (50 mL/60 g) low-fat quark
  or puréed cottage cheese
2 to 3 tbsp (30 to 45 mL) mineral
  water

1 Peel the kiwi and cut into wedges. Dip briefly into boiling water, then rinse in cold water and drain.

2 Finely grate the zest of the lemon and squeeze out the juice. Purée together the kiwi, ⅔ of the gooseberries, 1 tbsp (15 mL) lemon juice and sweetener to taste in a blender or with a potato masher.

3 Combine ricotta and quark with the mineral water, lemon zest, 2 tbsp (30 mL) lemon juice and sweetener to taste. Stir until creamy.

4 Spoon the ricotta mixture into two dessert dishes and top with fruit purée. Garnish with the remaining gooseberries.

Honey–Apple Crêpes

Carbohydrates	●●●◖	40 min.
Fat	++	
Fiber	●	

Per serving: approx. 425 calories
15 g protein · 21 g fat · 43 g carbohydrates

FOR 2 SERVINGS:
¾ cup (175 mL/75 g) coarsely
  ground whole wheat flour
2 tbsp (30 mL/15 g) all-purpose
  flour
½ cup (125 mL) low-fat milk
⅔ cup (150 mL) mineral water
Salt
Liquid sweetener
2 tbsp (30 mL) flaked almonds or
  chopped hazelnuts
2 extra-large eggs
6 tsp (30 mL) oil, divided
1 small apple
2 tbsp (30 mL) lemon juice
1 tsp (5 mL) liquid honey
½ tsp (2 mL) ground cinnamon

1 Stir together flour, milk, mineral water, 1 pinch of salt and 2 dashes of sweetener. Let stand for 30 minutes.

2 Toast almonds in a dry skillet (frying pan) until golden. Stir the eggs into the batter.

3 Preheat oven to 120°F (50°C). Cook 6 small crêpes. For each, heat 1 tsp (5 mL) of the oil and cook ⅙ of the batter on both sides until golden. Keep warm in the oven.

4 Core and slice the apple paper-thin and sprinkle immediately with lemon juice. Roll up the crêpes and arrange on a plate. Top with apple slices, drizzle with honey, and sprinkle with cinnamon and toasted nuts.

Cherry Pudding with Almonds

Carbohydrates	●●●●	35 min.
Fat	+	(+ 45 min.
Fiber	●●	baking)

Per serving: approx. 386 calories
13 g protein · 15 g fat · 47 g carbohydrates

FOR 2 SERVINGS:
Oil
Fine dry bread crumbs
4 slices bread
2 cups (about 10 oz/300 g) pitted
  sweet cherries
2 eggs
2⅓ tbsp (35 mL/30 g) sugar
1¼ cups (300 mL) low-fat milk
1 lemon
1 vanilla bean
2 tbsp (30 mL) chopped almonds

1 Oil a small ovenproof dish and coat with bread crumbs. Cut the bread slices into thirds and lay 4 pieces in the bottom of the dish. Top with ½ the cherries, then lay in 4 more pieces of bread, the remaining cherries and the remaining bread.

2 Combine the eggs, sugar and milk. Finely grate the lemon zest and squeeze out the juice. Slice the vanilla bean in half lengthwise and scrape out the seeds. Add the vanilla seeds, lemon zest and lemon juice to the custard mixture. Pour over the pudding and leave to soak for 5 minutes.

3 Preheat oven to 400°F (200°C). Sprinkle chopped almonds over the pudding and bake for 45 minutes.

Ricotta Cream with Kiwi–Gooseberry Purée, top Honey–Apple Crêpes, bottom left Cherry Pudding with Almonds, bottom right

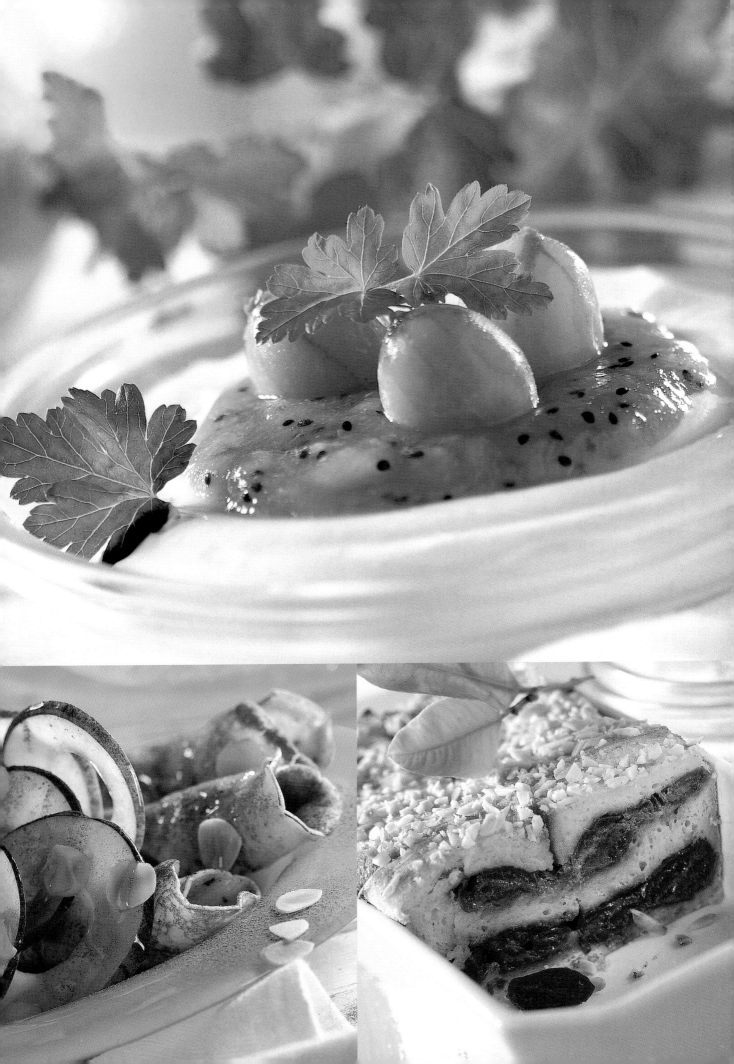

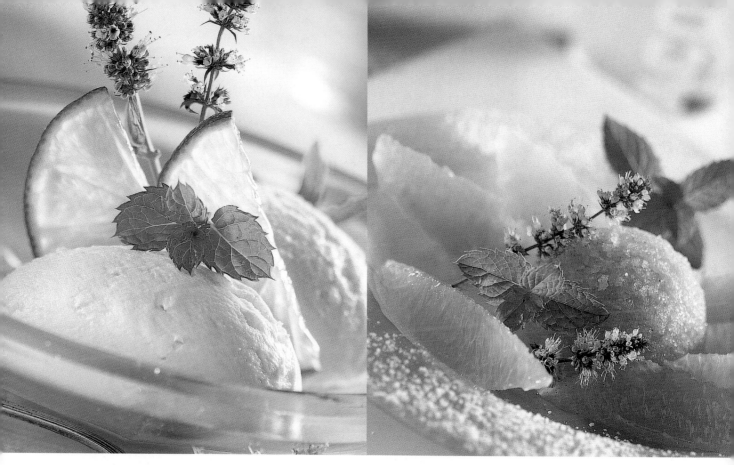

Buttermilk–Lime Ice Cream

Carbohydrates	–		30 min.
Fat	●●		(+ 3 to 4 hrs. freezing)
Fiber	–		

Per serving: approx. 90 calories
1 g protein · 8 g fat · 4 g carbohydrates

FOR 8 SERVINGS:
2 cups (500 mL) buttermilk
²/₃ cup (150 mL/150 g)
   crème fraîche or sour
   cream
Juice of 1½ limes
2 tsp (10 mL) lemon extract
2 tbsp (30 mL) icing (confectioner's) sugar
1 tsp (5 ml) liquid
   sweetener
Thin slices of lime
Mint sprigs or chopped
   lemon grass

1 Whisk together but-
termilk, crème
fraîche, lime juice, lemon
extract, icing sugar and
sweetener.

2 Place the mixture in
an ice cream maker
and churn-freeze (or
place in a metal or plastic
bowl in the freezer for 3
to 4 hours, stirring every
hour to keep it smooth).
Transfer to a freezer-safe
bowl and place in the
freezer. Before serving,
put two ice cream dishes
in the refrigerator.

3 Scoop the ice cream
into the chilled dishes.
Garnish with half-moons
of lime and a mint sprig
and serve.

Mango Sorbet on Marinated Oranges

Carbohydrates	●●◖		30 min.
Fat	–		(+ 15 to 20 min. freezing)
Fiber	●●		

Per serving: approx. 135 calories
2 g protein · 1 g fat · 27 g carbohydrates

FOR 2 SERVINGS:
1 large ripe mango
1 tbsp (15 mL) coconut milk
Juice of 1 lime
Liquid sweetener
½ tsp (2 mL) ground
   cinnamon
Pinch ground coriander
   seeds
2 medium oranges
½ tsp (2 mL) orange flower
   water
1 tsp (5 mL) orange liqueur
1 tsp (5 mL) icing (confectioner's) sugar
Mint sprigs

1 Cut the mango into
pieces and peel,
removing the pit and
reserving the juice.
Combine fruit and juice
with the coconut milk,
lime juice, sweetener,
cinnamon and coriander.
Purée and strain through
a sieve. Churn-freeze in
an ice cream maker for
15 to 20 minutes.

2 Peel and section the
oranges and combine
with orange flower water
and liqueur.

3 Sprinkle two plates
with icing sugar.
Arrange the oranges on
the plates. Make small
balls of sorbet and
arrange on top. Garnish
with mint leaves.

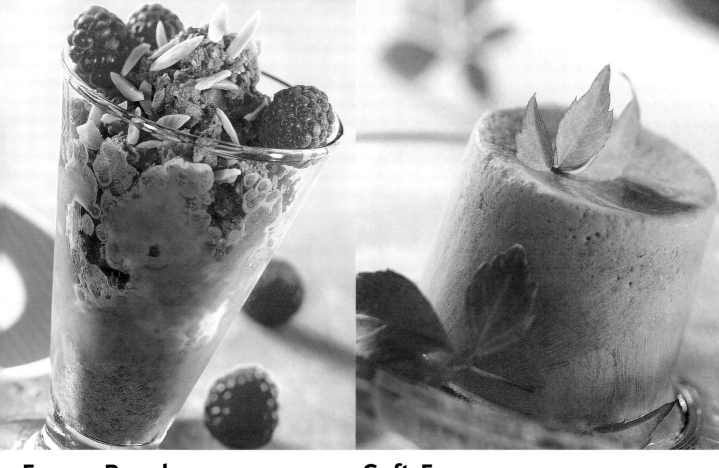

Frozen Raspberry Yogurt

Carbohydrates	●●	15 min.
Fat	●●●	(+ 2 hrs. freezing)
Fiber	●●	

Per serving: approx. 230 calories
17 g protein · 12 g fat · 21 g carbohydrates

FOR 2 SERVINGS:
2 cups (500 mL/250 g) raspberries
1 tsp (5 mL) raspberry brandy
1 tsp (5 mL) vanilla sugar
½ tsp (2 mL) lemon juice
1 tbsp (15 mL) slivered almonds
¾ cup (175 mL/175 g) yogurt
1 tbsp (15 mL) maple syrup
Pinch ground ginger
3 tbsp (45 mL/50 g) whipping (35%) cream

1 Set aside a few of the nicest raspberries. Combine the remainder with the brandy, vanilla sugar and lemon juice, and let stand for 10 minutes.

2 Toast the almonds until golden and leave to cool. Purée the raspberry mixture, then stir in the yogurt, maple syrup and ginger.

3 Whip the cream until stiff and fold into the raspberry mixture. Pour into a freezer-safe dish and freeze for 2 hours. Stir occasionally to prevent large ice crystals from forming.

4 Spoon into tall glasses. Garnish with the toasted almonds and remaining raspberries.

Soft-Frozen Cherry Yogurt

Carbohydrates	–	15 min.
Fat	●●	(+ 1? hrs. freezing)
Fiber	–	

Per serving: approx. 90 calories
1 g protein · 8 g fat · 4 g carbohydrates

FOR 2 SERVINGS:
3 tbsp (45 mL/50 g) whipping (35%) cream
Pinch vanilla
Liquid sweetener
½ cup (125 mL/100 g) pitted sour cherries
⅓ cup (75 mL/75 g) low-fat yogurt

1 Whip the cream until stiff, then stir in vanilla and a little sweetener.

2 Purée the cherries and their juice in a blender or with a potato masher. Combine with the yogurt in a small bowl, add 1 or 2 dashes of sweetener, then carefully fold in the whipped cream.

3 Spoon the mixture into two molds or ramekins and freeze for 1½ hours.

 TIP: Almond cookies go well with this dessert.

Ginger–Pear Granita

Carbohydrates ●	30 min.
Fat –	(+ 40 min. cooling)
Fiber ●	(+ 2 hrs. freezing)

Per serving: approx. 96 calories
1 g protein · 2 g fat · 10 g carbohydrates

FOR 2 SERVINGS:
1 lemon (organic preferred)
½ tsp (2 mL) grated fresh ginger
1 tsp (5 mL) fructose
¾ cup (175 mL) water, divided
1 ripe pear
Finely grated bittersweet chocolate
Lemon wedges

1 Use a zester to remove the lemon peel in thin strips. Cut into shorter lengths, if necessary. Squeeze out the juice.

2 In a small saucepan, bring lemon zest, ginger, fructose and ½ cup (125 ml) of the water to a boil. Simmer, uncovered, on low heat for 10 minutes, until syrupy.

3 Peel, core and slice the pear and combine with 2 tsp (10 mL) lemon juice and the remaining ¼ cup (50 mL) water in a small saucepan. Cook, covered, on low heat for 8 minutes.

4 Strain the lemon–ginger syrup through a fine-mesh strainer into a medium-sized metal bowl and leave to cool, covered, for 40 minutes.

5 Using a fork, crush the pear slices and stir into the syrup. Place the bowl in the freezer for 2 hours. Stir occasionally to prevent large ice crystals from forming.

6 Spoon into two glasses. Garnish with a bit of chocolate and lemon wedges and serve.

Walnut Ice Cream

Carbohydrates ◖	30 min.
Fat +	(+ freezing time)
Fiber –	

Per serving: approx. 180 calories
3 g protein · 15 g fat · 8 g carbohydrates

FOR 8 SERVINGS:
½ cup (125 mL/60 g) chopped walnuts
¾ cup (175 mL/200 g) cream or half-and-half
1¼ cups (300 mL/300 g) low-fat milk
½ vanilla bean
2 tbsp (30 mL) icing (confectioner's) sugar, plus a bit for the plates
2 egg yolks
5 tbsp (75 mL) walnut liqueur, plus a bit for the top
½ tsp (1 mL) ground cinnamon
Orange slices

1 Toast the walnuts in a dry skillet (frying pan) and leave to cool. Set aside ½ the nuts and grind the rest.

2 Combine cream and milk in a medium saucepan. Slice the vanilla bean in half lengthwise, scrape out the seeds, and add both the seeds and the pod to the mixture.

3 Stir in the icing sugar. Heat until almost boiling, then remove from heat. Whisk the egg yolks and stir in. Reheat, stirring constantly, until the mixture thickens. Leave to cool, stirring occasionally.

4 Stir in the ground nuts, liqueur and cinnamon. Churn-freeze in an ice cream maker.

5 Refrigerate two dessert plates. Sprinkle with icing sugar. Scoop ice cream onto each dish, sprinkle with remaining nuts, drizzle a little liqueur on top and garnish with half-moons of orange.

 TIP: Instead of walnuts, use blanched hazelnuts or almonds and substitute an almond liqueur.

Ginger–Pear Granita, top
Walnut Ice Cream, bottom

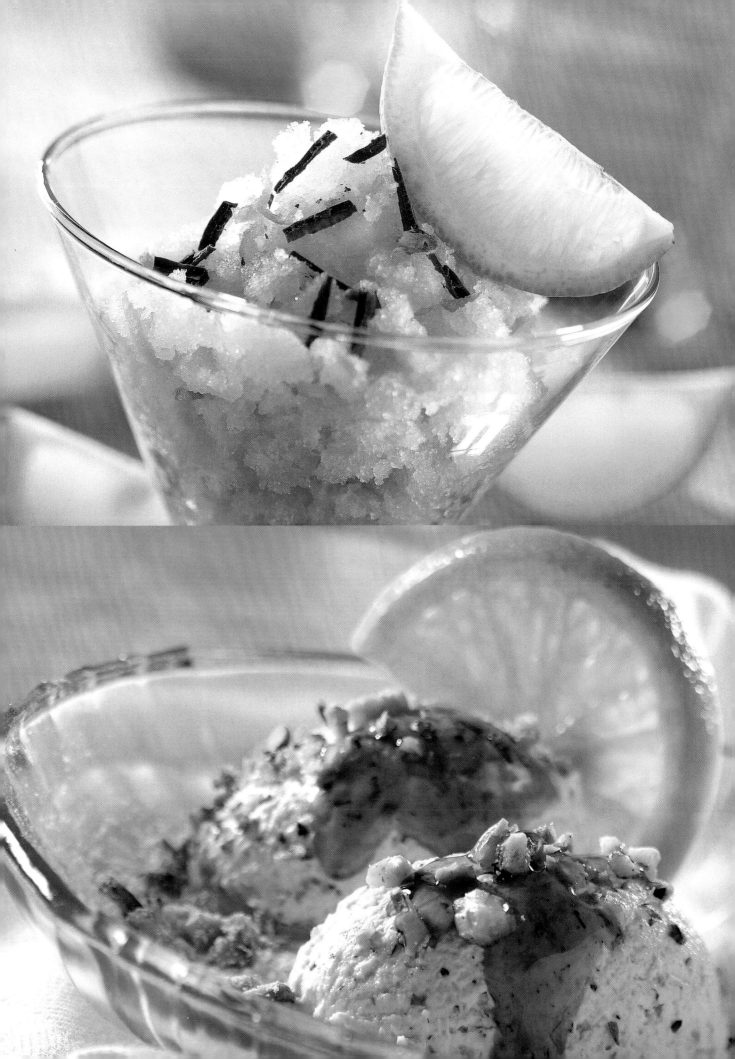

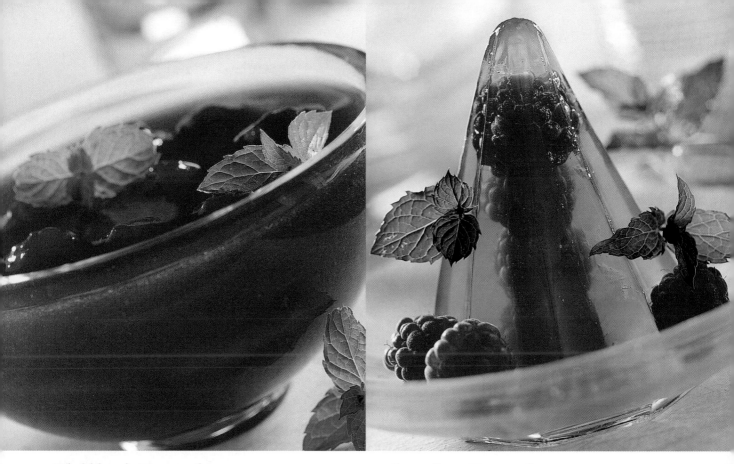

Chilled Raspberry–Champagne Cocktail

Carbohydrates ◖		20 min.
Fat —		(+ 2 to 3 hrs. chilling)
Fiber ●●		

Per serving: approx. 65 calories
2 g protein · 1 g fat · 8 g carbohydrates

FOR 2 SERVINGS:
2 cups (500 mL/250 g) raspberries
Liquid sweetener
¾ cup (175 mL) water
1 piece of lemon zest
1 tsp (5 mL) cornstarch
¼ cup (50 mL) dry champagne
Mint leaves

1 Combine about ⅓ of the raspberries with a little sweetener and set aside. Combine the remainder with the water and lemon zest. Simmer, uncovered, for 4 minutes. Strain while still hot.

2 Combine cornstarch with 1 tbsp (15 mL) cold water, stir into the strained raspberries and reheat. Cook until thickened. Add the remaining raspberries, the champagne and a little sweetener.

3 Refrigerate in two small bowls for 2 to 3 hours. Garnish with mint and serve.

Apple–Raspbery Jell

Carbohydrates ●●		15 min.
Fat —		(+ 4 hrs. chilling)
Fiber ●●		

Per serving: approx. 132 calories
5 g protein · 1 g fat · 22 g carbohydrates

FOR 2 SERVINGS:
1 (¼ oz/7 g/1 tbsp) envelope unflavored gelatin
1½ cups (300 mL) apple juice, divided
1⅔ cups (400 mL/200 g) fresh or frozen raspberries
1 tbsp (15 mL) mint tea
Mint leaves

1 Pour gelatin over ¼ cup (50 mL) of the apple juice. If raspberries are frozen, thaw and drain.

2 Combine mint tea and remaining 1 cup (250 mL) of apple juice, bring to a boil, then strain through a coffee filter. Dissolve the gelatin in the hot mixture. Stir in ½ of the raspberries. Pour into two cone-shaped or other decorative molds and refrigerate for 4 hours.

3 Dip the molds briefly into hot water and turn the jelly out onto two plates. Garnish with the remaining berries and a few mint leaves and serve.

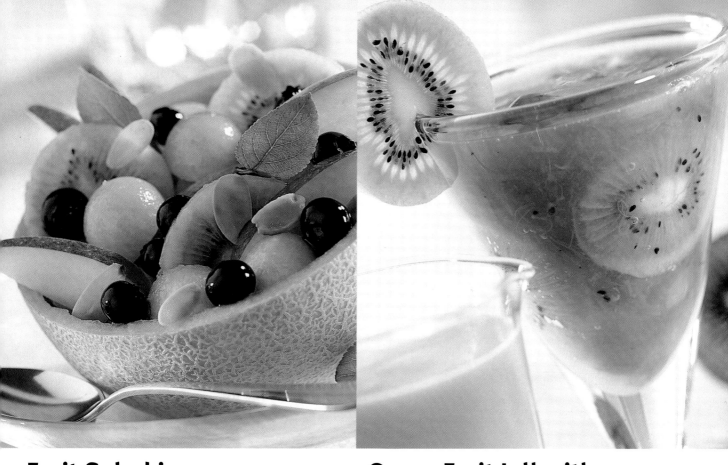

Fruit Salad in Melon Boats

Carbohydrates ●●		35 min.
Fat ●		
Fiber ●●		

Per serving: approx. 143 calories
3 g protein · 4 g fat · 22 g carbohydrates

FOR 2 SERVINGS:
½ small Galia or honeydew
   melon (1¼ cups/300 mL/
   200 g)
⅔ cup (150 mL/100 g) fresh
   or frozen blueberries
1 small apple
1 kiwi fruit
1 tbsp (15 mL) flaked
   almonds

1 Scoop out the seeds of the melon. Remove the fruit with a melon baller. Set aside the rind. Thaw and drain the blueberries, if frozen. Cut the apple in thin wedges, and peel and thinly slice the kiwi.

2 Gently combine berries, melon balls, apple and kiwi, and place in melon rind. Let stand for 10 minutes.

3 Toast the almonds in a dry nonstick skillet (frying pan) until golden and sprinkle over top.

Green Fruit Jell with Vanilla Sauce

Carbohydrates ●●		30 min.
Fat ●		
Fiber ●		

Per serving: approx. 126 calories
3 g protein · 3 g fat · 20 g carbohydrates

FOR 4 SERVINGS:
¾ cup (175 mL) apple juice
3 tbsp (50 mL/30 g) quick-
   cooking tapioca
½ tsp (2 mL) ground cloves
1⅓ cups (325 mL/200 g)
   green gooseberries
1 vanilla bean
2 kiwi fruit
⅔ cup (150 mL) low-fat milk
1 tsp (5 mL) cornstarch
1 egg yolk, lightly beaten
1 tbsp (15 mL) sugar

1 Combine the apple juice and ¾ cup (175 mL) water. Mix in the tapioca and let stand for 10 minutes. Bring the mixture to a boil and stir in ground cloves. Simmer, covered, on low heat for 20 minutes.

2 Add 1 tbsp (15 mL) water to the gooseberries and cook for 10 minutes, then add the tapioca mixture. Peel and slice the kiwi. Slice the vanilla bean in half and scrape out the seeds. Stir ½ the vanilla seeds and the kiwi into the fruit mixture. Pour into glasses and chill.

3 Bring the milk to a simmer and stir in the remaining vanilla seeds. Mix cornstarch with a little cold water and stir into the milk along with the egg yolk and sugar. Cook, stirring, until thickened. Leave to cool. Serve with the jelled fruit.

Yogurt Mousse with Marinated Figs

Carbohydrates	●◖	45 min.
Fat	+	(+ 2 to 3 hrs. chilling)
Fiber	–	

Per serving: approx. 266 calories
6 g protein · 16 g fat · 18 g carbohydrates

FOR 2 SERVINGS:
½ (¼ oz/7 g/1 tbsp) package unflavored gelatin
⅔ cup (150 mL/150 g) low-fat yogurt
1 tbsp (15 mL) lemon juice
1 tbsp (15 mL) orange flower water
Liquid sweetener
⅓ cup (75 mL/80 g) whipping (35%) cream
1 tsp (5 mL) vanilla sugar
Sunflower oil
¼ cup (50 mL) port
¼ cup (50 mL) freshly squeezed orange juice
Pinch orange zest
½ tsp (2 mL) honey
2 ripe figs
½ tsp (1 mL) cornstarch
Lemon balm leaves

1 Pour gelatin over ¼ cup (50 mL) cold water. Add ½ cup (50 ml) boiling water and stir until completely dissolved. Leave to cool slightly.

2 Combine yogurt, lemon juice and orange flower water, and stir until smooth. Add sweetener and set aside. Whip the cream with vanilla sugar until stiff.

3 Fold the gelatin into the whipped cream. Fold the whipped cream into the yogurt mixture. Lightly oil two molds, fill with the mousse and cover with plastic wrap. Refrigerate for 2 to 3 hours, until firm.

4 Heat the port, orange juice, orange zest and honey. Quarter and stir in the figs. Leave to cool, then marinate, covered, for 1 hour.

5 Drain the figs. Bring the marinade to a boil. Combine the cornstarch with 1 tbsp (15 mL) water and then stir into marinade. Stir until thick, then let cool. Turn the yogurt mousse out on dessert plates. Garnish with sauce, figs and lemon balm.

TIP: Instead of using the figs, peel, halve and core 1 pear. Slice the halves to form a fan. Marinate in the port as described above and serve with the mousse.

Red Fruit Jell with Yogurt Sauce

Carbohydrates	●●◖	35 min.
Fat	●●●	
Fiber	●●	

Per serving: approx. 224 calories
5 g protein · 12 g fat · 26 g carbohydrates

FOR 2 SERVINGS:
1⅔ cups (400 mL/350 g) mixed berries: blackberries, raspberries, blueberries, etc.
½ cup (125 mL) unsweetened cherry or red currant juice
1 tbsp (15 mL) coarsely ground buckwheat flour
¼ cup (50 mL) water
Liquid sweetener
1 tbsp (15 mL) flaked almonds
½ cup (125 mL/125 g) low-fat yogurt
½ tsp (2 mL) vanilla sugar
1 tsp (5 mL) lemon juice
3 tbsp (45 mL/50 g) whipping (35%) cream
Small mint leaves

1 Place ⅔ of the berries in a small saucepan. Add cherry juice and bring to a boil. Combine the flour with the water, stir into the berries and cook for 2 minutes, stirring constantly. Stir in sweetener to taste.

2 Fold the remaining berries into the mixture, pour into two dessert bowls and refrigerate.

3 Toast the almonds in a dry nonstick skillet (frying pan) until golden, then turn out on a plate to cool.

4 Combine yogurt, vanilla sugar and lemon juice. Whip the cream until stiff and fold into the yogurt. Top each dish of fruit with a dollop of the yogurt mixture, and garnish with almonds and mint leaves.

 TIP: You can save 6 g of fat by using low-fat milk instead of cream in the sauce.

Yogurt Mousse with Marinated Figs, top
Red Fruit Jell with Yogurt Sauce, bottom

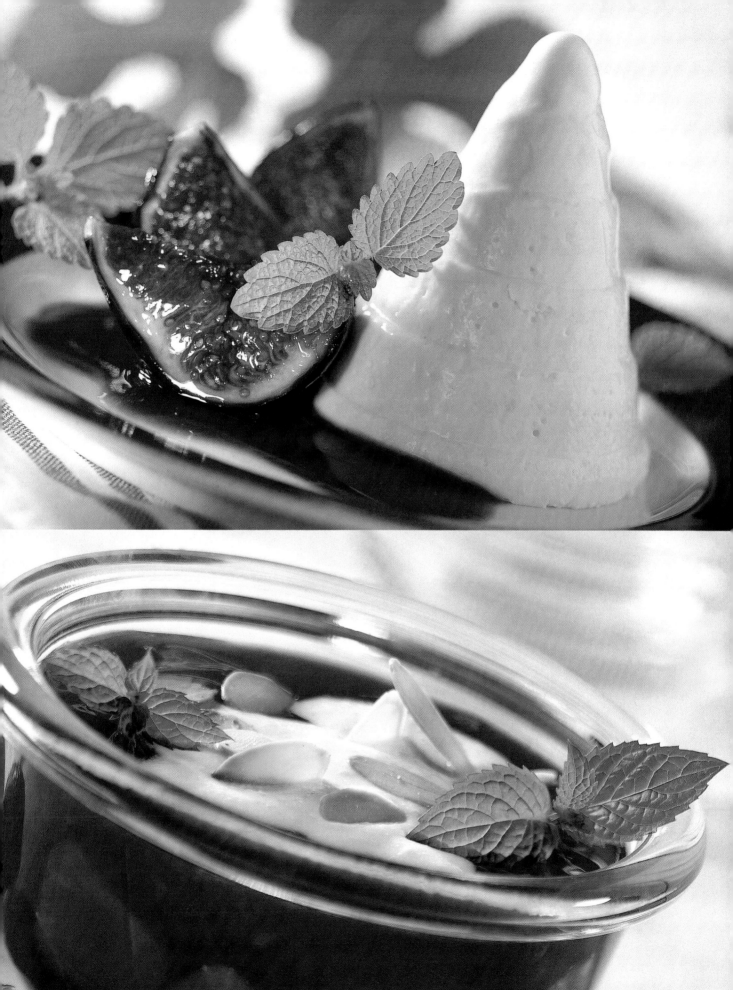

Exotic Rice Pudding

Carbohydrates	●●●●	30 min.
Fat	–	
Fiber	●	

Per serving: approx. 235 calories
5 g protein · 2 g fat · 48 g carbohydrates

FOR 4 SERVINGS:
1 cup (250 mL) low-fat milk
½ cup (125 mL) unsweetened
   coconut milk
1 (4-serving/120 g) package rice
   pudding mix
1 small papaya
1 vanilla bean
1 pineapple, or 1 (19-oz/540 mL) can
   pineapple pieces
2 bananas

1 Combine milk and coconut milk and bring to a boil. Add the rice pudding mix and cook, uncovered, on medium heat until sauce begins to thicken, about 10 minutes.

2 Scoop out the papaya seeds. Peel and slice finely. Slice the vanilla bean lengthwise and scrape out the seeds. Chop the pineapple and slice the bananas.

3 Combine vanilla seeds, papaya, pineapple and banana, and stir into the pudding.

 TIP: This can be served as a sweet main dish.

Apple–Quark Yogurt

Carbohydrates	●	20 min.
Fat	–	
Fiber	–	

Per serving: approx. 137 calories
19 g protein · 2 g fat · 11 g carbohydrates

FOR 2 SERVINGS:
1 large apple
1 cup (250 mL/250 g) low-fat quark
   or puréed cottage cheese
3 to 4 tbsp (45 to 60 mL) mineral
   water
Juice of ½ lemon or lime
1 tsp (5 mL) vanilla sugar
⅓ cup (75 mL) low-fat yogurt
1 tbsp (15 mL) chopped almonds

1 Peel, core and dice the apple. In a small saucepan, cover the apple with a little water and cook on low heat until tender.

2 Combine quark, mineral water, lemon juice and vanilla sugar. Stir until smooth.

3 Fold the yogurt into the quark mixture and spoon into two dessert dishes. Top with the apple, sprinkle with almonds and serve.

TIPS: You can omit the lemon juice and season the quark with ground cinnamon. And in place of an apple, choose another fresh fruit—or grate the apple and combine it with the quark.

Millet Pudding with Apricots and Dried Cranberries

Carbohydrates	●●●◖	30 min.
Fat	●	(+ 1 hr.
Fiber	●	chilling)

Per serving: approx. 217 calories
6 g protein · 4 g fat · 37 g carbohydrates

FOR 2 SERVINGS:
1 cup (250 mL) low-fat milk
¼ cup (50 mL/50 g) millet
2 tbsp (25 mL/30 g) cream
1 tsp (5 mL) orange zest, divided
Liquid sweetener
5 or 6 apricots
¼ cup (50 mL) unsweetened apricot
   juice
2 tbsp (30 ml) dried cranberries
1 small cinnamon stick
Dash lemon juice

1 Pour the milk into a small saucepan. Grind millet finely and stir into the milk. Bring to a boil, stirring constantly, and cook, uncovered, for 2 minutes.

2 Stir in the cream, ½ the orange zest and sweetener to taste. Remove from heat and allow to thicken for 5 minutes. Rinse two small molds or bowls in cold water. Spoon in the millet mixture, spreading smoothly, and refrigerate for 1 hour.

3 Quarter and pit the apricots. Simmer the apricots, apricot juice, dried cranberries and cinnamon stick on low heat for 20 minutes. Stir in lemon juice and a little sweetener and leave to cool.

4 Turn the puddings out on two plates. Garnish with apricots and remaining orange zest.

Exotic Rice Pudding, top
Apple–Quark Yogurt, bottom left
Millet Pudding with Apricots and
Dried Cranberries, bottom right

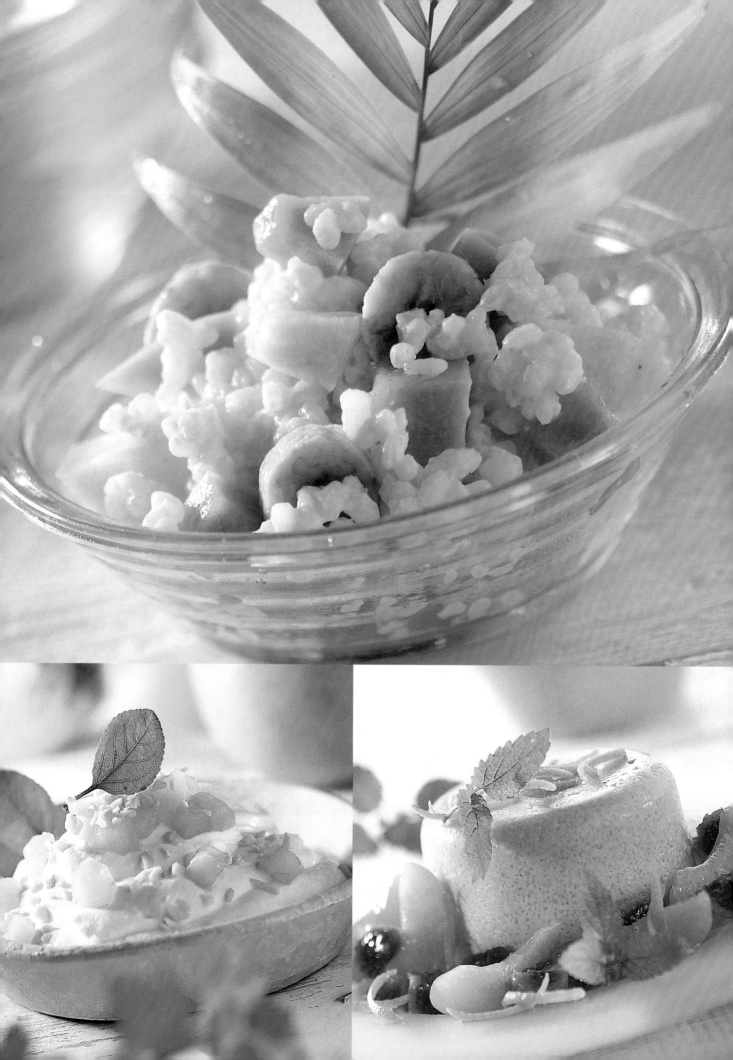

Savory Baked Goods, Breads, Rolls, Cakes and Pies

Delicious baked goods for guests and fests

Would you like to bring a leisurely dinner to a fitting end with a delicious dessert? Spoil your guests—and yourself—with a scrumptious cake or a pie? Look no further than the many recipes in the pages that follow. No one will describe *these* treats as "diabetic" baking.

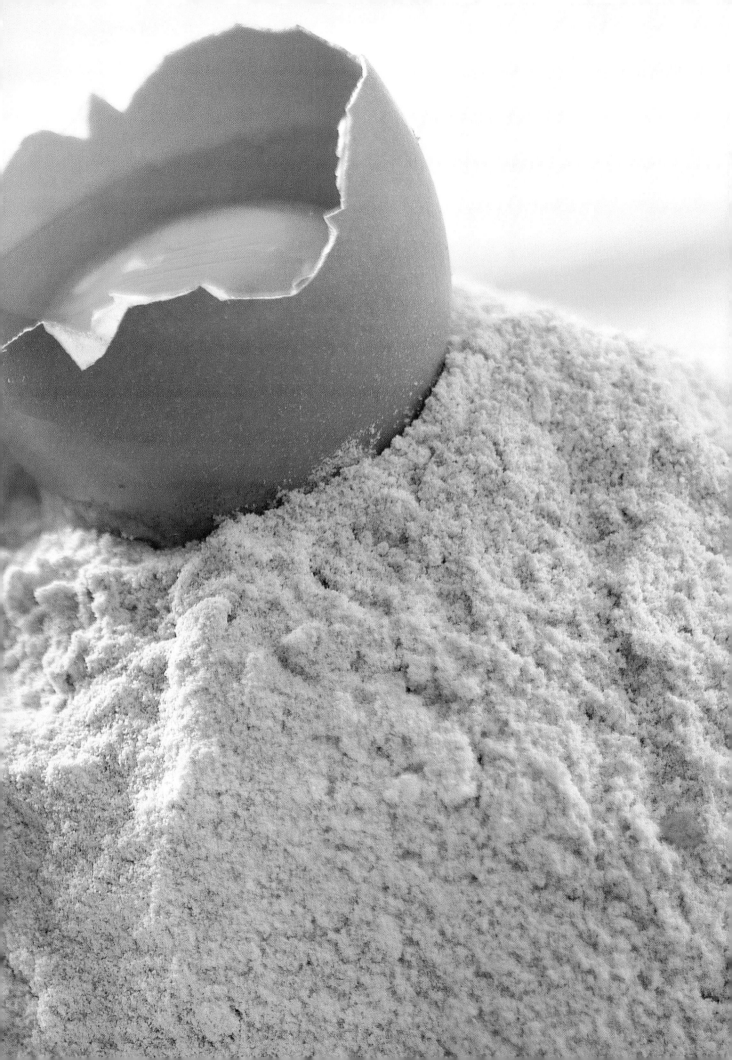

Granola Buns

Carbohydrates ●●	30 min
Fat　　　　　　●●	(+ 50 min. resting)
	(+ 30 to 35 min. baking)

Per serving: approx. 210 calories
9 g protein · 4 g fat · 35 g carbohydrates

FOR 8 BUNS:
2 cups (500 mL/250 g) coarsely ground whole wheat
　　flour
½ tsp (2 mL) salt
Grated zest of ½ lemon
2 (¼ oz/7 g/2¼ tsp) envelopes active dry yeast
⅔ cup (150 mL) lukewarm milk
1 egg
1 cup (250 mL/100 g) unsweetened granola or muesli
　　with raisins and nuts
Old-fashioned rolled oats
Milk for glazing

1 Sift the flour into a large bowl. Stir in salt and lemon zest. Stir the yeast into the milk until smooth and let stand until frothy, about 10 minutes. Stir the egg and the yeast mixture into the flour. Knead until smooth and elastic. Cover and leave to rise in a warm place for 30 minutes.

2 Knead the dough again, stretching it a little; sprinkle with granola and work in. Divide the dough into 8 pieces and shape into rolls. Sprinkle a fine layer of rolled oats on the work surface and roll the balls of dough over it, gently pressing in the oats.

3 Preheat the oven to 325°F (160°C). Arrange the buns on a baking sheet lined with parchment paper. Brush with milk and leave to stand, covered, for 20 minutes. Bake for 30 to 35 minutes.

 TIP: The buns can be frozen and baked as needed. Thaw, then bake in a preheated 325°F (160°C) oven.

 TIP. These tasty rolls make a good snack as is, or you can spread them with a thin layer of butter or margarine.

Quick Quark Rolls

Carbohydrates ●●	30 min.
Fat　　　　　　●●	(+ 15 min. resting)
	(+ 20 to 25 min. baking)

Per serving: approx. 159 calories
7 g protein · 5 g fat · 23 g carbohydrates

FOR 8 ROLLS:
½ cup (125 mL/125 g) low-fat quark or puréed cottage
　　cheese
2 tbsp (30 mL) sunflower oil
5 tbsp (75 mL) milk
1 egg
½ tsp (2 mL) salt
2 cups (500 mL/230 g) coarsely ground whole wheat
　　flour
1½ tsp (7 mL) baking powder
Milk for glazing

1 Combine quark, oil, milk, egg and salt, and stir until smooth. Combine the flour and baking powder, then sift into the quark mixture gradually, stirring. When the dough becomes too stiff to stir, knead in the remaining flour. Shape the dough into a rope. Leave to rest for 15 minutes. If it still sticks to your fingers, add a little more flour and knead.

2 Preheat the oven to 350°F (180°C). Divide the dough into 8 pieces, shape into balls and arrange on a baking sheet lined with parchment paper. Brush with milk and cut across the top with a sharp knife. Bake for 20 to 25 minutes, until golden.

TIPS: These rolls taste best freshly baked, but you can also freeze them. Arrange the rolls to form a wheel, brush with egg yolk, sprinkle with poppy seeds and chopped nuts or sesame seeds, as desired, and bake.

Granola Buns, top
Quick Quark Rolls, bottom

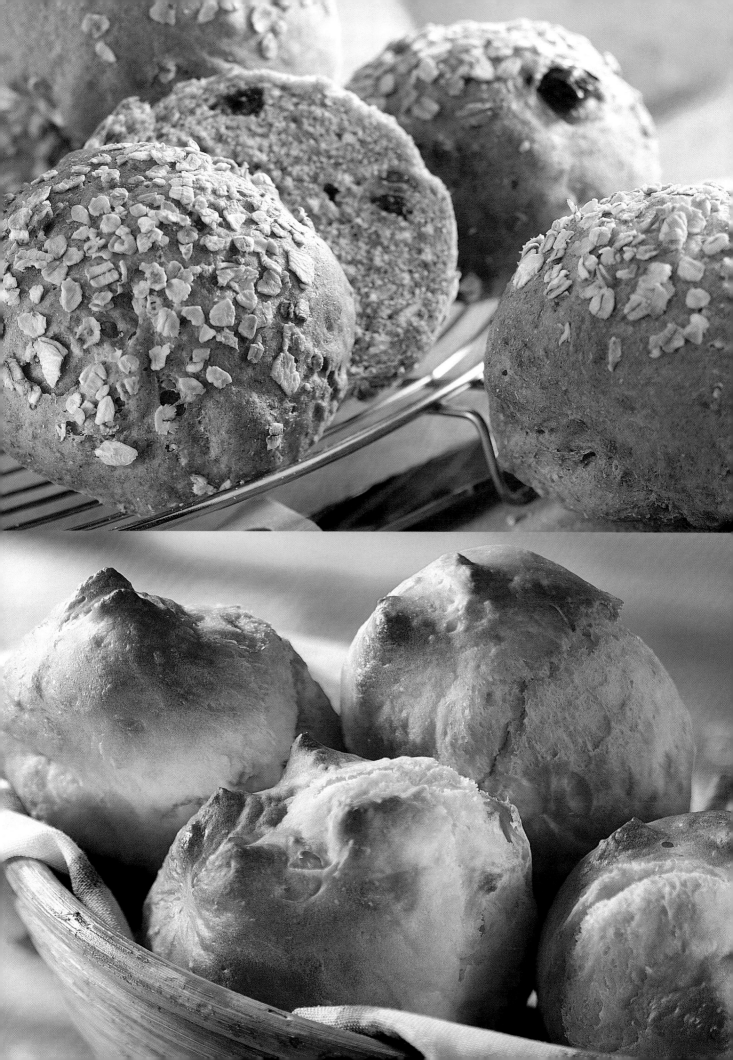

Pumpkin-Seed Rings

Carbohydrates ●●◖	1 hr.
Fat ●●	(+ 30 min.
resting) (+20 to 30 min. baking)	

Per serving: approx. 213 calories
9 g protein · 8 g fat · 26 g carbohydrates

FOR 6 SMALL RINGS:
2 cups (500 mL/250 g) coarsely
   ground whole wheat flour
1/2 tsp (2 mL) salt
1 (1/4 oz/7 g/2 1/4 tsp) envelope
   active dry yeast
1/2 cup (125 mL) lukewarm water
1 tsp (5 mL) sugar
1 1/2 tbsp (22 mL/20 g) melted
   cooled butter
2 tbsp (30 mL) milk
2 tbsp (30 mL) pumpkin seeds
2 tbsp (30 mL) sunflower seeds

1 Sift the flour into a bowl and sprinkle with salt. Dissolve sugar in water and sprinkle in yeast. Let stand for 10 minutes, or until frothy. Stir into the flour with the butter. Oil your hands, knead the dough and leave to rise, covered, in a warm place for 30 minutes.

2 Preheat the oven to 350°F (180°C). Knead the dough again and divide into 6 pieces. Oil your hands and roll each piece of dough into a thin rope 12 to 14 inches (30 to 35 cm) long. Shape into rings and press the ends together. Briefly dip the rings into a bowl of warm water, drain slightly, then arrange on a baking sheet lined with parchment paper. Brush with milk. Sprinkle with the pumpkin and sunflower seeds, and press lightly into the dough. Leave to rest, covered, for 10 minutes. Bake for 20 to 30 minutes, until light brown.

Spelt–Walnut Bread

Carbohydrates ●◖	30 min.
Fat —	(+ 50 min.
resting) (+ 40 min. baking)	

Per serving: approx. 114 calories
4 g protein · 3 g fat · 17 g carbohydrates

FOR 1 LOAF:
2 tsp (10 mL) sugar
1 1/2 cups (375 mL) lukewarm water
4 cups (1 L/500 g) spelt flour
2 (1/4 oz/7 g/2 1/4 tsp) envelopes
   active dry yeast
2 tsp (10 mL) salt
1 tsp (5 mL) ground cardamom
1/2 cup (125 mL/60 g) chopped
   walnuts
2 tbsp (30 mL) walnut oil
Flour

1 Dissolve sugar in water, sprinkle yeast over and let stand for 10 minutes, or until frothy. Put the flour in another bowl, make a well in the center and pour in the yeast mixture. Stir in the salt, cardamom, walnuts and oil, adding water as needed if dough is too stiff. Knead until smooth and elastic. Let stand in a warm place, covered, for 30 minutes.

2 Oil a 10- x 6-inch (25 x 15 cm) loaf pan. Knead the dough once more on a floured work surface, shape into a loaf and place in the pan. Leave to rise for 20 minutes.

3 Preheat the oven to 350°C (180°F). Place a pan of hot water in the bottom of the oven. Lightly brush or spray the bread with water and bake for 40 minutes.

Ciabatta with Thyme

Carbohydrates ●●●	40 min.
Fat —	(+ 1 hr. 15 min.
resting) (+ 45 min. baking)	

Per serving: approx. 163 calories
5 g protein · 3 g fat · 28 g carbohydrates

FOR 1 LARGE ROUND LOAF
OR 12 SMALL ROLLS:
3 1/3 cups (825 mL/400 g) coarsely
   ground whole wheat flour
1 cup (250 mL/100g) light rye flour
Salt
2 tbsp (30 mL) olive oil, divided
2 tsp (10 mL) sugar
1 1/4 cups (300 mL) lukewarm water
2 (1/4 oz/7 g/2 1/4 tsp) envelopes
   active dry yeast
2 tbsp (30 mL) dried thyme, divided

1 Sift both types of flour into a large bowl. Sprinkle with 1/2 tsp (2 mL) salt and add 1 tbsp (15 mL) of the oil. In a small bowl, dissolve the sugar in the water, sprinkle the yeast over and let stand for 10 minutes, or until frothy. Slowly stir into the flour, then knead. Cover and leave the dough to rise in a warm place for 45 minutes.

2 Cover a baking sheet with parchment paper and sprinkle 1 tbsp (15 mL) of the thyme in the center. Knead the dough again, shape into a thick, round loaf or 12 small rolls and place on the baking sheet. Combine the remaining 1 tbsp (15 mL) oil and thyme and 2 pinches of salt and brush generously on the dough. Leave to rise for 30 minutes.

3 Preheat the oven to 350°F (180°C). Bake for 15 minutes. Reduce the heat to 325°F (160°C) and bake for a further 30 minutes.

Pumpkin-Seed Rings, top
Spelt–Walnut Bread, bottom left
Ciabatta with Thyme, bottom right

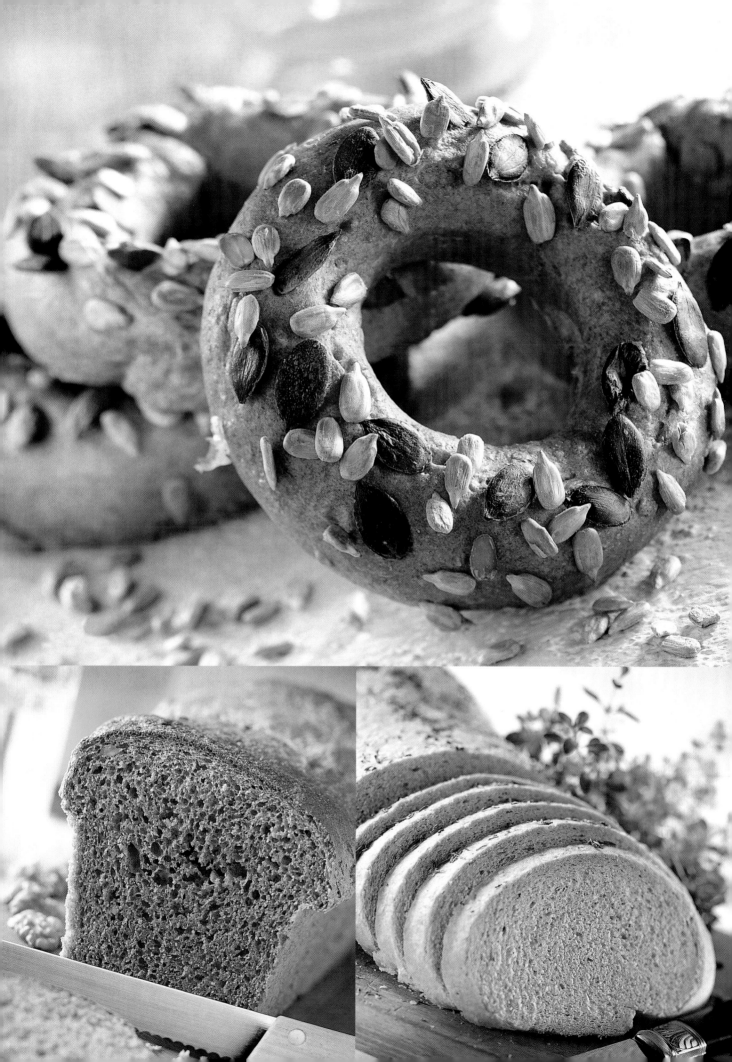

Ham Crescents

Carbohydrates ●◖	45 min.
Fat ●	(+ 30 min. resting)
	(+ 15 min. baking)

Per serving: approx. 117 calories
6 g protein · 4 g fat · 14 g carbohydrates

FOR 12 CRESCENTS:
FOR THE PASTRY:
1 mealy (floury) potato, cooked the previous day
1²/₃ cup (400 mL/200 g) coarsely ground whole wheat
   flour
²/₃ cup (150 mL/150 g) low-fat quark or puréed cottage
   cheese
2 tbsp (30 mL/30 g) soft margarine
1 small egg
Pinch nutmeg
Salt
FOR THE FILLING:
1 bunch green (spring) onions
2 oz (60 g) lean smoked ham
2 tbsp (30 mL/30 g) margarine
1 tbsp (15 ml) flour
2 tbsp (30 mL/30 g) sour cream
2 to 3 tbsp (30 to 45 ml) water
1 tbsp (15 mL) chopped fresh parsley
1 tsp (5 mL) chopped fresh marjoram, or ½ tsp (2 mL) dried
Freshly ground pepper
½ cup (50 mL) milk
Pinch turmeric
1 to 2 tbsp (15 to 30 mL) caraway seeds

1 Peel the potato and press through a ricer or grate finely. Combine with the flour, quark, margarine, egg, nutmeg and salt. Knead until smooth. Cover and leave in a cool place to rest for at least 30 minutes.

2 Slice the green onions and finely dice the ham. Slightly heat the margarine, stir in the green onions and ham, and brown on medium heat for 1 to 2 minutes. Sprinkle with the flour and cook 1 minute more. Remove from heat, stir in the sour cream, water, parsley, marjoram and a little pepper. Set aside.

3 Thoroughly knead the dough. Roll out to form a 12- x 16-inch (30 x 40 cm) rectangle and cut 12 squares. Place a little of the ham mixture in the center of each. Starting in one corner, roll up and turn the outer ends to form a crescent. Place seam side down on a baking sheet covered with parchment paper.

5 Preheat the oven to 400°F (200°C). Whisk the milk and turmeric, brush on the crescents and sprinkle with caraway. Bake for 15 minutes, or until golden.

Black Olive and Sun-Dried Tomato Loaves

Carbohydrates ●◖	30 min.
Fat –	(+ 1 hr. resting)
	(+ 35 min. baking)

Per serving: approx. 124 calories
4 g protein · 3 g fat · 19 g carbohydrates

FOR 2 LOAVES:
3¹/₃ cups (825 mL/400 g) coarsely ground whole wheat
   flour
1²/₃ cups (400 mL/200 g) freshly ground amaranth
   (health-food stores)
1 tsp (5 mL) dried oregano
1 tsp (5 mL) sugar
1½ cups (375 mL) lukewarm water
1 (¼ oz/7 g/2¼ tsp) envelope active dry yeast
3 tbsp (45 mL) olive oil, divided
¾ cup (175 mL/100 g) pitted black olives
2 oz (60 g) sun-dried tomatoes in oil

1 Sift the flour and amaranth together and stir in the oregano. In a large bowl, dissolve sugar in water, sprinkle yeast on top and let stand for 10 minutes, or until frothy. Gradually add the flour and 2 tbsp (30 mL) of the oil, adding water as needed if dough is too dry. Knead until smooth and elastic. Cover and leave in a warm place to rise for 30 minutes.

2 Chop the olives and sun-dried tomatoes and knead into the dough. Divide in 2 pieces and shape into oval loaves. Place on a baking sheet covered with parchment paper. Leave to rise, covered, for 30 minutes.

3 Preheat the oven to 350°F (180°C). Brush the loaves with the remaining 1 tbsp (15 mL) of olive oil and score the top. Bake for 35 minutes. Cool on a cake rack.

 TIP: If the dough remains sticky after rising, add a little wheat germ and knead, then leave to rest for another 5 to 10 minutes. Wheat germ soaks up a lot of liquid, so don't add a lot—it can make the dough dry.

TIP: This bread tastes heavenly served with quark, cheese, ham or nothing at all. It can also be frozen.

180

Ham Crescents, top
Black Olive and Sun-Dried Tomato Loaves, bottom

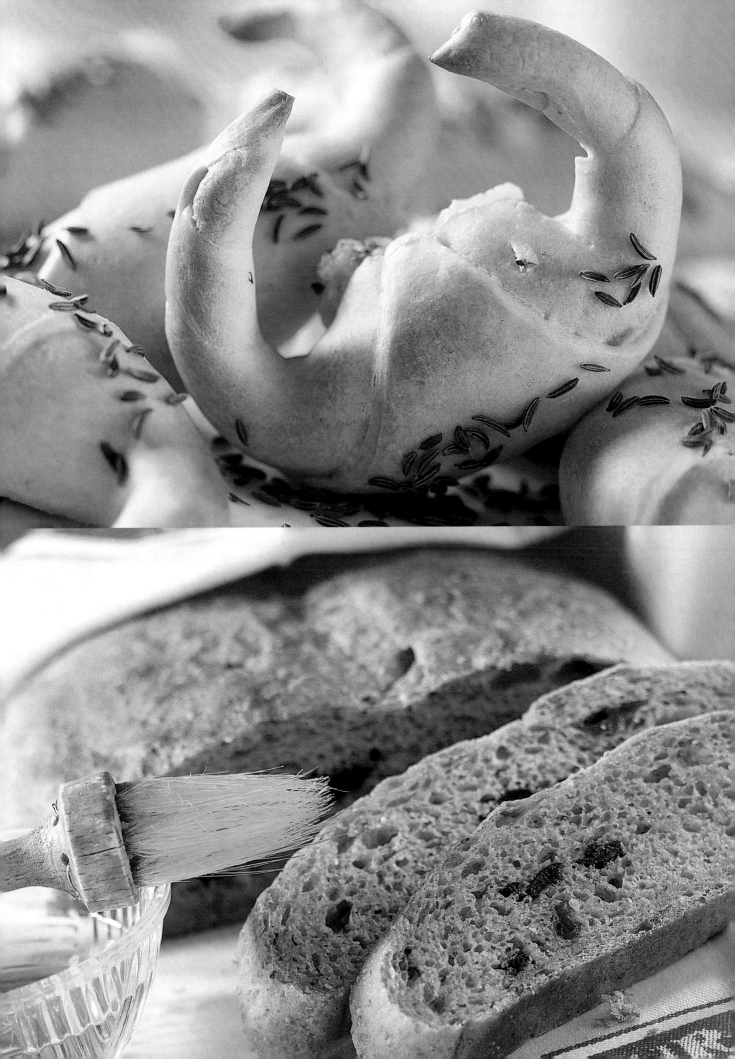

Caraway Bread Sticks

Carbohydrates ●●◖	1 hr.
Fat –	(+ 40 min. resting)
	(+ 20 to 25 min. baking)

Per serving: approx. 165 calories
6 g protein · 2 g fat · 29 g carbohydrates

FOR 6 STICKS:
1²⁄₃ cups (400 mL/200 g) coarsely ground whole wheat flour
½ cup (125 mL/50 g) rye flour
½ tsp (2 mL) salt
Pinch freshly ground pepper
1 (¼ oz/7 g/2¼ tsp) envelope active dry yeast
½ cup (125 mL) lukewarm low-fat milk
Caraway seeds
1 egg yolk

1 Sift both types of flour with salt and pepper. Sprinkle yeast over the milk and let stand for 10 minutes, or until frothy. Gradually stir into the flour. Knead the dough for at least 5 minutes, then leave to rise in a warm place, covered, for 40 minutes.

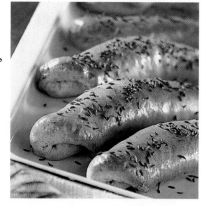

2 Thoroughly knead the dough again. Form into a rope, divide into 6 pieces and shape into balls. Roll the balls into 2- x 5-inch (5 x 12 cm) rectangles, sprinkle lightly with caraway seeds and shape into sticks. Place on a baking sheet covered with parchment paper.

3 Preheat the oven to 350°F (180°C). Whisk the egg yolk with 1 tbsp (15 mL) water, brush the sticks and sprinkle with more caraway seeds. Bake for 20 to 25 minutes.

TIP: Garnish with sesame seeds or grated Emmenthal cheese before baking.

Savory Galette

Carbohydrates ●●●	50 min.
Fat +	(+ 40 min. resting)
	(+ 30 min. baking)

Per serving: approx. 380 calories
21 g protein · 18 g fat · 33 g carbohydrates

FOR 6 TO 8 SERVINGS:
FOR THE CRUST:
1²⁄₃ cups (400 mL/200 g) coarsely ground whole wheat flour
Salt
1 (¼ oz/7 g/2¼ tsp) envelope active dry yeast
½ cup (125 mL) lukewarm milk
FOR THE TOPPING:
3½ oz (100 g) rindless cooked ham
1 tbsp (15 mL) olive oil
2 green (spring) onions
1 clove garlic
5 cups (1.25 L) sliced Savoy or Chinese (Napa) cabbage
2 tomatoes
Freshly ground pepper
Freshly grated nutmeg
4 sprigs fresh basil
2 tbsp (30 mL/30 g) sour cream
½ cup (125 mL/60 g) grated provolone or Gouda cheese

1 Sift the flour into a large bowl and add a little salt. Sprinkle the yeast over the milk and let stand 10 minutes, or until frothy. Gradually stir into the flour. Knead until smooth. Cover and leave the dough to rise in a warm place for 30 minutes.

2 Cut the ham into ¾-inch (2 cm) strips. Slice the green onions and chop the garlic. Heat the oil, stir in onions and garlic, and gently sauté until translucent. Score, blanch, peel and dice the tomatoes and stir in. Stir in the cabbage and season with salt. Cook, uncovered, for 5 minutes, until most of the liquid has evaporated. Grate in pepper and nutmeg. Chop the basil and stir in with the sour cream.

3 Preheat the oven to 350°F (180°C). Oil a 10-inch (25 cm) springform pan. Knead the dough, roll out and place in the pan to cover the bottom and a bit up the sides. Fill with the topping and sprinkle with cheese. Leave to rise for 10 minutes, then bake for 30 minutes.

Savory Galette, right

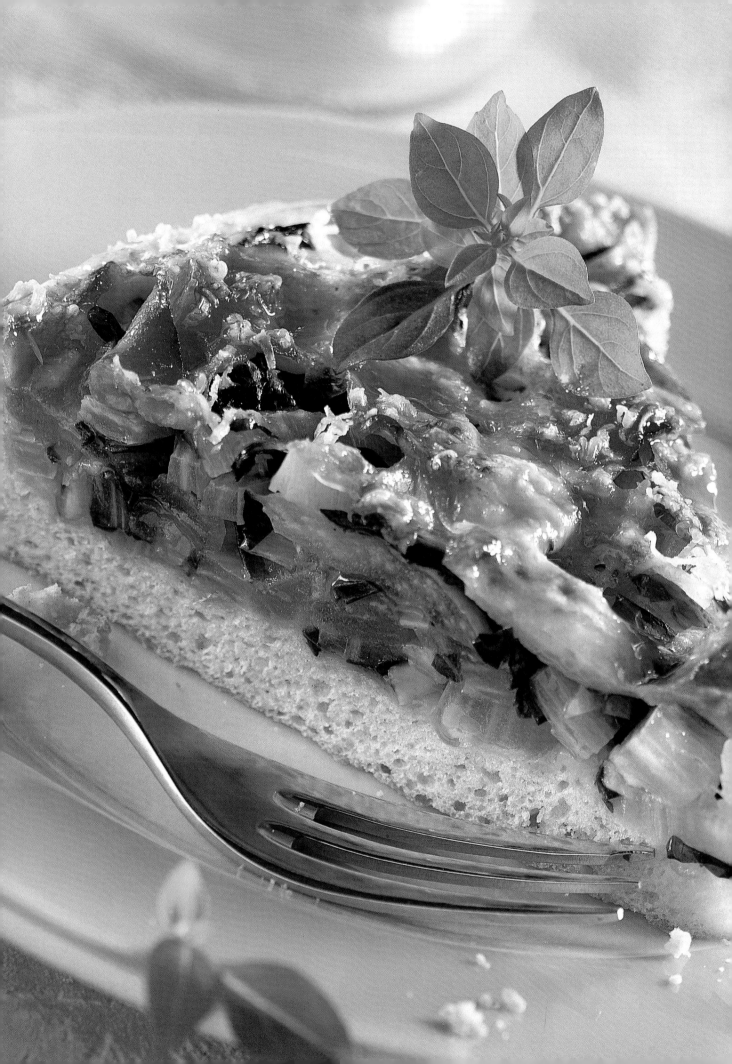

Leek Turnovers

Carbohydrates ●●	1 hr.
Fat ●●●	(+ 30 min. resting)
	(+ 20 min. baking)

Per serving: approx. 247 calories
11 g protein · 12 g fat · 24 g carbohydrates

FOR 8 TURNOVERS:
FOR THE PASTRY:
2 cups (500 mL/250 g) coarsely ground whole wheat
    flour
1 tsp (5 mL) salt
½ tsp (2 mL) dried oregano
1 egg yolk
3 tbsp (45 mL) olive oil
½ cup (125 ml) water
FOR THE FILLING:
2 leeks
2 oz (60 g) turkey salami
2½ oz (75 g) low-fat cheese
2 tsp (10 mL) dried oregano
3 tbsp (45 mL) whole sunflower seeds
Salt and freshly ground pepper
2 tbsp (30 mL) milk
1 egg white
¼ tsp (1 mL) turmeric
3 tbsp (45 mL) chopped sunflower seeds

1 Combine flour, salt, ½ tsp (2 mL) oregano, egg yolk, oil and water. Knead until smooth. Wrap in plastic wrap and refrigerate for 30 minutes.

2 Slice the leek lengthwise, wash thoroughly and slice into strips. Place in saucepan, cover with a little water and cook on medium heat for 5 minutes. Drain. Finely dice the salami and cheese. Combine with the leeks, oregano, whole sunflower seeds, salt and pepper.

3 Thoroughly knead the dough again and divide into 8 pieces. Roll each piece out into a 6-inch (15 cm) circle and put some of the leek mixture in the center. Brush the edges with egg white, fold over to form semicircles, and press edges together with a fork to seal. Arrange on a baking sheet lined with parchment paper.

4 Preheat oven to 400°F (200°C). Whisk together milk and turmeric and brush on the turnovers. Sprinkle with chopped sunflower seeds. Bake for 20 minutes, until golden.

Spelt Brioches

Carbohydrates ●●●●◖	20 min.
Fat ●●●	(+ 1 hr. 5 min. resting)
	(+ 20 min. baking)

Per serving: approx. 216 calories
7 g protein · 10 g fat · 51 g carbohydrates

FOR 2 BRIOCHES:
1¼ cups (300 mL/160 g) spelt flour
½ tsp (2 mL) salt
1 tsp (5 mL) sugar
7 tbsp (100 ml) lukewarm water
1 (¼ oz/7 g/2¼ tsp) envelope active dry yeast
1 tbsp (15 mL) olive oil
½ tsp (2 mL/2 g) butter
Flour

1 Combine flour and salt in a large bowl. Dissolve the sugar in the water and sprinkle yeast over. Let stand 10 minutes, or until frothy. Make a well in the flour and pour yeast mixture into the center. Pour the oil around the edge of the flour. Knead the dough from the center, then shape into a ball. Cover and leave to rise for 45 minutes, until doubled in size.

2 Grease two 1-cup (250ml) brioche molds or four ½-cup (125 mL) ramekins with the butter. Using floured hands, knead the dough again and divide in half or quarters. Divide each piece into 2 balls, one larger than the other. Place the large balls in the molds. Make an indentation in the center of each with your fingertips and set a smaller ball on top. Cover and leave to rise for 20 minutes.

3 Preheat the oven to 350°F (180°C). Bake for 20 minutes, until golden. Turn the brioches out on a wire rack and cool.

 TIPS: These brioches are excellent with Spinach Gratin (see recipe on page 80).

Leek Turnovers, top
Spelt Brioches, bottom

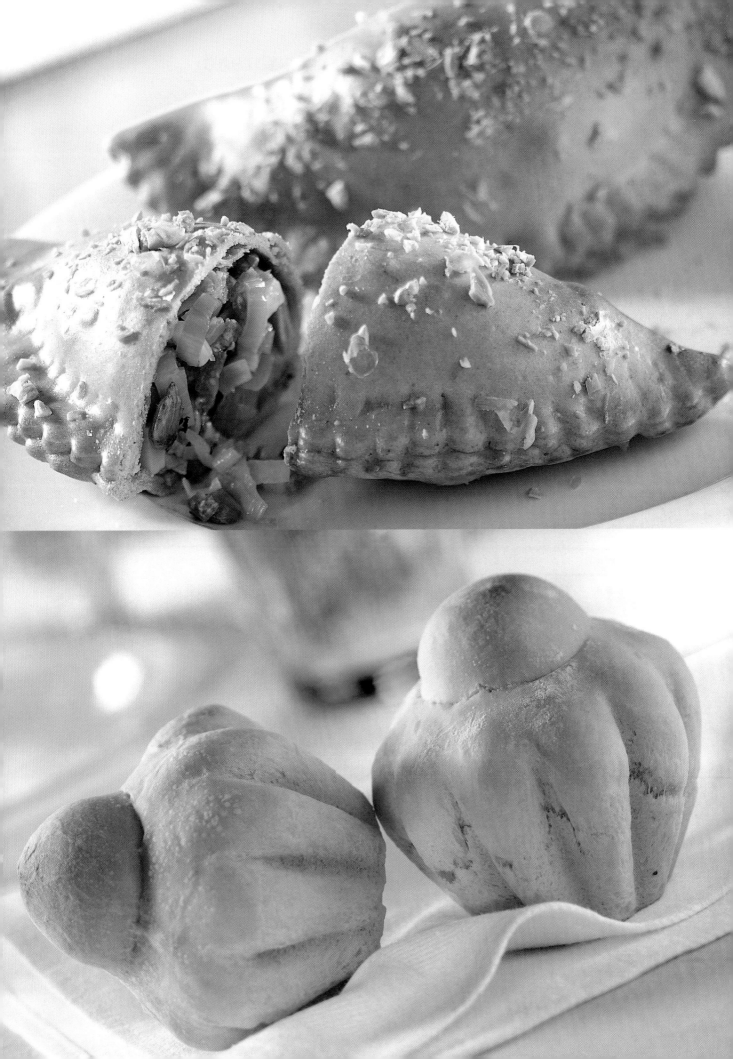

Spinach–Feta Tarts

Carbohydrates ●●●◖	45 min.
Fat ●●●	(+ 20 min. baking)

Per serving: approx. 341 calories
17 g protein · 13 g fat · 40 g carbohydrates

FOR 4 TARTS:
FOR THE PASTRY:
1²⁄₃ cups (400 mL/200 g) whole wheat flour
½ tsp (2 mL) baking powder
Salt
½ cup (125 mL/100 g) low-fat quark or puréed cottage
 cheese
3 to 4 tbsp (45 to 60 mL) milk
FOR THE FILLING:
2 tbsp (30 mL) olive oil
1 small onion
10 oz (300 g) spinach
1 clove garlic
Salt and freshly ground pepper
Pinch ground allspice
½ tsp (2 mL) sweet paprika
1 egg
2 tbsp (30 mL) chopped fresh parsley
¾ cup (175 mL/100 g) halved cherry tomatoes
¾ cup (175 mL/100 g) crumbled feta

1 Oil four 5-inch (12 cm) tart molds. Combine
 flour, baking powder, a little salt, quark and
milk. Knead into a smooth dough. Divide into 4
pieces and roll out. Place in molds to cover bottom
and sides.

2 Chop the onion, garlic and spinach. Heat the oil,
 stir in the onion and garlic, and sauté until
translucent. Stir in spinach and cook on high heat
until the liquid evaporates. Season with salt, pepper, allspice and paprika. Leave to cool.

3 Preheat the oven to 350°F (180°C). Whisk
 together egg and parsley, combine with the
spinach, and fill the tarts with this mixture.
Arrange the cherry tomatoes on top, cut side down,
and sprinkle feta over all. Bake for 20 minutes.

 TIP: If you're using frozen spinach, a 10-oz
(300 g) package is a good size. Stir in with
the browned onion and garlic and thaw,
covered, then take off the cover and let the liquid
evaporate.

Crispbread Pizzas

Carbohydrates ●●◖	25 min.
Fat +++	(+ 15 min. baking)

Per serving: approx. 522 calories
29 g protein · 33 g fat · 27 g carbohydrates

FOR 2 SERVINGS:
6 rye crispbreads, such as Ryvita
2 tbsp (30 mL/30 g) sour cream
1½ oz (40 g) paper-thin rindless prosciutto
2 tbsp (30 mL) olive oil, divided
2 small onions
1 clove garlic
2 tbsp (30 mL) dry white wine
Salt and freshly ground pepper
¼ cup (50 mL/30 g) freshly grated Parmesan cheese
1¼ cups (300 mL/150 g) grated mozzarella cheese
10 cherry tomatoes
1 tsp (5 mL) dried oregano

1 Preheat the oven to 350°F (180°C). Arrange the
 crispbreads on a baking sheet and spread with
sour cream. Arrange the prosciutto on top.

2 Thinly slice the onion and chop the garlic. Heat
 1 tbsp (15 mL) of the oil. Stir in the onions and
garlic, and gently sauté on low heat until translucent. Stir in the wine and cook for 2 minutes. Add
salt and pepper, stir in the Parmesan, and spread on
the crispbreads. Sprinkle mozzarella on top.

3 Halve the tomatoes and arrange, cut side up, on
 the mozzarella. Sprinkle with salt, pepper,
oregano and the remaining 1 tbsp (15 mL) oil. Bake
for 15 minutes.

 TIP: Slice a fennel bulb very finely, cook
with the onion and garlic, and arrange on
the crispbreads with the other ingredients.

SAVORY BAKED GOODS, BREADS, ROLLS, CAKES AND PIES

Spinach–Feta Tarts, top
Crispbread Pizzas, bottom

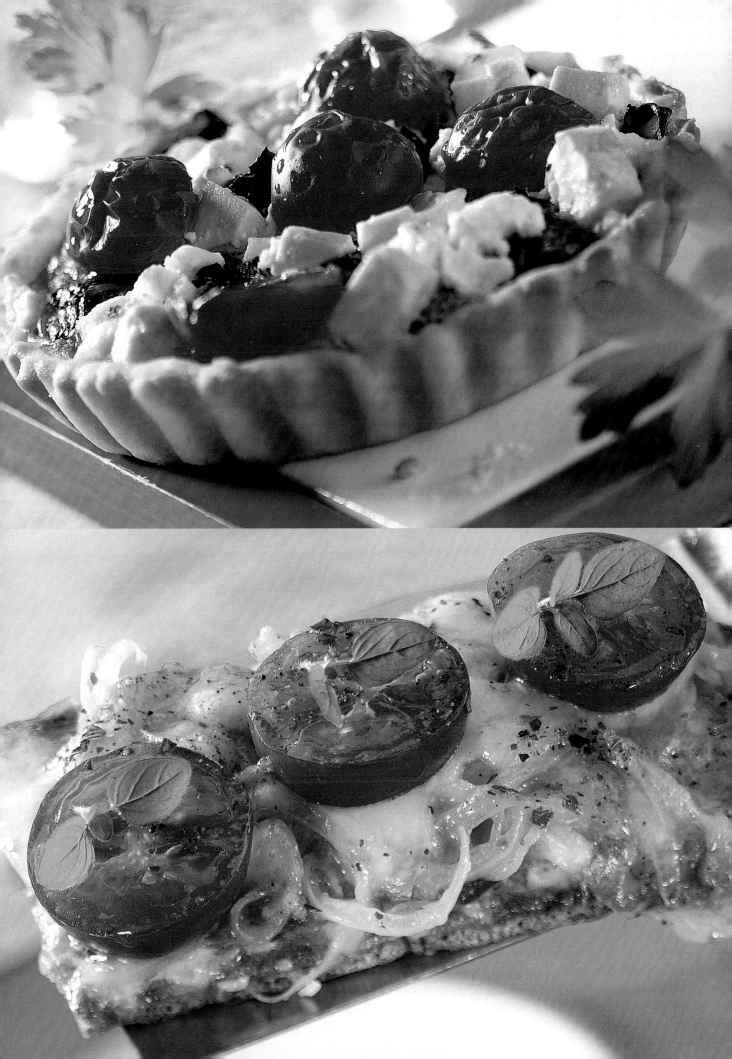

Berry–Buttermilk Tarts

Carbohydrates ●●	1 hr. 15 min.
Fat ●●●	(+ 30 min. resting)
	(+ chilling to set) (+ 15 min. baking)

Per serving: approx. 229 calories
7 g protein · 12 g fat · 22 g carbohydrates

FOR 6 TARTS:
FOR THE PASTRY:
1 cup (250 mL/125 g) coarsely ground whole wheat flour
⅓ cup (75 mL/65 g) cold margarine
1 small egg yolk
1 tbsp (15 mL) icing (confectioner's) sugar
FOR THE FILLING:
1 (¼ oz/7 g/1 tbsp) envelope unflavored gelatin
Zest and juice of ½ lemon
1 cup (250 mL/250 g) buttermilk
Liquid sweetener
Vanilla
FOR THE TOPPING:
½ (¼ oz/7 g/1 tbsp) envelopes unflavored gelatin
½ cup (125 mL) unsweetened berry or apple juice
1½ cups (375 mL/200 g) mixed berries
¼ cup (50 mL/20 g) chopped pistachios

1 Combine flour, margarine, egg yolk and icing sugar. Knead until smooth. Wrap in plastic wrap and refrigerate for 30 minutes.

2 Preheat the oven to 350°F (180°C). Divide the dough into 6 balls of equal size. Roll each into a circle between layers of plastic wrap. Press into a 4-inch (10 cm) tart mold and bake for 15 minutes, until golden. Cool on a wire rack.

3 Pour 1 envelope gelatin over 2 tbsp (30 mL) water and let sit for 1 minute. Combine the lemon zest and juice with the buttermilk and a few dashes of sweetener and vanilla. Add 2 tbsp (30 mL) boiling water to the gelatin and stir to dissolve. Stir into the buttermilk. Carefully remove the pastry from the molds. Wash the molds, rinse in cold water and pour in the buttermilk mixture. Refrigerate immediately and leave until set.

4 Soak ½ envelope gelatin in 2 tbsp (30 mL) cold water. Combine with ½ the fruit juice in a pan and bring to a boil. Add remaining fruit juice. Refrigerate, but don't allow to set completely. Unmold buttermilk jelly and place in the pastry shells. Sprinkle with pistachio nuts and arrange berries on top. Carefully pour on the partly gelled fruit juice. Refrigerate until set.

TIP: These tarts may be best for experienced bakers—this pastry can be tricky to make.

Fruit Tarts

Carbohydrates ●●●●	40 min.
Fat +	(+ 30 min. resting)
	(+ 15 min. baking) (+ 1 hr. 15 min. chilling)

Per serving: approx. 376 calories
7 g protein · 18 g fat · 46 g carbohydrates

FOR 4 TARTS:
FOR THE PASTRY:
1¼ cups (300 mL/150 g) coarsely ground whole wheat flour
3 tbsp (45 mL) unsweetened flaked or shredded coconut
2 tbsp (30 mL) sugar
Pinch salt
2½ tbsp (37 mL/40 g) butter
1 egg yolk
3 to 4 tbsp (45 to 60 mL) milk
FOR THE FILLING:
2 slices fresh or canned pineapple (about 5 oz/150 g)
8 red grapes
1 ripe fig
½ banana
1 small kiwi fruit
1 tangerine
2 tbsp (30 mL/30 g) crème fraîche or sour cream
2 tbsp (30 mL/30 g) low-fat yogurt
1 tsp (5 mL) lemon juice
Liquid sweetener
Finely chopped pistachios (optional)

1 Combine flour, coconut, sugar, salt, butter, egg yolk and milk. Knead thoroughly, wrap in plastic wrap and refrigerate for 30 minutes.

2 Preheat the oven to 350°F (180°C). Oil four 4- to 5-inch (10 to 12 cm) tart molds. Divide the dough into 4 equal pieces, roll into thin circles between layers of plastic wrap and press into the molds. Prick the bottom of the pastry in several places with a fork and cover with parchment paper and pie weights. Bake for 15 minutes. Leave to cool, then remove weights and paper.

3 Peel, chop and slice fruit into attractive small pieces, fill the pastries, and refrigerate for 1 hour.

4 Combine crème fraîche, yogurt, lemon juice and sweetener. Top the tarts with this mixture and garnish with pistachios, if desired.

Berry–Buttermilk Tarts, top
Fruit Tarts, bottom

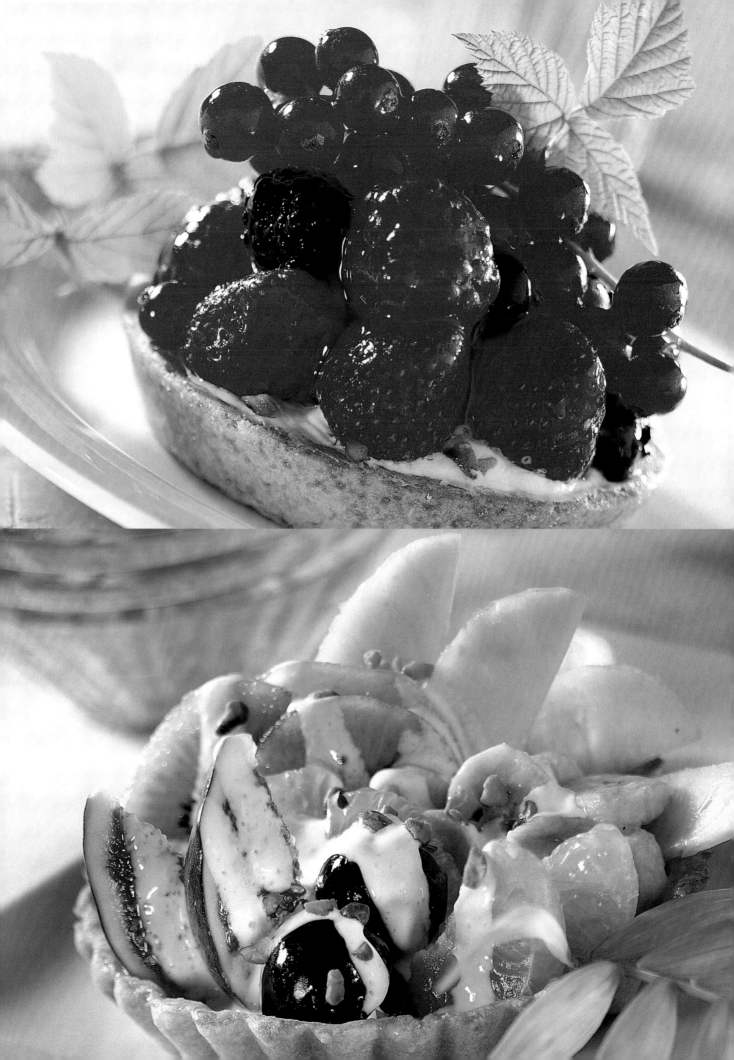

Raisin Scones

Carbohydrates ●●◐	30 min.
Fat ●	(+ 15 min. baking)

Per serving: approx. 163 calories
2 g protein · 5 g fat · 26 g carbohydrates

FOR 10 SCONES:
2 cups (500 mL/250 g) coarsely
   ground whole wheat flour
1 tsp (5 mL) baking powder
1 tbsp (15 mL) sugar
Salt
¼ cup (50 mL/50 g) margarine
½ cup (125 mL) cold low-fat milk
3 tbsp (45 mL/20 g) raisins
Milk for glazing

1 Combine the flour with the baking powder, sugar and a pinch of salt. Lightly mix in the margarine. Create a well in the center of the dough, pour in the milk, and knead lightly. Wash the raisins in hot water, blot dry, chop finely and knead into the dough.

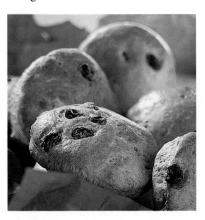

2 Preheat the oven to 325°F (160°C). On a floured surface, roll out the dough to a thickness of ½ inch (1 cm). Cut out 3-inch (8 cm) circles. Arrange on a baking sheet covered with parchment paper and brush with a little milk. Bake for 15 minutes, until golden.

Blueberry Muffins

Carbohydrates ●◐	20 min.
Fat ●	(+ 20 min. baking)

Per serving: approx. 144 calories
4 g protein · 7 g fat · 18 g carbohydrates

FOR 12 MUFFINS:
⅓ cup (75 mL/75 g) margarine
¼ cup (50 mL/50 g) sugar
Liquid sweetener
2 small eggs
½ tsp (2 mL) vanilla
Pinch salt
1¾ cups (425 mL/220 g) coarsely
   ground whole wheat flour
2 tsp (10 mL) baking powder
¾ cup (175 mL/180 g) buttermilk
1¼ cups (300 mL/170 g) blueberries

1 Preheat the oven to 325°F (160°C). Line the cups of a muffin tin with paper cups.

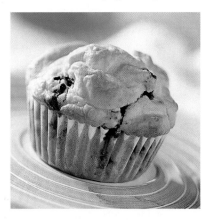

2 Beat margarine and sugar together until fluffy and light. Stir in a few dashes of sweetener, the eggs, vanilla and salt. Combine the flour with baking powder and stir into the batter alternately with the buttermilk. Gently fold blueberries into the batter.

3 Spoon into muffin cups and bake for 20 to 25 minutes.

‼ TIP: You can use frozen blueberries. Thaw and drain before folding them in.

Carrot–Nut Muffins

Carbohydrates ●◐	30 min.
Fat ●	(+ 20 min. baking)

Per serving: approx. 116 calories
3 g protein · 6 g fat · 13 g carbohydrates

FOR 12 MUFFINS:
3 small eggs, separated
2 large carrots
½ cup (125 mL/90 g) sugar
3 tbsp (45 ml) warm water
Pinch ground cloves
Pinch ground cinnamon
1 cup (250 mL/75 g) ground
   hazelnuts
1 tsp (5 mL) baking powder
⅔ cup (150 mL/75 g) coarsely
   ground whole wheat flour

1 Preheat the oven to 325°F (160°C). Place paper cups in a muffin tin. Grate the carrots. Beat egg whites until stiff and refrigerate.

2 Beat the egg yolks, sugar and water until smooth. Stir in the carrots. Combine cloves, cinnamon, nuts, baking powder and flour. Fold into the batter alternately with the beaten egg whites.

3 Spoon immediately into muffin cups. Bake for 20 minutes. Leave to cool in the tin.

‼ TIP: These muffins are particularly moist, and they taste just as good if you cut the sugar to ⅓ cup (75 mL/70 g).

Carrot–Nut Muffins, right

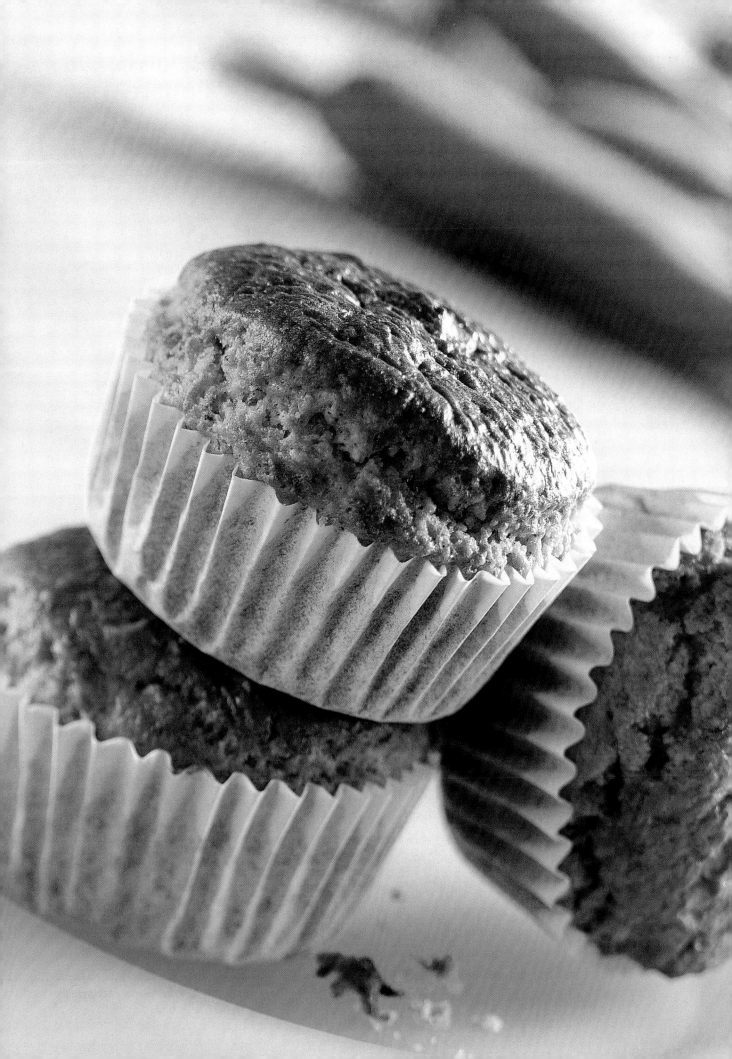

Raspberry Cream Puffs

Carbohydrates ●	40 min.
Fat ●	(+ 30 min. baking)

Per serving: approx. 110 calories
5 g protein · 6 g fat · 9 g carbohydrates

FOR 10 CREAM PUFFS:
FOR THE FILLING:
1 tsp unflavored gelatin (⅓ of a ¼ oz/7 g/1 tbsp envelope)
1¼ cups (300 mL/150 g) raspberries
½ cup (125 mL/100 g) low-fat quark or puréed cottage cheese
FOR THE CHOUX PASTRY:
1 cup (250 mL) water
¼ cup (50 mL/50 g) butter
1 tsp (5 mL) sugar
Pinch salt
1 cup (250 mL/150 g) flour
3 eggs
1 tsp (5 mL) baking powder

1 Soak the gelatin in 1 tbsp (15 mL) cold water for 10 minutes. Combine the raspberries and quark. Heat the gelatin in a small saucepan and dissolve. Add a little of the raspberry mixture to the gelatin, then quickly stir the gelatin into the raspberries. Refrigerate.

2 Preheat the oven to 350°F (180°C). Combine the water, butter, sugar and salt, and bring to a boil. Remove from heat, stir in flour, and beat until smooth. Heat again quickly, stirring constantly, then pour into a bowl. Gradually beat in baking powder and eggs, one at a time, until the batter is shiny and forms long, stiff peaks.

3 Put the batter in a pastry bag with a large nozzle and pipe 10 small mounds of dough onto a baking sheet lined with parchment paper. Bake for 30 minutes, until golden. Remove from the oven, cut in half and leave to cool. Fill the lower halves with the raspberry mixture and top with the upper halves.

Quark–Apple Turnovers

Carbohydrates ●●●	45 min.
Fat ●●●	(+ 20 min. resting) (+ 25 min. baking)

Per serving: approx. 248 calories
6 g protein · 10 g fat · 32 g carbohydrates

FOR 6 TURNOVERS:
FOR THE PASTRY:
⅓ cup (75 mL/60 g) low-fat quark or puréed cottage cheese
2½ tbsp (37 mL) oil
2 tbsp (30 mL) milk
2 tbsp (30 mL) sugar
1 egg yolk
1 cup (250 mL/100 g) pastry flour
½ tsp (2 mL) baking powder
FOR THE FILLING:
3 tbsp (45 mL/30 g) raisins
1 tbsp (15 mL) each rum and water
2 tart apples
1½ tsp (7 mL/10 g) butter
1 small piece of lemon zest
1 tsp (5 mL) honey
8 drops liquid sweetener
¼ tsp (1 mL) ground cinnamon
2 tbsp (30 mL) ground hazelnuts
2 tbsp (30 mL) fine dry bread crumbs
1 egg, separated

1 Combine quark, oil, milk, sugar, egg yolk, flour and baking powder. Knead until smooth. Shape into a rope and let rest, covered, for 20 minutes.

2 Soak the raisins in the rum and water. Peel and core the apples. Combine apples, butter, lemon zest and raisin–rum mixture and cook for 5 minutes. Leave to cool, then remove the lemon zest. Stir in all remaining ingredients except the egg.

3 Preheat the oven to 350°F (180°C). Roll the dough into six 5-inch (2 cm) circles. Spoon a little filling into the center of each. Brush the edges with egg white. Fold and pinch together with a fork. Arrange on a baking sheet lined with parchment paper and brush with egg yolk. Bake for 25 minutes.

Apple–Raisin Turnovers

Carbohydrates ●◀	40 min.
Fat ●	(+ 1 hr. resting) (+ 25 min. baking)

Per serving: approx. 134 calories
4 g protein · 5 g fat · 19 g carbohydrates

FOR 12 TURNOVERS:
FOR THE PASTRY:
1⅔ cups (400 mL/200 g) coarsely ground whole wheat flour
1 (¼ oz/7 g/2¼ tsp) envelope active dry yeast
1 tsp (5 mL) sugar
½ cup (125 mL) lukewarm milk
¼ cup (50 mL/60 g) soft margarine
Pinch salt
FOR THE FILLING:
½ cup (125 mL/125 g) low-fat quark or puréed cottage cheese
Liquid sweetener
¼ tsp (1 mL) ground cinnamon
⅓ cup (75 mL/50 g) raisins
2 large apples
2 tbsp (30 mL) lemon juice

1 Sift the flour into a large bowl and make a well in the center. Dissolve sugar in a little of the milk and sprinkle in yeast. Let stand until frothy. Combine with remaining pastry ingredients. Knead until smooth. Cover and let rise for 40 minutes.

2 Combine quark, a little sweetener and cinnamon. Stir in the raisins. Peel, core and finely dice the apples, sprinkle with lemon juice, and stir in.

3 Knead and form the dough into 12 balls. Roll into 5-inch (12 cm) circles. Spoon in a little of the apple–quark mixture, fold over and press down the edges.

4 Preheat the oven to 350°F (180°C). Arrange the turnovers on a baking sheet lined with parchment paper, cover and rise for 10 minutes. Bake for 20 to 25 minutes, until golden.

Raspberry Cream Puffs, top right
Quark–Apple Turnovers, bottom left
Apple–Raisin Turnovers, bottom right

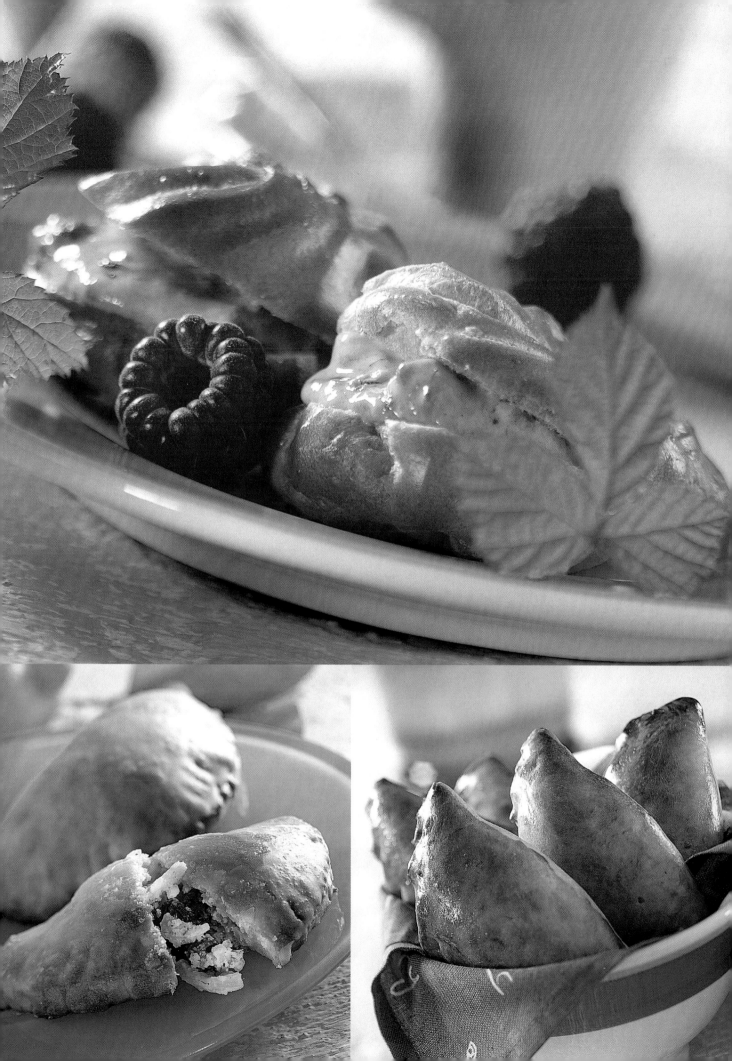

Strawberry–Cream Cheese Waffles

Carbohydrates ●●◕		45 min.
Fat ++		(+ 15 min. baking)

Per serving: approx. 374 calories
12 g protein · 22 g fat · 31 g carbohydrates

FOR 4 LARGE WAFFLES:
1½ cups (375 mL/250 g) strawberries
¾ cup (175 mL/200 g) low-fat cream cheese
Sweetener
½ cup (125 mL/100 g) whipping (35%) cream
2 tbsp (30 mL/30 g) soft butter
2 tbsp (30 mL) sugar
Pinch salt
1 egg, separated
1 tsp (5 mL) rum
1 tsp (5 mL) grated lemon zest
1 cup (250 mL/100 g) pastry flour
Pinch baking powder

1 Quarter and set aside a few strawberries and purée the rest. Mix the purée with cream cheese and stir in a little sweetener. Beat whipping cream until stiff, fold into the strawberry mixture and refrigerate.

2 Combine butter, sugar, salt, egg yolk, rum and lemon zest. Combine the flour and baking powder, sift into the butter and sugar mixture, and mix well. Beat the egg white until stiff and fold into the batter.

3 Heat a waffle iron and bake 4 large waffles. Leave to cool. (Don't stack the waffles—they'll get soft.) Spoon on the strawberry mixture and garnish with remaining strawberries.

Phyllo Fruit Baskets

Carbohydrates ●●●		35 min.
Fat ++		(+ 3 to 4 min. baking)

Per serving: approx. 398 calories
5 g protein · 27 g fat · 34 g carbohydrates

FOR 4 BASKETS:
FOR THE PASTRY CUPS:
3 sheets phyllo
1½ tbsp (22 mL/20 g) melted butter
FOR THE FILLING:
1 nectarine
1 pear
¾ cup (175 mL/100 g) raspberries
¼ cup (50 mL/50 g) mascarpone cheese
Seeds of ¼ vanilla bean
Liquid sweetener
3 tbsp (45 mL) milk
Mint leaves

1 Preheat the oven to 325°F (160°C). Butter four 4- to 5-inch (10 to 12 cm) molds. Stack the sheets of phyllo and cut into 4 squares. Brush the top layer of each with melted butter, place in the molds and press down. Trim the overhanging pastry with kitchen shears. Bake for 3 to 4 minutes, until golden. Leave to cool slightly, then carefully turn out of the molds.

2 Peel, core and dice the nectarine and pear, and combine with the raspberries. Mix together mascarpone, vanilla seeds, sweetener and milk, then combine with the fruit. Fill the baskets with the fruit mixture just before serving and garnish with mint.

Strawberry Cream–Cheese Waffles, top
Phyllo Fruit Baskets, bottom

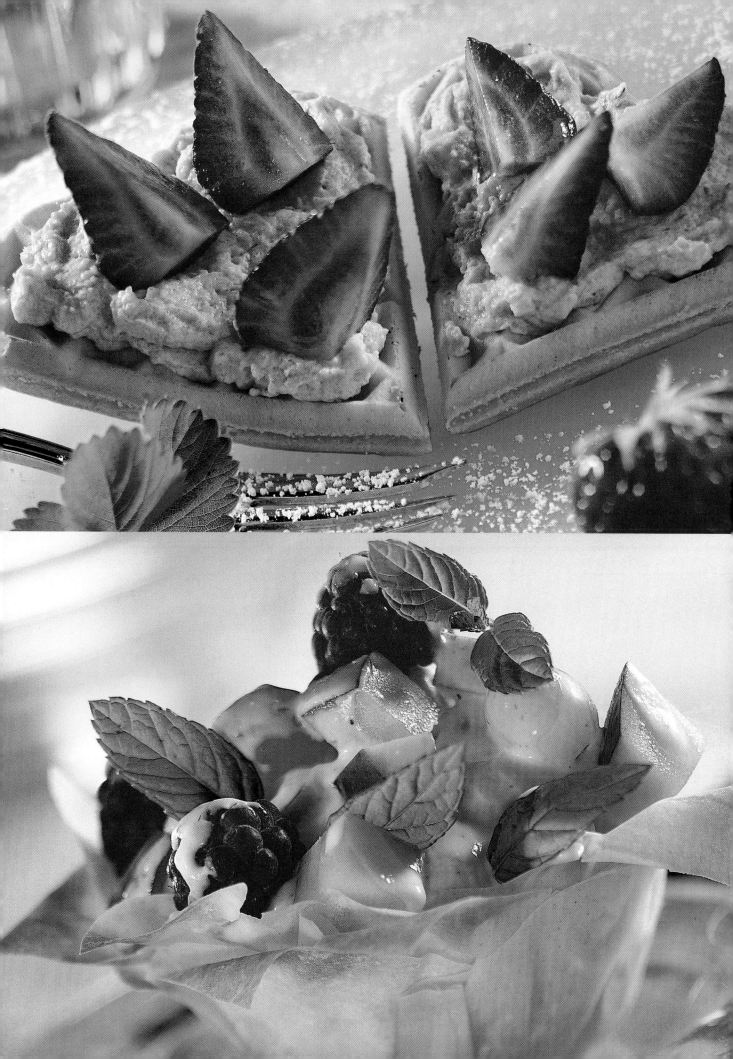

Clafoutis

| Carbohydrates ●◖ | 15 min. |
| Fat ●● | (+ 30 to 35 min. baking) |

Per serving: approx. 182 calories
10 g protein · 8 g fat · 17 g carbohydrates

FOR 4 CLAFOUTIS:
2¾ cups (675 mL/400 g) blueberries
4 eggs
1 tbsp (15 mL) icing (confectioner's) sugar
Seeds of ½ vanilla bean
Pinch salt
½ cup (125 mL) milk
⅓ cup (75 mL/40 g) pastry flour

1 Preheat the oven to 400°F (200°C). Oil four 5-inch (13 cm) ovenproof dishes or molds and arrange the blueberries in the bottom.

2 Beat the eggs with the icing sugar, vanilla seeds and salt until frothy. Stir in the milk, sift the flour on top and combine. Spoon the batter into the dishes. Bake for 30 to 35 minutes and serve warm.

TIP: You can prepare this baked pudding with other berries or cherries. If you're using frozen berries, fold them into the batter unthawed.

Mini-Panettones

Carbohydrates ●●●●	45 min.
Fat ●●●	(+ 50 min. resting)
	(+ 20 to 30 min. baking)

Per serving: approx. 339 calories
9 g protein · 12 g fat · 49 g carbohydrates

FOR 6 SMALL PANETTONES:
2½ cups (625 mL/300 g) pastry flour
2 tbsp (30 mL) sugar, divided
1 (¼ oz/7 g/2¼ tsp) envelope active dry yeast
½ cup (125 mL) lukewarm milk
¼ cup (50 mL/50 g) melted cooled butter
2 medium eggs
Freshly grated nutmeg
Pinch salt
Grated zest of 1 lemon (organic preferred)
¼ cup (50 mL/30 g) currants

1 In a large bowl, dissolve 1 tsp (5 mL) of the sugar with the milk and sprinkle in the yeast. Let stand for 10 minutes, or until frothy. Stir in the flour and remaining sugar until smooth. Whisk together the butter, eggs, a pinch of nutmeg and salt and the lemon zest, and mix into the flour. Add currants and knead. Leave to rise, covered, in a warm place for 30 minutes.

2 Thoroughly knead the dough again. On a floured work surface, stretch dough to form a flat patty. Oil 6 small molds, 4 to 5 inches (10 to 12 cm) tall. Shape the dough into 6 balls and place in the molds. Leave to rise, covered, for 20 minutes.

3 Preheat the oven to 325°F (160°C). Bake for 20 to 30 minutes, until puffed and golden on top. Leave to cool slightly, then turn out of the molds. Panettones are best eaten fresh, but they'll keep for 2 or 3 days after baking.

Clafoutis, top
Mini-Panettones, bottom

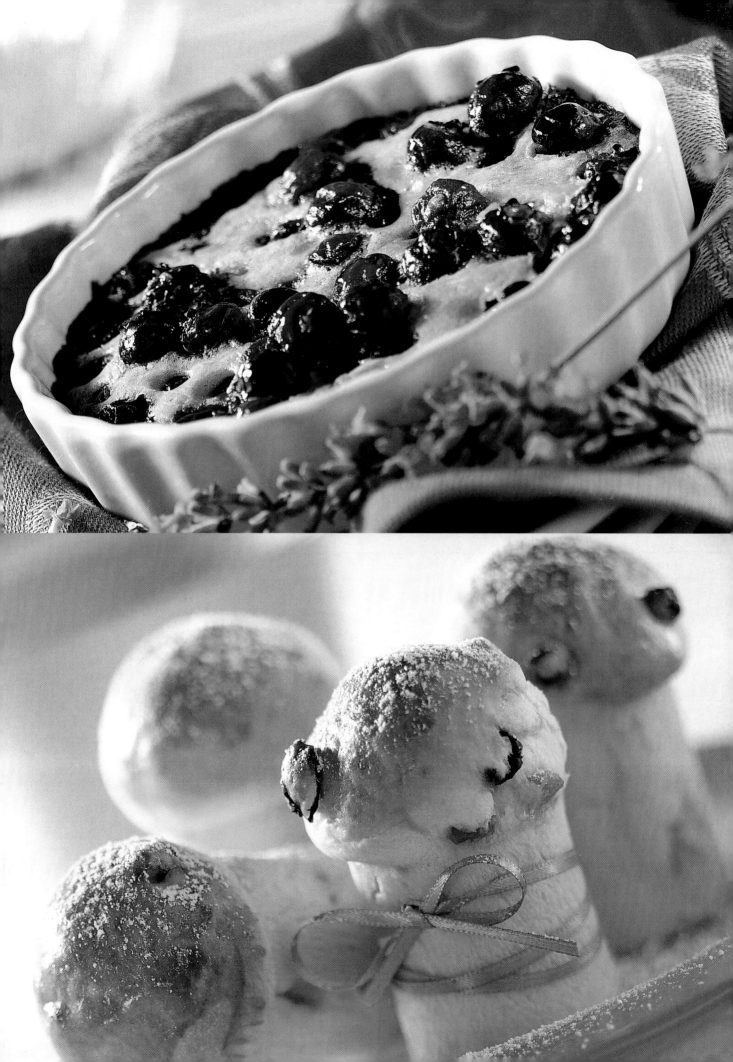

Nut Crescents

Carbohydrates ●●●	45 min.
Fat +	(+ 20 to 25 min. baking)

Per serving: approx. 298 calories
8 g protein · 15 g fat · 33 g carbohydrates

FOR 8 CRESCENTS:
FOR THE PASTRY:
1¾ cups (425 mL/200 g) pastry flour
Salt
1 tsp (5 mL) sugar
½ tsp (2 mL) grated orange zest
½ (¼ oz/7 g/2¼ tsp) envelope active dry yeast
⅓ cup (75 mL) lukewarm milk
1 egg yolk
1½ tbsp (22 mL/20 g) melted cooled butter
FOR THE FILLING:
⅓ cup (75 mL/70 g) mixed chopped nuts
1½ tsp (7 mL) sugar
¼ tsp (1 mL) ground cinnamon
¼ tsp (1 mL) unsweetened cocoa powder
3 tbsp (45 mL) water
1 egg yolk
2 tbsp (30 mL) blanched chopped almonds

1 Sift the flour into a large bowl with a pinch of salt, the sugar and the orange zest. Sprinkle yeast into milk; let stand for 10 minutes, or until frothy. Stir yeast mixture, then stir into the flour along with the egg yolk and butter. Knead to form a smooth dough. Leave to rise, covered, in a warm place for 30 minutes.

2 Combine the mixed nuts with the sugar, cinnamon, cocoa and water.

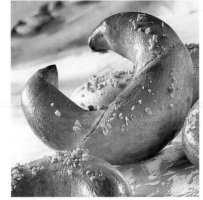

3 Preheat oven to 350°F (180°C). Knead the dough again and cut in half. On a floured surface, roll out each half to form a 10- x 10-inch (25 x 25 cm) square and cut into 4 smaller squares. Spread the nut mixture on a corner of each. Starting with that corner, roll the dough, curving the ends to form a crescent. Arrange on a baking sheet lined with parchment paper and brush with the egg yolk. Sprinkle with almonds and bake for 20 to 25 minutes, until golden.

Spiced Plum–Nut Danishes

Carbohydrates ●●●◖	40 min.
Fat ●●●	(+ 50 min. resting)
	(+ 25 min. baking)

Per serving: approx. 302 calories
7 g protein · 11 g fat · 41 g carbohydrates

FOR 6 PASTRIES:
2 cups (500 mL/250 g) flour
¼ cup (50 mL/50 g) butter
½ cup (125 mL) lukewarm milk
3 tbsp (45 mL) sugar, divided
1 (¼ oz/7 g/2¼ tsp) envelope active dry yeast
1 egg yolk
5 plums (about 10 oz/300 g)
4 to 6 whole cloves
3 tbsp (45 mL) water
Liquid sweetener
1 tsp (5 mL) ground cinnamon
3 tbsp (45 mL) chopped almonds

1 Sift the flour into a bowl. Melt ½ the butter and leave to cool. Combine milk and 2 tbsp (30 mL) of the sugar and sprinkle in yeast. Let stand for 10 minutes, or until frothy. Stir until smooth. Pour the butter and egg yolk onto the flour, then gradually add the yeast mixture. Knead until smooth and elastic. Leave to rise, covered, in a warm place for 30 minutes.

2 Pit and quarter the plums. Heat the cloves in the water, stir in the plums and simmer on medium heat until the liquid has evaporated. Remove the cloves, stir in sweetener and leave to cool.

3 On a floured surface, knead and roll out the dough to form an 8- x 12-inch (20 x 30 cm) rectangle. Combine the remaining 1 tbsp (15 mL) sugar, the cinnamon and the almonds. Sprinkle evenly over the dough and spread with the plum compote. Starting with the long side, roll up the pastry, then slice into 6 rounds. Arrange on a baking sheet lined with parchment paper and leave to rise, covered, for 20 minutes.

4 Preheat the oven to 350°F (180°C). Melt the remaining butter and brush on the pastries. Bake for 25 minutes.

Spiced Plum—Nut Danishes, right

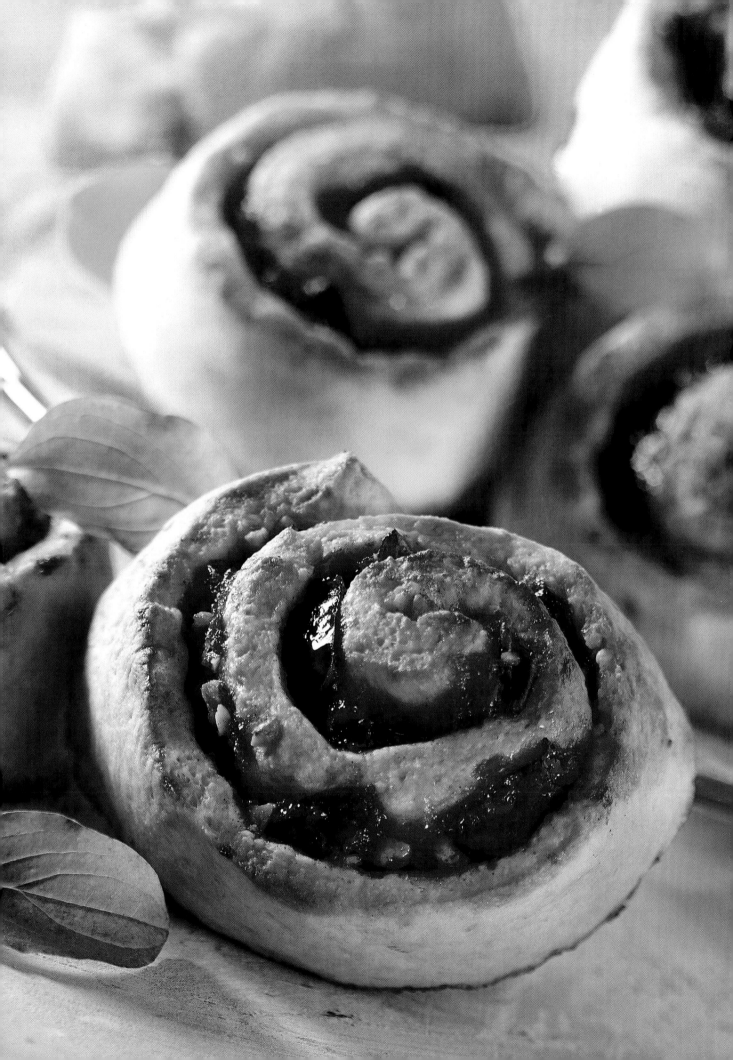

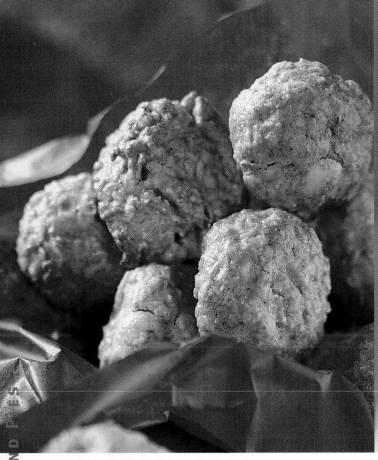

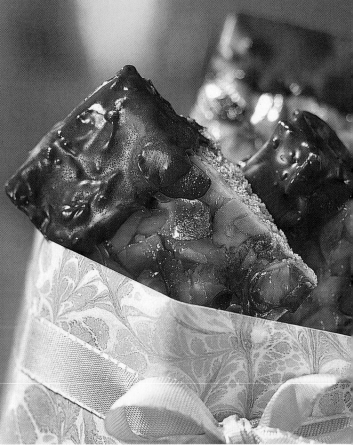

Oatmeal Macaroons

Carbohydrates ◖	30 min.
Fat ●	(+ 10 to 12 min. baking)

Per serving: approx. 47 calories
1 g protein · 3 g fat · 4 g carbohydrates

FOR 32 MACAROONS:
¼ cup (50 mL/60 g) butter
1¼ cups (300 mL/100 g) old-fashioned rolled oats
1 egg
⅓ cup (75 mL/50 g) sugar
Seeds of ½ vanilla bean
Pinch salt
½ tsp (2 mL) ground cinnamon
½ tsp (2 mL) unsweetened cocoa powder
½ cup (125 mL/50 g) coarsely ground whole wheat flour
⅓ cup (75 mL/50 g) chopped unsalted peanuts, hazelnuts or walnuts

1 Preheat the oven to 350°F (180°C). Melt the butter in a small saucepan, stir in the rolled oats and toast until light brown; set aside. Beat the egg, sugar, vanilla, salt, cinnamon and cocoa until fluffy. Stir in the flour, toasted rolled oats and nuts.

2 Drop teaspoonfuls of dough 1½ inches (4 cm) apart on a baking sheet lined with parchment paper. Bake for 10 to 12 minutes, until golden.

Spiced Almond Bars

Carbohydrates ●	30 min.
Fat ●●	(+ 30 min. baking)

Per serving: approx. 121 calories
2 g protein · 8 g fat · 12 g carbohydrates

FOR 20 BARS:
1¼ cups (300 mL/150 g) coarsely ground whole wheat flour
1 tsp (5 mL) baking powder
½ cup (125 mL) sugar, divided
½ tsp (2 mL) grated orange zest
½ tsp (2 mL) ground ginger
½ tsp (2 mL) ground coriander seeds
Pinch salt
1 egg
½ cup (125 mL/90 g) cold butter, divided
2 tbsp (30 mL) milk
¾ cup (175 mL/100 g) slivered almonds
2 (1-oz/30 g) squares bitter-sweet chocolate

1 Combine the flour, baking powder, ½ the sugar, orange zest, ginger, coriander and salt. Stir in the egg and ⅔ of the butter and knead until smooth. Preheat the oven to 325°F (160°C). Line a baking sheet with parchment paper. Roll the dough into an 8- x 12-inch (20 x 30 cm) rectangle. Bake for 20 minutes.

2 Combine remaining sugar and butter, the milk and almonds, and bring to a boil. Spread over the dough and bake for another 10 minutes. Cool and cut into 20 bars. Melt the chocolate and dip in one end of each bar. Chill until firm.

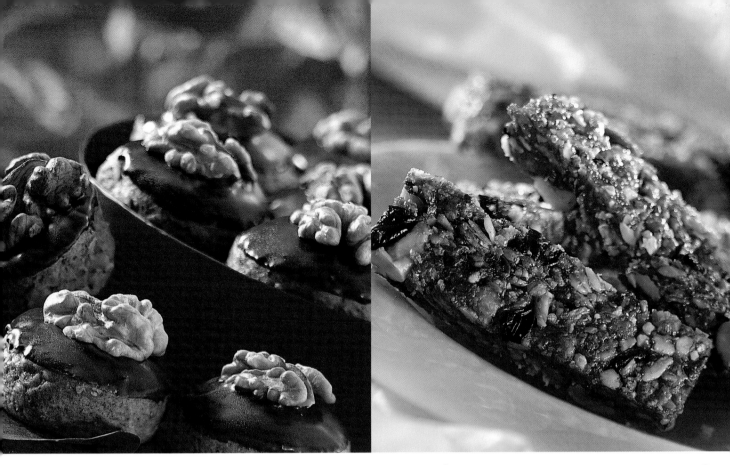

Walnut–Ginger Cakes

Carbohydrates ●	30 min.
Fat ● ●	(+ 1 night resting)
	(+ 15 to 20 min. baking)

Per serving: approx. 113 calories
2 g protein · 7 g fat · 9 g carbohydrates

FOR 20 CAKES:
¼ cup (50 mL) sugar
2 tbsp (30 mL/30 g) butter
¾ tsp (4 mL) baking soda
1 tbsp (15 mL) rum
1 egg
1¼ cups (300 mL/150 g) whole wheat flour
⅔ cup (150 mL/75 g) finely chopped walnuts
Pinch each ground cinnamon, cloves, mace, allspice and cardamom
1 tsp (5 mL) grated lemon zest
Pinch salt
2 (1-oz/30 g) squares bittersweet chocolate
20 walnut halves

1 Combine sugar and butter. Combine baking soda, rum and egg. Combine flour, nuts, spices, lemon zest and salt. Knead all these together, wrap in plastic wrap and let rest overnight.

2 Roll the dough into a rope, divide into 20 pieces and form into balls. Roll out to rounds ½ inch (1 cm) thick.

3 Preheat the oven to 325°F (160°C). Place a sheet of parchment paper on a baking sheet and arrange the rounds on the paper. Bake for 15 to 20 minutes. Melt the chocolate and use as a topping with the walnut halves.

Granola Bars

Carbohydrates ●	15 min.
Fat ● ●	(+ 1½ hrs. resting)
	(+ 1 hr. baking)

Per serving: approx. 106 calories
2 g protein · 7 g fat · 9 g carbohydrates

FOR 24 BARS:
¼ cup (50 mL/50 g) butter
¾ cup (175 mL/200g) cream
¼ cup (50 mL) milk
¼ cup (50 mL) sugar
1 tsp (5 mL) ground cinnamon
½ tsp (2 mL) ground ginger
Pinch ground cardamom
2⅓ cups (575 mL/250 g) unsweetened muesli with raisins and nuts
⅓ cup (75 mL/40 g) pastry flour
½ cup (125 mL/50 g) chopped hazelnuts

1 Melt the butter. Stir in the cream, milk, sugar, cinnamon, ginger and cardamom. Stirring constantly, bring to a boil and cook until thickened. Add the muesli and flour and cook until it becomes a thick porridge. Remove from heat and let stand, covered, for 30 minutes.

2 Roll out the dough to a thickness of ¼ inch (0.5 cm) and place on a baking sheet lined with parchment paper. Sprinkle with nuts and leave to dry for 1 hour.

3 Preheat oven to 325°F (160°C). Bake for 1 hour, leave to cool slightly, then slice into 24 bars. Cool, then carefully separate and leave to dry on a wire rack.

Hazelnut Squares

Carbohydrates	◖	30 min.
Fat	++	(+ 15 min. baking)
		(+ 1 hr. 20 min. cooling)

Per serving: approx. 304 calories
1 g protein · 27 g fat · 7 g carbohydrates

FOR 10 SQUARES:
FOR THE BASE:
2½ tbsp (37 mL/40 g) soft butter
2 eggs, separated
3 tbsp (45 mL) sugar
¼ cup (50 mL/60 g) cream
2⅓ cups (575 mL/200 g) ground hazelnuts
1 tsp (5 mL) ground cinnamon
1 tsp (5 mL) unsweetened cocoa powder
Seeds of ½ vanilla bean
Salt
FOR THE FROSTING:
½ cup (125 mL/100 g) low-fat yogurt
8 oz (250 g/250 g) mascarpone cheese
1 tsp (5 mL) grated orange zest
2 tbsp (30 mL) orange liqueur
Sweetener
1 (¼ oz/7 g/1 tbsp) envelope unflavored gelatin
¼ cup (50 mL) freshly squeezed orange juice
½ cup (125 mL/50 g) blanched skinned chopped
   hazelnuts

1 Preheat the oven to 325°F (160°C). Beat butter, egg yolks and sugar until creamy and smooth. Stir in cream, hazelnuts, cinnamon, cocoa and vanilla seeds. Beat the egg whites with a pinch of salt until stiff and fold into the mixture. Line a 9- x 13-inch (23 x 33 cm) baking pan with parchment paper. Pour in the batter and smooth with a spatula. Bake for 15 minutes, then leave to cool in the pan.

2 Meanwhile, combine the yogurt, mascarpone, orange zest, liqueur and sweetener. Pour gelatin over orange juice and heat to dissolve the gelatin. Stir in a little of the yogurt mixture, then stir the gelatin into the yogurt combination. Refrigerate for 20 minutes.

3 Frost the cake with the yogurt mixture and refrigerate for 1 hour. Before serving, sprinkle with chopped hazelnuts and cut into 10 squares.

Crunchy Apple Slices

Carbohydrates	●●◖	45 min.
Fat	●●	(+ 1 hr. resting)
		(+ 20 min. baking)

Per serving: approx. 214 calories
4 g protein · 9 g fat · 28 g carbohydrates

FOR 8 SLICES:
FOR THE BASE:
1⅔ cups (400 mL/200 g) coarsely ground whole wheat
   flour
1 tsp (5 mL) sugar
½ cup (125 mL) lukewarm milk
1 (¼ oz/7 g/2¼ tsp) envelope active dry yeast
¼ cup (50 mL/50 g) soft margarine
Salt
FOR THE FILLING:
4 small tart apples
3 tbsp (45 mL) lemon juice
¼ cup (50 mL/40 g) pine nuts
Pinch ground cinnamon
FOR THE GLAZE:
2 tbsp (30 mL) apricot jam (at least 40% fruit)
2 tbsp (30 mL) water

1 Put the flour in a bowl and make a well in the center. Dissolve sugar in the milk and sprinkle in the yeast. Let stand for 10 minutes, or until frothy. Pour the yeast mixture into the well along with the margarine and a pinch of salt. Knead from the center out to form a smooth dough. Leave to rise, covered, in a warm place for 40 minutes.

2 Peel the apples, quarter, core and cut into thin wedges. Sprinkle with lemon juice. Knead the dough again on a floured surface and roll out to form an 8- x 12-inch (20 x 30 cm) rectangle.

3 Line a baking sheet with parchment paper. Place dough on top, make an edge all around the dough and notch decoratively. Arrange overlapping wedges of apple on the dough and sprinkle with pine nuts and cinnamon. Let rise, covered, for 10 minutes.

4 Preheat the oven to 350°F (180°C). Bake for 20 minutes. Warm the apricot jam, thin with water and spread over the cake. Cut into 8 slices.

Hazelnut Squares, top
Crunchy Apple Slices, bottom

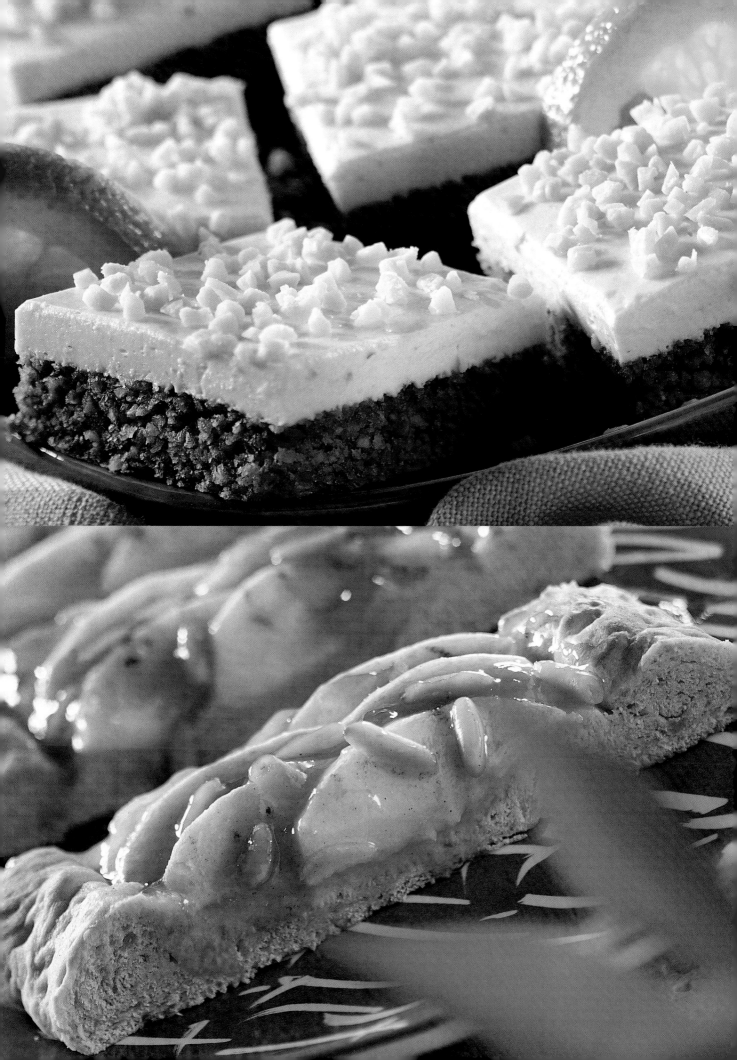

Apricot Galette

Carbohydrates ●	25 min.
Fat —	(+ 30 min. resting) (+ 1 hr. baking)

Per serving: approx. 67 calories
2 g protein · 2 g fat · 11 g carbohydrates

FOR 10 SERVINGS:
FOR THE BASE:
1 (¼ oz/7 g/2¼ tsp) envelope active dry yeast
2 tbsp (30 mL) sugar
¼ cup (50 mL) lukewarm milk
¾ cup (175 mL/75 g) pastry flour
1 tbsp (15 mL) soft butter
Pinch cinnamon
Pinch salt
FOR THE TOPPING:
6 apricots
⅓ cup (75 mL) buttermilk
2 tbsp (30 mL) sugar
2 tbsp (30 mL/30 g) cream
1 tbsp (15 mL) cornstarch

1 Sprinkle yeast into milk and let stand for 10 minutes, or until frothy. Combine with the sugar, flour, butter, cinnamon and salt. Knead until smooth. Leave to rise, covered, in a warm place for 30 minutes.

2 Grease an 8-inch (20 cm) springform pan. Knead the dough again, roll out to fit, and line the pan with the dough, creating an edge along the sides. Quarter and pit the apricots and arrange on the dough.

3 Preheat the oven to 350°F (180°C). Combine the sugar, buttermilk, cream and cornstarch, and pour over the apricots. Bake for 1 hour. Cut into 10 wedges and serve.

 TIP: You can use the same amount of peaches instead of the apricots.

Pear Tarte Tatin

Carbohydrates ●◖	30 min.
Fat ●●●	(+ 20 min. resting) (+ 30 to 35 min. baking)

Per serving: approx. 162 calories
3 g protein · 9 g fat · 17 g carbohydrates

FOR 12 SERVINGS:
FOR THE PASTRY:
1⅓ cups (325 mL/150 g) pastry flour
Salt
¼ cup (50 mL/50 g) butter
1 egg
2 to 3 tbsp (30 to 45 mL) milk
2 tbsp (30 mL) sugar
Seeds of ½ vanilla bean
FOR THE FILLING:
5 medium-sized half-ripe pears
1½ tbsp (22 mL/20 g) butter
2 tbsp (30 ml) sugar
1 tsp (5 mL) ground cinnamon
½ cup (125 mL) chopped walnuts
Icing (confectioner's) sugar (optional)

1 Knead together the flour, salt, butter, egg, milk, sugar and vanilla seeds until a firm dough is achieved. Wrap in plastic wrap and leave to rest for 20 minutes.

2 Peel, halve and core pears. Grease a 10-inch (25 cm) springform pan with the butter. Sprinkle sugar, cinnamon and walnuts on the bottom of the pan and arrange the pears, sliced side down.

3 Preheat the oven to 350°F (180°C). Roll out the dough so it's slightly larger than the pan. Gently press over the fruit and tuck into the sides of pan. Prick with a fork in a few places. Bake for 30 to 35 minutes. Leave to cool slightly in the pan. Invert onto a large plate and leave to cool completely. Cut into 12 pieces and serve with a little icing (confectioners) sugar dusted over the top, if desired.

Apple–Pear Tart

Carbohydrates ●◖	20 min.
Fat ●●	(+ 1 hr. chilling) (+ 1 hr. baking)

Per serving: approx. 125 calories
2 g protein · 8 g fat · 13 g carbohydrates

FOR 10 SERVINGS:
FOR THE PASTRY:
¾ cup (175 mL/100 g) flour
1 tsp (5 mL) sugar
⅓ cup (75 mL/70 g) butter
1 egg yolk
Salt
FOR THE FILLING:
1 large apple
1 pear
1 egg yolk
FOR THE GLAZE:
1 tbsp (15 mL) apricot jam

1 Knead together flour, sugar, butter, egg yolk and salt to form a smooth dough. Wrap in plastic wrap and refrigerate for 1 hour.

2 Preheat the oven to 350°F (180°C). Grease an 8-inch (20 cm) springform pan. Roll out the dough so it's slightly larger than the pan and line the pan and a bit up the sides with it. Peel, core and slice the apple and pear and arrange in a fan-like formation on top of the dough. Brush with the egg yolk. Bake for 1 hour.

3 Warm the apricot jam with a little water, stirring, and brush on the tart while still hot. Cut into 10 pieces and serve.

Apricot Galette, top
Pear Tarte Tatin, bottom left
Apple–Pear Tart, bottom right

SAVORY BAKED GOODS, BREADS, ROLLS, CAKES AND PIES

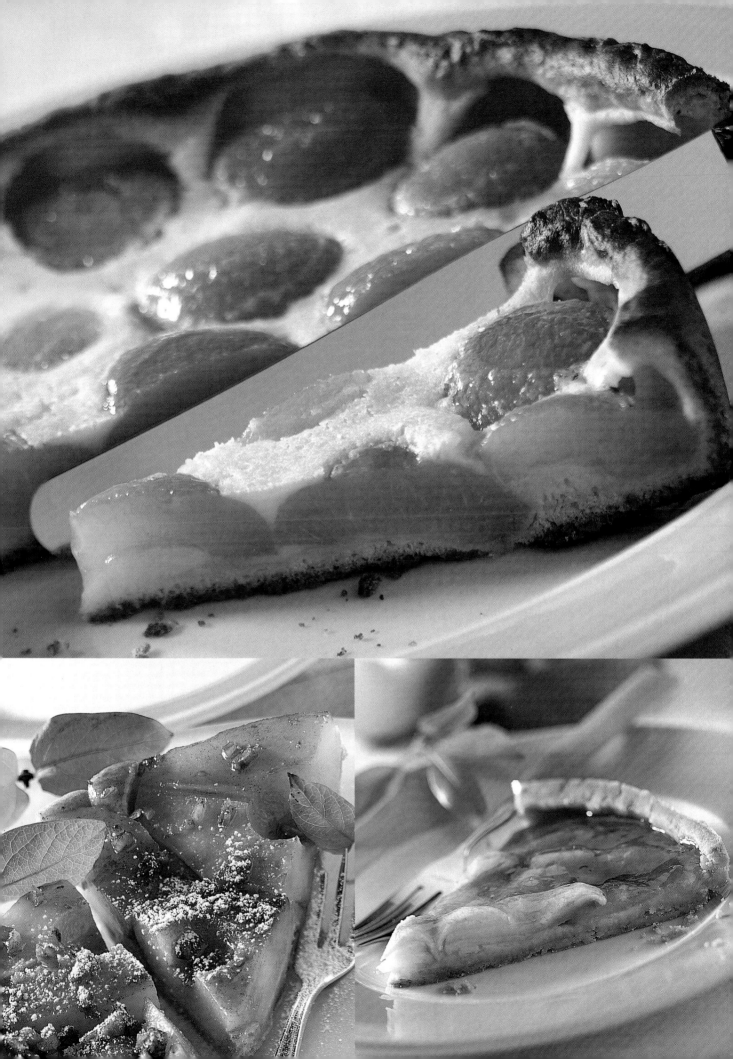

English Teacake

| Carbohydrates ●◖ | 45 min. |
| Fat ●●● | (+ 50 min. baking) |

Per serving: approx. 206 calories
4 g protein · 14 g fat · 16 g carbohydrates

FOR 10 SERVINGS:
⅓ cup (75 mL/70 g) butter
¼ cup (50 mL) sugar
2 eggs
Juice and zest of ½ lemon
¾ cup (175 mL/75 g) coarsely ground whole wheat flour
½ cup (125 mL/50 g) cornstarch
¾ cup (175 mL/100 g) dried apricots
¾ cup (175 mL/100 g) chopped almonds
1 tsp (5 mL) baking powder
Salt

1 Preheat the oven to 325°F (160°C). Finely chop the apricots. Cream the butter, then gradually beat in sugar and eggs until smooth. Fold in lemon juice, lemon zest, flour, cornstarch, apricots, almonds, baking powder and a little salt.

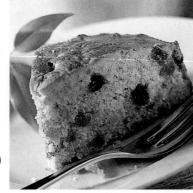

2 Grease an 8-inch (20 cm) springform pan. Pour in batter and bake for 50 minutes. Turn out onto a wire rack to cool. Cut into 10 pieces and serve.

Carrot–Potato Cake

| Carbohydrates ●◖ | 25 min. |
| Fat ● | (+ 1 hr. baking) |

Per serving: approx. 100 calories
4 g protein · 4 g fat · 14 g carbohydrates

FOR 10 SERVINGS:
1 small cooked potato
1 carrot
¾ cup (175 mL/100 g) coarsely ground whole wheat flour
1 tsp (5 mL) baking powder
2 tbsp (30 mL/15 g) raisins
2 eggs, separated
2 tbsp (30 mL/30 g) butter
3 tbsp (45 mL) sugar
½ tsp (2 mL) ground cinnamon
Grated zest and juice of 1 lemon
Freshly grated nutmeg

1 Peel and grate the potato and carrot. Mix with the flour, baking powder and raisins.

2 Preheat the oven to 350°F (180°C). Grease an 8-inch (20 cm) springform pan. Beat the egg whites until stiff. Combine the egg yolks with the butter, sugar, cinnamon, lemon juice, lemon zest and nutmeg. Fold into the potato–carrot mixture. Fold in egg whites. Pour the batter into the pan and bake for 1 hour. Leave to cool in the pan. Cut into 10 pieces and serve.

 TIP: Instead of a potato, you can use grated zucchini or pumpkin and combine as above. The cake will be very moist.

Carrot–Potato Cake, right

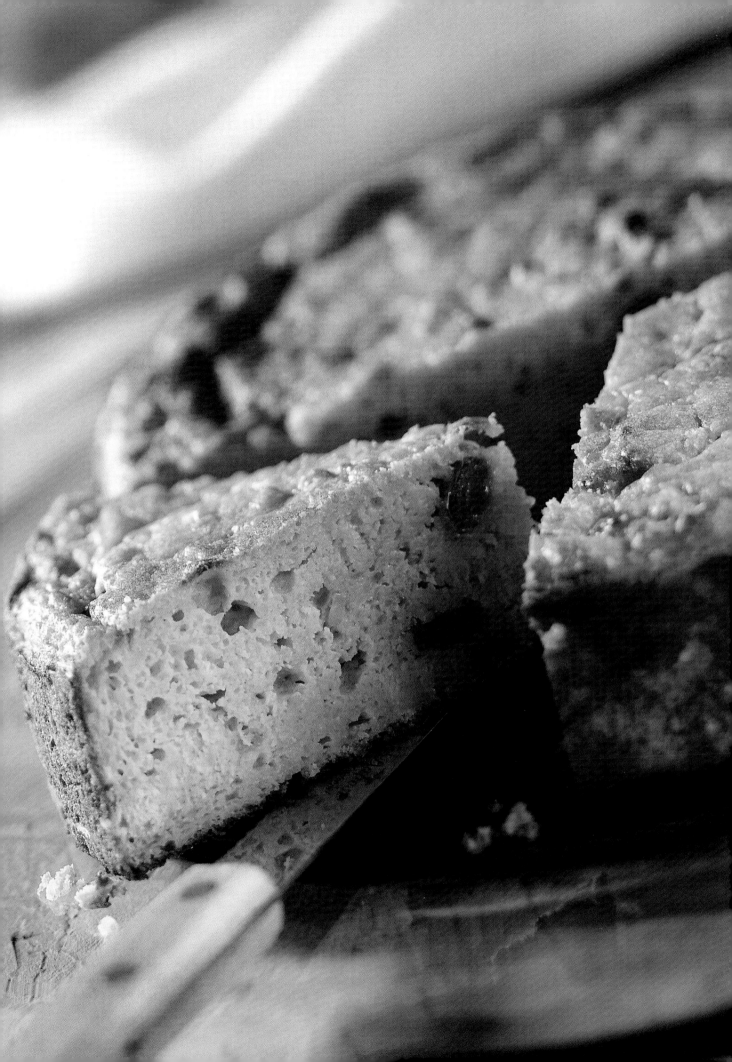

Yogurt Cake with Fresh Figs

| Carbohydrates ●● | 20 min. |
| Fat ●● | (+ 45 to 50 min. baking) |

Per serving: approx. 175 calories
5 g protein · 7 g fat · 23 g carbohydrates

FOR 12 SERVINGS:
1 cup (250 mL/250 g) yogurt
2 eggs
¼ cup (50 mL) sugar
1 vanilla bean
Salt
1 tsp (5 mL) grated orange zest
1 tbsp (15 mL) rum
¼ cup (50 mL/60 g) melted cooled butter
1⅓ cups (325 mL/250 g) durum wheat semolina
1½ tsp (7 mL) baking powder
Fine dry bread crumbs
6 ripe fresh figs

1 Preheat the oven to 325°F (160°C). Split the vanilla bean lengthwise and scrape out the seeds. Mix yogurt, eggs, sugar, vanilla seeds, a pinch of salt, orange zest, rum and butter. Combine the semolina and baking powder and stir into the mixture.

2 Grease a 10-inch (25 mL) springform pan and sprinkle with bread crumbs. Pour in the batter. Quarter the figs, lay them on top and let them sink into the batter. Bake for 45 to 50 minutes, until golden. Leave to cool in the pan, then remove and cut into 12 pieces.

!! **TIP:** Replace the fresh figs with dried ones. Before using, soak for 1 hour in water or a little more rum, then drain, blot dry and cut into quarters.

Dark Pound Cake

| Carbohydrates ●◖ | 20 min. |
| Fat ●●● | (+ 45 min. baking) |

Per serving: approx. 166 calories
3 g protein · 11 g fat · 15 g carbohydrates

FOR 12 SERVINGS:
Fine dry bread crumbs
½ cup (125 mL/125 g) butter
2 tbsp (30 mL) sugar
2 eggs
1¼ cups (300 mL/150 g) flour
2 tsp (10 mL) baking powder
⅓ cup (75 mL/100 g) whole-berry cranberry sauce, preferably not sweetened with sugar
1 tsp (5 mL) unsweetened cocoa powder
Juice and zest of 1 lemon
Ground cinnamon

1 Preheat the oven to 325°F (160°C). Oil an 8-inch (20 cm) round cake or Bundt pan and sprinkle with bread crumbs. Beat together butter, sugar and eggs until creamy and smooth. Combine the flour and baking powder and fold in along with the cranberry sauce. Stir in cocoa, lemon zest, lemon juice and a little cinnamon.

2 Bake on a rack two positions from the bottom of the oven for 45 minutes. Let the cake cool for 5 minutes, then remove from the pan and leave to cool completely on a wire rack. Cut into 12 pieces and serve.

!! **TIP:** Allowing this cake to sit for a day before slicing will deepen the cranberry flavor. When it's cool, store it in a cake plate with a top or a cake tin, or wrap it well to keep it moist.

Yogurt Cake with Fresh Figs, top
Dark Pound Cake, bottom

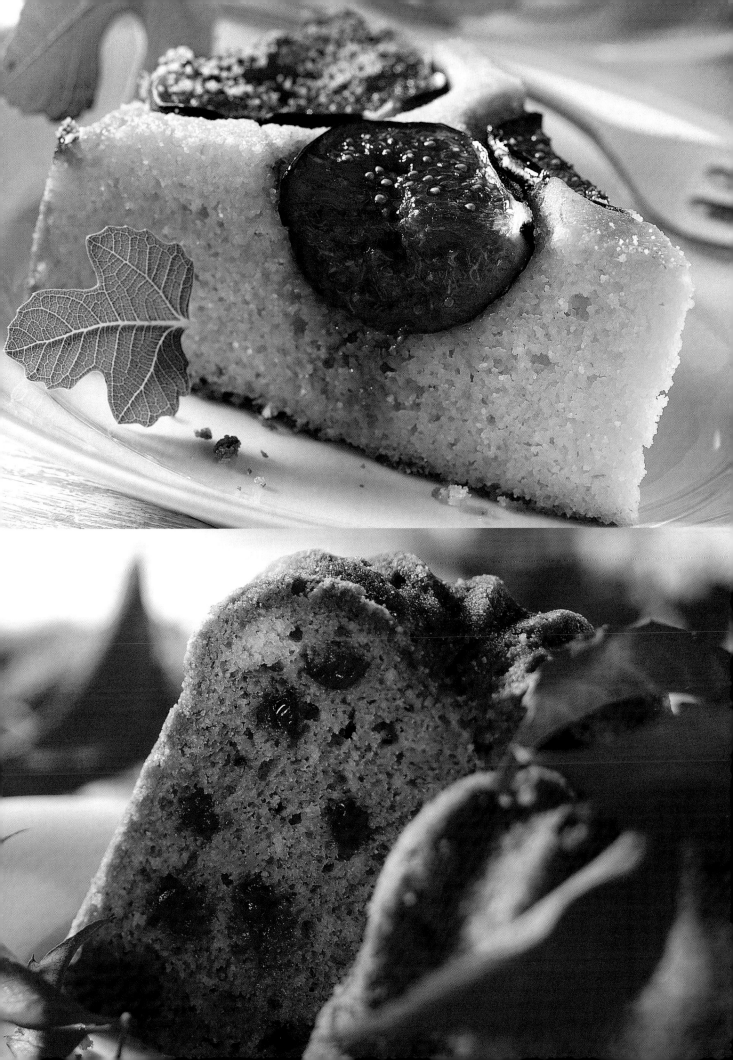

Rhubarb Flan

Carbohydrates ●●◖	20 min.
Fat +	(+ 1 hr. resting)
	(+ 45 to 50 min. baking)

Per serving: approx. 290 calories
8 g protein · 15 g fat · 21 g carbohydrates

FOR 12 SERVINGS:
FOR THE CRUST:
2 cups (500 mL/250 g) coarsely ground whole wheat
    flour
½ tsp (2 mL) baking powder
3 tbsp (45 mL) sugar
Pinch salt
½ cup (125 mL/125 g) margarine
½ tsp (2 mL) grated lemon zest
1 large egg
FOR THE FILLING:
⅔ cup (150 mL/750 g) finely sliced rhubarb
½ cup (125 mL/150 g) strawberry jam (60% fruit)
2 eggs, separated
⅓ cup (75 mL/100 g) liquid honey
½ cup (125 mL/125 g) low-fat quark or puréed cottage
    cheese
1½ cups (325 mL/100 g) ground almonds
Pinch ground cinnamon

1 Combine flour, baking powder, sugar, salt, margarine, lemon zest and whole egg. Knead, wrap in plastic wrap and refrigerate for 1 hour.

2 Combine rhubarb and strawberry jam and set aside. Beat the egg whites until stiff and refrigerate. Whisk the egg yolks with the honey until frothy. Stir in quark, almonds and cinnamon.

3 Preheat the oven to 325°F (160°C). On a floured surface, roll out the dough until thin. Cut out a 10-inch (25 cm) circle and place in a 10-inch (25 cm) springform pan. Roll the remaining dough into a rope and press into the sides of the pan. Distribute the rhubarb mixture over the dough. Fold the egg whites into the quark mixture and spread smoothly on top. Bake for 40 to 45 minutes. Leave to cool, then cut into 12 pieces.

Buckwheat Torte with Red Currants

Carbohydrates ●◖	20 min.
Fat ●	(+ 40 min. baking)
	(+ 3 hrs. 15 min. chilling)

Per serving: approx. 115 calories
5 g protein · 5 g fat · 13 g carbohydrates

FOR 12 SERVINGS:
FOR THE CAKE:
3 eggs, separated
Salt
4 tbsp (60 mL/50 g) sugar
Zest and juice of ½ lemon
½ cup (125 mL/60 g) buckwheat flour
FOR THE FILLING AND TOPPING:
1½ (¼ oz/7 g/1 tbsp) envelopes unflavored gelatin
¼ cup (50 mL) cold water
1¼ cups (300 mL) red currants
1 tbsp (15 mL) sugar
1⅔ cups (400 ml/400 g) low-fat yogurt
Sweetener
½ cup (125 mL/100 g) whipping (35%) cream

1 Preheat the oven to 325°F (160°C). Beat the egg whites and a pinch of salt until stiff and refrigerate. Combine egg yolks and sugar and beat until creamy and thick. Combine lemon zest, 3 tbsp (45 mL) lemon juice and the flour. Carefully fold the beaten egg whites into the batter.

2 Cover the bottom of an 8-inch (20 cm) springform pan with parchment paper and pour in the batter. Bake for 15 minutes. Cover with aluminum foil and bake for another 25 minutes. Using a sharp knife, carefully remove the cake from the pan and turn out onto a wire rack. Leave to cool.

3 Sprinkle the the gelatin over the cold water and dissolve it by placing it over hot water. Combine ⅔ of the red currants with the sugar and stir into the yogurt. Stir a little of the yogurt mixture into the gelatin, then stir the gelatin into the yogurt. Add sweetener to taste. Whip the cream and fold in. Refrigerate for 15 minutes.

4 Cut the cake in two horizontally and place one layer on a cake plate. Spread it with ½ the yogurt mixture. Lay on the second layer of cake and cover with the remaining yogurt mixture. Refrigerate for 2 to 3 hours. Garnish with the remaining currants and cut into 12 pieces.

Rhubarb Flan, top
Buckwheat Torte with Red Currants, bottom

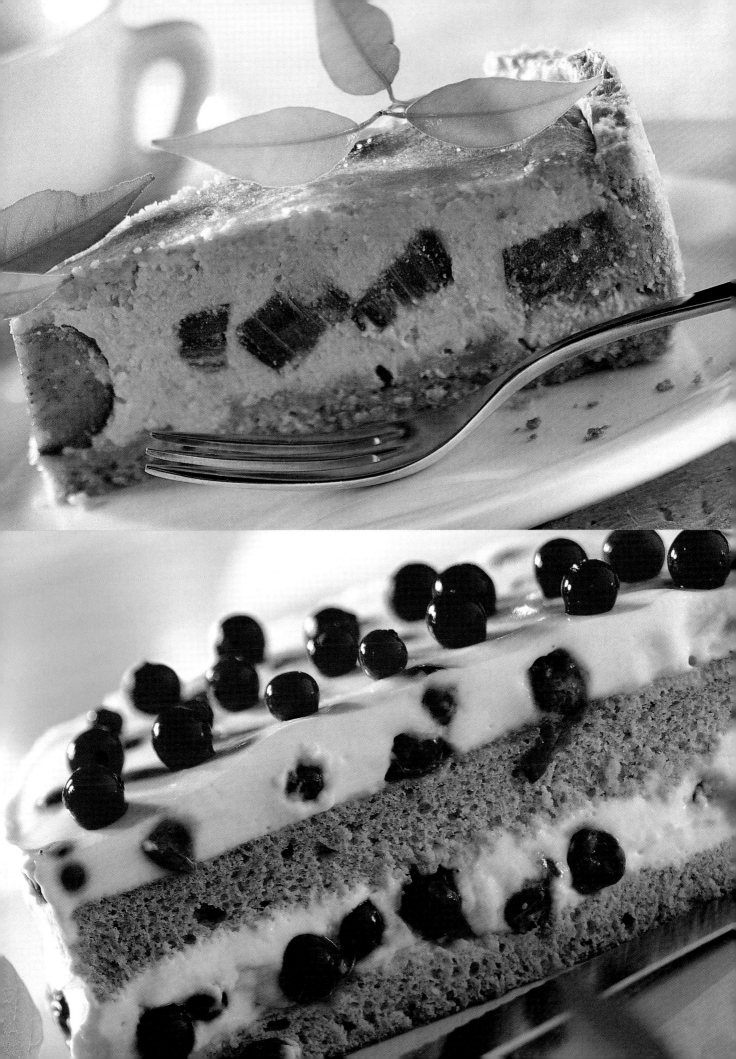

Apricot Creams

Carbohydrates ●●	40 min.
Fat ●	(+ 1 hr. 50 min. resting)
	(+ 25 to 30 min. baking)

Per serving: approx. 148 calories
4 g protein · 5 g fat · 21 g carbohydrates

FOR 10 PASTRIES:
FOR THE PASTRY:
2 cups (500 mL/250 g) whole wheat flour
3 tbsp (45 mL) sugar, divided
1 (¼ oz/7 g/2¼ tsp) envelope active dry yeast
2 tbsp (30 mL) vegetable oil
1 tsp (5 mL) melted margarine
¼ cup (50 mL/25 g) chopped hazelnuts
FOR THE PASTRY CREAM:
½ cup (125 mL) low-fat milk
1 tsp (5 mL) cornstarch
1 vanilla bean
1 egg yolk
Sweetener
FOR THE TOPPING:
5 small apricots

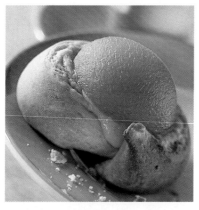

1 Sift the flour into a large bowl and make a well in the center. Dissolve 1 tbsp (15 mL) of the sugar in about ⅓ cup (75 mL) lukewarm water. Sprinkle in yeast; let stand 10 minutes, or until frothy. Stir until smooth. Pour into the well and combine with the flour. Add the remaining sugar and the oil, and knead until smooth. Leave to rise, covered, for 1½ hours.

2 Heat the milk on low heat. Mix cornstarch and 1 tbsp (15 mL) cold water. Split, scrape and stir in the seeds of the vanilla bean. Stir into the milk and bring to a boil. Remove from the heat and stir in the egg yolk and a little sweetener. Leave to cool.

3 Thoroughly knead the dough again and roll out to form an 8- x 12-inch (20 x 30 cm) rectangle. Spread with margarine and sprinkle with hazelnuts. Starting with the short side, roll up and cut into 10 slices. Place on a baking sheet lined with parchment paper and leave to rise, covered, for 20 minutes.

4 Preheat the oven to 325°F (160°C). Cut the apricots in half and remove the pits. Create a depression in the center of each pastry. Place 1 tsp (5 mL) of the pastry cream and 1 apricot half, cut side down, over each. Bake for 25 to 30 minutes.

Choux Ring with Tropical Fruit

Carbohydrates ●●	40 min.
Fat +	(+ 25 to 30 min. baking)

Per serving: approx. 280 calories
10 g protein · 17 g fat · 23 g carbohydrates

FOR 6 SERVINGS:
½ cup (125 mL) water
Scant 2 tbsp (25 mL/25 g) butter
Salt
1 tsp (5 mL) sugar
⅔ cup (150 mL/75 g) flour
2 eggs
1 ripe papaya
1 small banana
1 small orange
1 star fruit
Lemon juice
½ cup (125 mL/100 g) low-fat quark or puréed cottage cheese
Sweetener
½ cup (125 mL/100 g) whipping (35%) cream
Icing (confectioner's) sugar

1 Preheat the oven to 400°F (200°C). Bring the water, butter, a pinch of salt and the sugar to a boil in a large saucepan on medium heat. Beat in the flour, stirring constantly, and continue to cook and stir until the dough leaves the side of the pan and a skin forms on the bottom of the saucepan. Put the dough in a bowl and cool slightly. Beat in the eggs one by one until a smooth, shiny batter forms.

2 Using a pastry bag with a large star-shaped nozzle, shape a ring 3 inches (7.5 cm) thick and 8 inches (20 cm) in diameter on a baking sheet lined with parchment paper. Bake for 25 to 30 minutes. Leave to cool, then cut in two horizontally, separate the two halves and let stand.

3 Peel and cut the fruit attractively and sprinkle with lemon juice.

4 Combine quark, sweetener and a few dashes of lemon juice, and stir until smooth. Whip the cream until stiff and fold into the quark mixture. Spread the bottom half of the ring with the quark mixture. Top with the upper half and dust with icing sugar, if desired. Arrange fruit in the center. Cut into 6 pieces and serve immediately.

 TIP: You can use fresh seasonal fruit of any kind in this recipe.

Choux Ring with Tropical Fruit, right

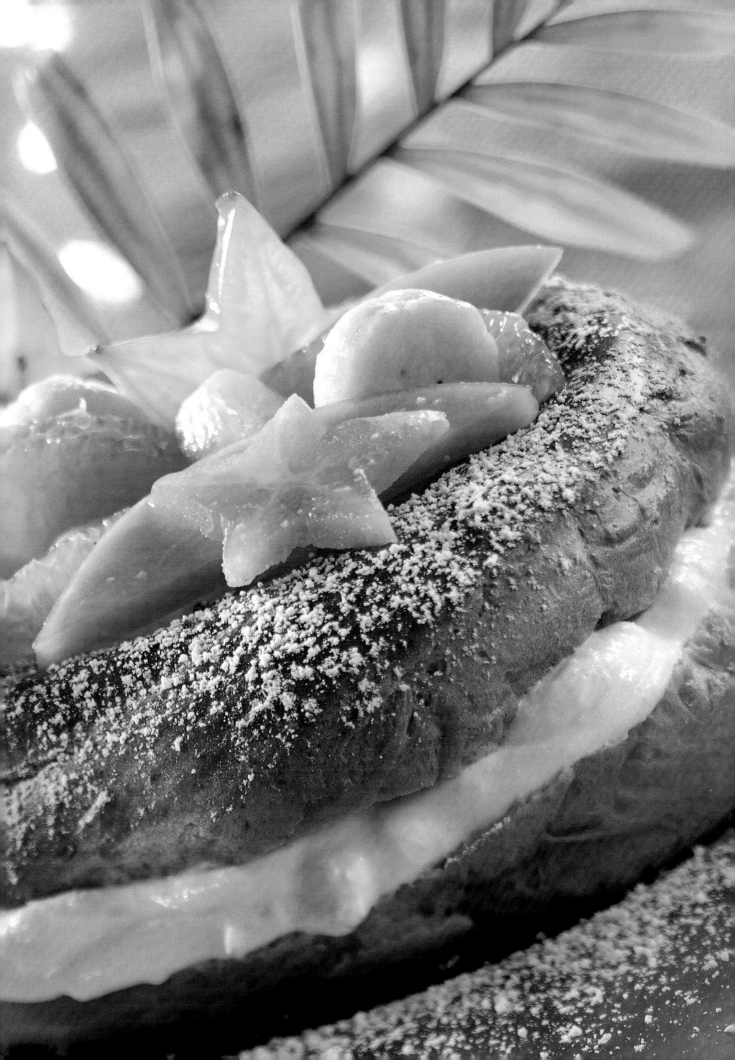

Lime–Almond Flan

Carbohydrates ●◖	20 min.
Fat ●●●	(+ 3 hrs. 20 min. chilling)
	(+ 40 min. baking)

Per serving: approx. 186 calories
6 g protein · 10 g fat · 18 g carbohydrates

FOR 12 SERVINGS:
FOR THE CRUST:
1¼ cups (300 mL/150 g) coarsely ground whole wheat flour
¼ cup (50 mL/50 g) sugar
Salt
1 egg yolk
7 tbsp (100 mL/100 g) cold margarine
½ cup (125 mL/60 g) ground almonds
FOR THE FILLING:
1½ (¼ oz/7 g/1 tbsp) envelopes unflavored gelatin
½ cup (125 mL) cold water
7 tbsp (100 mL/100 g) low-fat quark or puréed cottage cheese
2 cups (500 mL) buttermilk
Juice and grated zest of 1 lime
Sweetener
Lemon balm sprigs

1 Combine flour, sugar and a pinch of salt. Make a well in the center and slip in the egg yolk.. Place small pieces of margarine on top. Knead together quickly, then wrap in plastic wrap and refrigerate for 1 hour. Brown the almonds in a dry skillet (frying pan) and leave to cool.

2 Preheat the oven to 350°F (180°C). On a floured work surface, roll out the dough until thin. Use a 10-inch (25 cm) springform pan to cut the dough. Line the bottom of the pan and pierce in several places with a fork. Shape the remaining dough into a rope and press into the sides of the pan. Bake for 10 minutes. Leave to cool on a wire rack for 45 minutes.

3 Soak the gelatin in the cold water for 5 minutes, then dissolve over hot water. Stir in the quark, buttermilk, lime juice and lime zest until smooth. Add sweetener and refrigerate for 20 minutes, until the gelatin starts to set.

4 Place the pastry on a cake plate and fill with the quark mixture. Refrigerate for at least 2 hours. Garnish with lemon balm, cut into 12 pieces and serve.

Berry Cake with Vanilla Whipped Cream

Carbohydrates ●●●	25 min.
Fat ✢	(+ 35 to 40 min. baking)

Per serving: approx. 230 calories
5 g protein · 16 g fat · 15 g carbohydrates

FOR 12 SERVINGS:
4 eggs, separated
3 tbsp (45 mL) sugar
3 tbsp (45 mL) rum
7 tbsp (100 mL/100 g) melted cooled butter
Salt
1¼ cups (300 mL/150 g) all-purpose flour
Pinch baking powder
3¼ cups (800 mL/500 g) mixed berries: strawberries, raspberries, blueberries, etc.
¾ cup (175 mL/200 g) whipping (35%) cream
Seeds of ½ vanilla bean
1 tsp (5 mL) icing (confectioner's) sugar
Sweetener
1 tbsp (15 mL) flaked almonds

1 Beat the egg yolks with sugar and rum until frothy. Stir in the butter. Beat the egg whites with a pinch of salt until stiff and place over the egg yolks. Sift the flour and baking powder over top and fold in.

2 Preheat the oven to 325°F (160°C). Cover the bottom of a 10-inch (25 cm) springform pan with parchment paper. Divide the batter in half. Fold about ⅓ of the berries into one half, pour into the pan and spread smooth. Pour the remaining batter on top and spread smooth. Bake for 35 to 40 minutes. Cool slightly. Slide onto a wire rack.

3 Whip the cream until soft peaks form. Beat in the vanilla seeds and icing sugar. Whip until stiff and add sweetener. Toast the almonds in a dry skillet (frying pan) until golden and leave to cool. Fold the remaining fruit into the whipped cream and cover the cake, or arrange the fruit over the cream. Sprinkle with almonds. Cut into 12 pieces and serve.

 TIP: Sprinkle with grated bittersweet chocolate instead of almonds.

Lime–Almond Flan, top
Berry Cake with Vanilla Whipped Cream, bottom

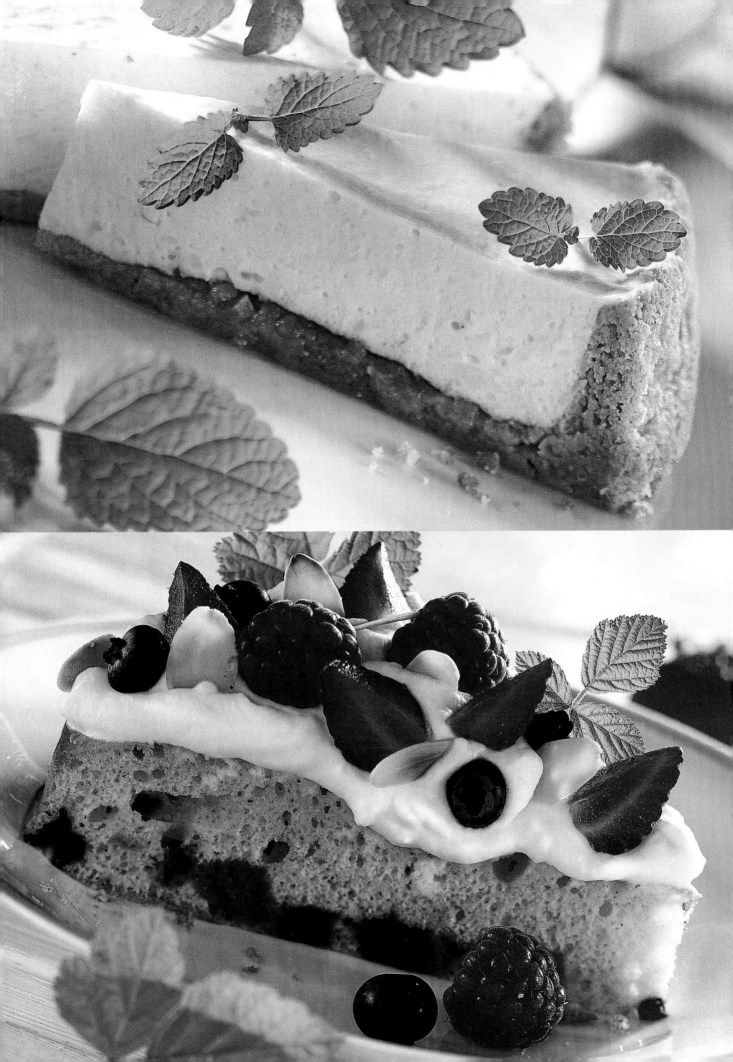

Cherry–Quark Strudel

Carbohydrates ●●●	50 min.
Fat ●●●	(+ 30 to 40 min. baking)

Per serving: approx. 266 calories
10 g protein · 10 g fat · 34 g carbohydrates

FOR 4 SERVINGS:
¾ cup (175 mL/175 g) low-fat quark or puréed cottage
  cheese
1 egg yolk
½ tsp (2 mL) vanilla sugar
Sweetener
14-oz (398 mL) can water-packed sour cherries
1½ tbsp (22 mL/20 g) butter
3½-oz (100 g) package strudel dough or phyllo sheets
¼ cup (50 mL) zwieback or fine dry bread crumbs
½ tsp (2 mL) ground cinnamon
2 tbsp (30 mL) sugar

1 Combine quark, egg yolk, vanilla sugar and
 sweetener. Drain the cherries. Melt the butter.
Roll the strudel dough out onto a tea towel.
Remove any cornstarch with a brush. Brush a little
butter on the dough.

2 Preheat the oven to 400°F (200°C). Combine
 crumbs, cinnamon and sugar, and sprinkle over
the dough. Spread the quark mixture on top, then
cover with cherries. Use the tea towel to assist in
rolling up the strudel. Place seam side down on a
baking sheet lined with parchment paper. Tuck in
the ends.

3 Bake for 30 to 40 minutes, until golden. Brush
 with butter while still hot and cut into 4 pieces.
Serve warm or cold.

TIPS: In cherry season, boil pitted Morello
or other sour cherries with a few dashes of
sweetener. Drain and use as above. The
strudel can also be frozen and reheated in a 350°F
(180°C) oven for 15 minutes.

Apricot Cheesecake

Carbohydrates ●	20 min.
Fat ●●●	(+ 50 min. baking)

Per serving: approx. 171 calories
9 g protein · 10 g fat · 12 g carbohydrates

FOR 10 SERVINGS:
½ cup (125 mL/100 g) soft butter
2 eggs
¼ cup (50 mL) sugar
Seeds of ½ vanilla bean
½ tsp (2 mL) grated orange zest
1 tbsp (15 mL) rum
2 cups (500 mL/500 g) low-fat quark or puréed cottage
  cheese
⅓ cup (75 mL/50 g) durum wheat semolina
¾ cup (175 mL/100 g) dried apricots (unsulphured
  preferred)

1 Preheat the oven to 325°F (160°C). Cream the
 butter. Beat in the eggs and sugar until creamy
and thick. Stir in the vanilla, orange peel, rum,
quark and semolina.

2 Grease an 8-inch (20 cm) springform pan and
 sprinkle with a little semolina. Spoon in the batter and spread evenly. Quarter the apricots and
distribute evenly over the top, pressing lightly into
the batter. Spread the top smooth.

3 Bake for 50 minutes. Turn off the heat and leave
 the cake to cool with the oven door open. Cut
into 10 pieces and serve.

TIP: Dried fruits are high in minerals and
fiber, but also in sugar. This cake will taste
just as good with 1 cup (250 mL) fresh fruit,
such as pears or tangerines. If you use preserved
cherries, blueberries, peaches or apricots, drain
well first.

SAVORY BAKED GOODS, BREADS, ROLLS, CAKES AND PIES

Cherry–Quark Strudel, top
Apricot Cheesecake, bottom

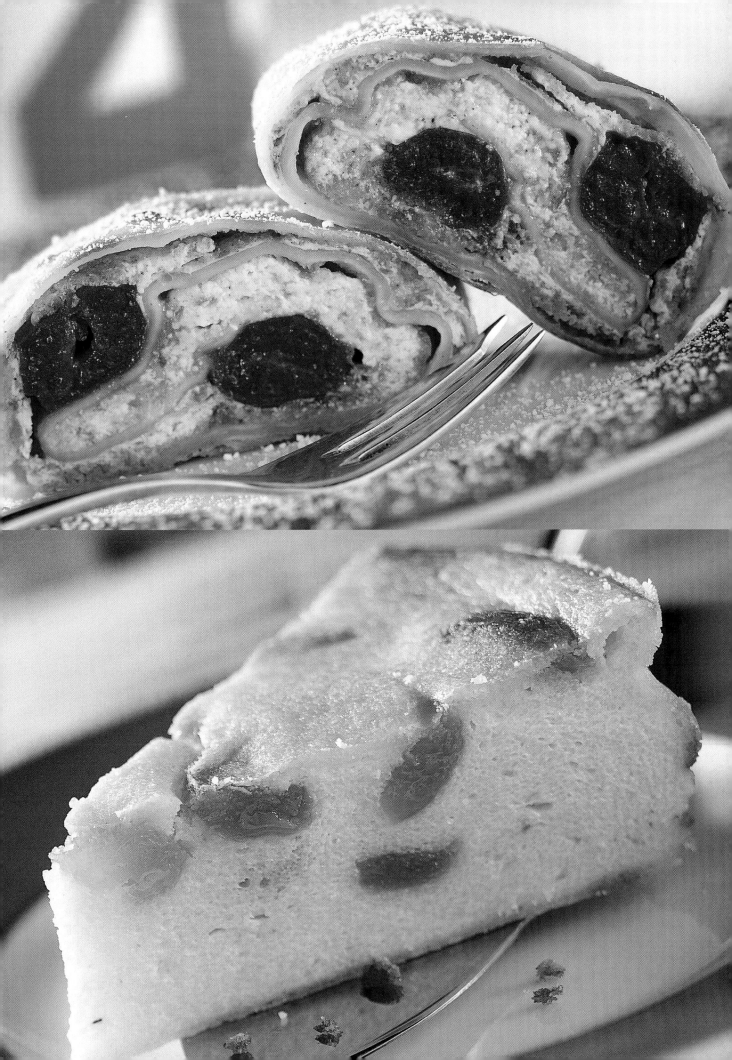

Blueberry–Semolina Cake

Carbohydrates ●◖	25 min.
Fat ●	(+ 1 hr. baking)

Per serving: approx. 106 calories
13 g protein · 4 g fat · 14 g carbohydrates

FOR 10 SERVINGS:
1¼ cups (300 mL) low-fat milk
5 whole cloves
½ cup (125 mL/75 g) durum wheat semolina
2 tbsp (30 mL) butter
3 tbsp (45 mL) sugar
1 tsp (5 mL) vanilla sugar
2 eggs, separated
Zest and juice of 1 lemon
1⅓ cups (325 mL/200 g) blueberries

1 Preheat the oven to 325°F (160°C). Grease an 8-inch (20 cm) springform pan and sprinkle with flour. Bring the milk and cloves to a boil. Remove from the heat and take out the cloves. Sprinkle in the semolina and simmer on low heat until thick. Leave to cool slightly.

2 Beat butter, sugar and vanilla sugar until creamy and pale. Beat in the egg yolks, lemon juice and lemon zest. Stir in the lukewarm semolina mixture.

3 With clean beaters, in a bowl free of grease, beat the egg whites until stiff. Carefully fold the blueberries and egg whites into the batter. Pour into the prepared pan and bake for 1 hour. Cut into 10 pieces and serve.

!! TIP: Wild blueberries taste better and are sweeter than the more common cultured blueberries. If you're using wild blueberries, omit the vanilla sugar.

Orange–Rice Flan

Carbohydrates ●●	2 hrs.
Fat ●●●	(+ 30 min. resting)
	(+ 18 min. baking) (+ 2 hrs. chilling)

Per serving: approx. 208 calories
5 g protein · 11 g fat · 24 g carbohydrates

FOR 12 SERVINGS:
FOR THE CRUST:
⅓ cup (75 mL/80 g) cold margarine
1¼ cups (300 mL/150 g) coarsely ground whole wheat flour
Sugar
FOR THE FILLING:
2 cups (500 mL) milk
Salt
1 tsp (5 mL) vanilla
⅔ cup (150 mL/130 g) brown rice
1 (¼ oz/7 g/1 tbsp) envelope unflavored gelatin
¼ cup (50 mL) cold water
¼ cup (50 mL) boiling water
Grated zest and juice of 2 oranges
⅔ cup (150 mL/150 g) low-fat yogurt
Sweetener
½ cup (125 mL/125 g) whipping (35%) cream
2 oranges for garnishing

1 Cut the margarine into small pieces and knead into the flour with a little sugar. Add a few drops of cold water if the dough is too crumbly (it should not become sticky). Wrap in plastic wrap and refrigerate for 30 minutes.

2 Combine milk, a pinch of salt and the vanilla, and bring to a boil. Sprinkle in the rice and cook, covered, on low heat for 50 to 60 minutes. Leave to cool.

3 Preheat the oven to 350°F (180°C). Roll out the dough to fit a 10-inch (25 cm) springform pan and place in the pan. Pierce in several places with a fork. Bake for 18 minutes, until golden. Slide onto a wire rack.

4 Sprinkle gelatin over the cold water. Pour in the boiling water and stir until completely dissolved. Combine with the orange zest and juice, yogurt, cooked rice and sweetener. Whip cream until stiff and fold in.

5 Distribute the rice mixture evenly over the crust and refrigerate for at least 2 hours, until firm. Garnish the flan with sections and zest of 2 oranges. Cut into 12 pieces and serve.

Blueberry–Semolina Cake, top
Orange–Rice Flan, bottom

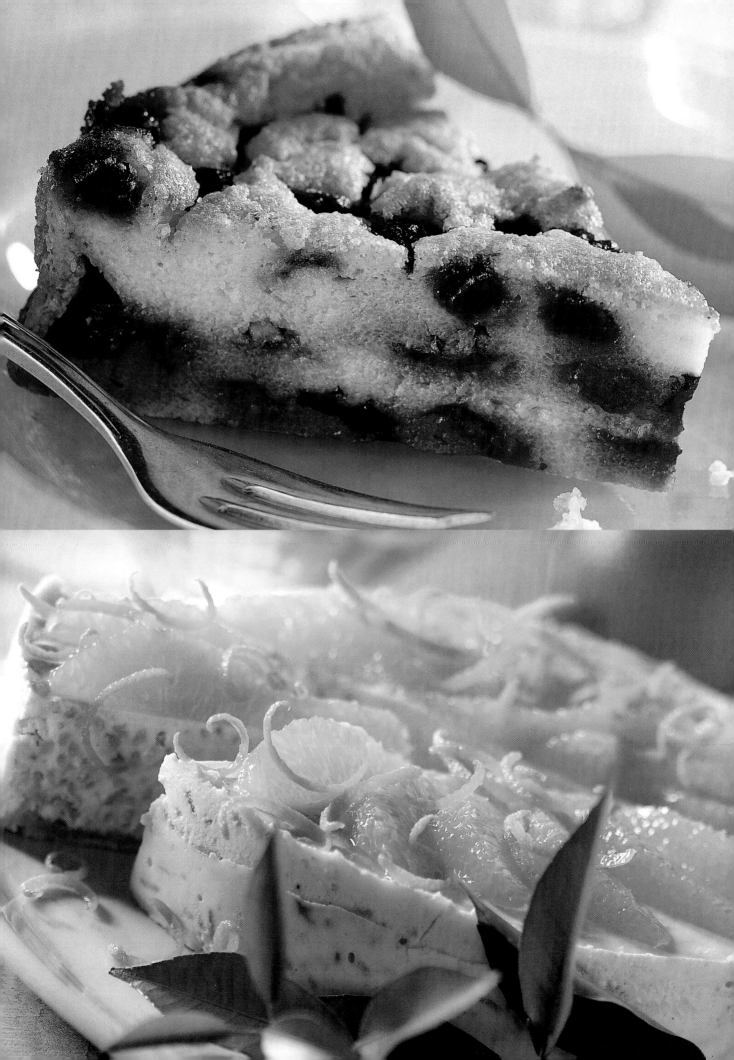

Mandarin Cheesecake

Carbohydrates ●◖	20 min.
Fat ●●●	(+ 30 min. resting)
	(+ 18 to 20 min. baking) (+ 1½ hrs. chilling)

Per serving: approx. 208 calories
6 g protein · 14 g fat · 16 g carbohydrates

FOR 10 SERVINGS:
FOR THE CRUST AND THE TOP:
1 cup (250 mL/100 g) pastry flour
1¼ cup (300 mL/100 g) blanched ground almonds
3 tbsp (45 mL) sugar
Salt
½ tsp (2 mL) grated orange zest
¼ cup (50 mL/50 g) butter
1 egg
FOR THE FILLING:
11-oz (310 mL) can mandarin oranges
½ cup (125 mL/100 g) low-fat cream cheese
½ tsp (2 ml) grated orange zest
Sweetener
½ cup (125 mL/100 g) whipping (35%) cream
1½ (¼ oz/7 g/1 tbsp) envelopes unflavored gelatin

1 Knead together flour, almonds, sugar, a pinch of salt, orange zest, butter and egg until firm. Wrap in plastic wrap and leave to rest for 30 minutes.

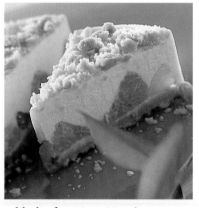

2 Preheat the oven to 350°F (180°C). Roll out 2 circles of dough, each 8 inches (20 cm) in diameter. Place on a baking sheet lined with parchment paper and bake for 18 to 20 minutes. Cool. Crumble one of the pastries and set aside.

3 Place the remaining pastry on a cake plate and put a cake ring around it. Drain mandarin oranges, reserving the juice. Combine cream cheese, mandarin juice, orange zest and a little sweetener, and stir until smooth. Whip the cream until stiff and fold in.

4 Soak the gelatin in ¼ cup (50 mL) cold water. Pour in ¼ cup (50 mL) boiling water and stir to dissolve. Stir in a little of the cream mixture, then stir the gelatin into the cream. Refrigerate for 30 minutes, until partially set. Arrange mandarin sections over the crust. Spread the gelatin mixture on top. Refrigerate for 1 hour, then sprinkle with the reserved crumbs. Cut into 10 pieces.

Grape Cheesecake

Carbohydrates ●◖	30 min.
Fat ●●	(+ 30 minutes resting)
	(+ 20 min. baking) (+ 2 hrs. chilling)

Per serving: approx. 209 calories
7 g protein · 11 g fat · 19 g carbohydrates

FOR 12 SERVINGS:
FOR THE CRUST:
1 cup (250 mL/100 g) pastry flour
⅔ cup (150 mL/50 g) blanched ground almonds
1 tbsp (15 mL) sugar
Pinch salt
¼ cup (50 mL/50 g) butter
1 small egg
FOR THE FILLING:
1 cup (250 mL/250 g) low-fat quark or puréed cottage cheese
2 tbsp (30 mL) icing (confectioner's) sugar
1 tsp (5 mL) grated orange zest
Sweetener
¾ cup (175 mL/200 g) whipping cream
1½ (¼ oz/7 g/1 tbsp) envelopes unflavored gelatin
¼ cup (50 mL) cold water
¼ cup (50 mL) boiling water
3 cups (750 mL/300 g) assorted seedless and seeded grapes
2 tbsp (30 mL) orange liqueur
Lemon balm sprigs (optional)

1 Knead together flour, almonds, sugar, salt, butter and egg until smooth. Wrap in plastic wrap and refrigerate for 30 minutes.

2 Preheat the oven to 350°F (180°C). Grease a 10-inch (25 cm) springform pan. Roll out the dough and place in the pan. Place parchment paper and pie weights on top and bake for 20 minutes, until golden. Leave to cool, then remove the weights and paper.

3 Combine quark, icing sugar, orange zest and a little sweetener. Whip the cream until stiff and fold in. Sprinkle the gelatin over the cold water. Pour in the boiling water and stir constantly until completely dissolved. Stir in the liqueur. Stir a little of the quark mixture into the gelatin, then quickly combine the gelatin with the rest of the quark. Set 12 grapes aside. Spread ½ the filling on the pastry, top with grapes, and spread the remaining filling over them. Refrigerate for 2 hours, until firm. Garnish with the reserved grapes, and a sprig of lemon balm, if desired, and cut into 12 pieces.

Grape Cheesecake, right

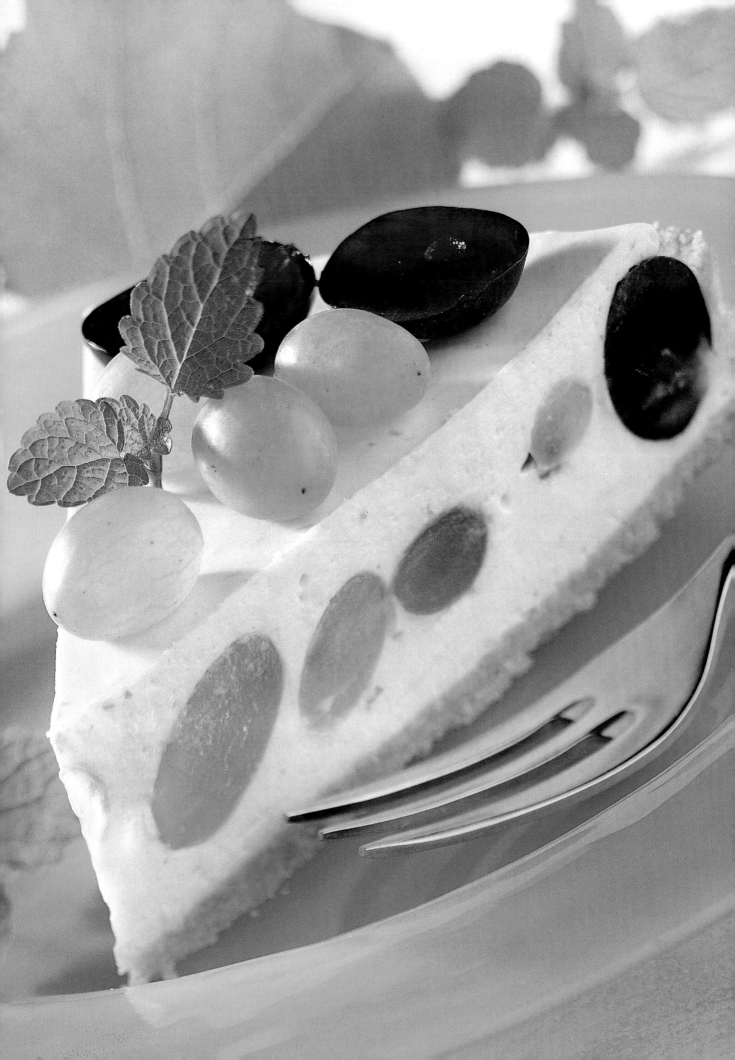

Nectarine–Strawberry Yogurt Flan

Carbohydrates ●◖		45 min.
Fat ●●●		(+ 15 min. baking)
		(+ 40 min. chilling)

Per serving: approx. 190 calories
4 g protein · 12 g fat · 16 g carbohydrates

FOR 12 SERVINGS:
FOR THE CRUST:
1 cup (250 mL/125 g) pastry flour
Pinch baking powder
Pinch salt
Seeds of ½ vanilla bean
3 tbsp (45 mL) sugar
¼ tsp (1 mL) grated orange zest
¼ cup (50 mL/50 g) butter
1 egg yolk
FOR THE FILLING:
1⅔ cups (400 mL/400 g) yogurt
1 tsp (5 mL) grated lemon zest
2 tbsp (30 mL) lemon juice
Sweetener
2 (¼ oz/7 g/1 tbsp) envelopes unflavored gelatin
¾ cup (175 mL/200 g) whipping (35%) cream
¼ cup (50 mL) freshly squeezed orange juice
1 tbsp (15 mL) strawberry jam
2 nectarines
1⅓ cups (325 mL/200 g) strawberries

1 Knead together the flour, baking powder, salt, vanilla, sugar, orange zest, butter and egg yolk until smooth. Wrap and refrigerate for 30 minutes. Preheat oven to 350°F (180°C). Grease a 10-inch (25 cm) springform pan. Roll out the dough and line the bottom and partway up the sides. Pierce a few times with a fork. Place parchment paper and pie weights on top. Bake for 15 minutes. Leave to cool, then remove the weights and paper but leave the ring.

2 Stir yogurt, lemon zest and lemon juice until smooth and add sweetener. Soak 1½ envelopes gelatin in ¼ cup (50 mL) cold water. Pour in ¼ cup (50 mL) boiling water and stir to dissolve. Stir in a little of the yogurt mixture, then combine the gelatin with the rest of the yogurt. Refrigerate until it starts to set.

3 Whip the cream until stiff and fold into the yogurt. Spread over the crust. Refrigerate for 30 minutes, until firm. Soak the remaining gelatin in 2 tbsp (30 mL) cold water. Combine orange juice and strawberry jam until smooth, then heat. Dissolve the gelatin in the orange mixture. Cool slightly, then spread on top of the cake and refrigerate. To serve, peel and slice the nectarines and quarter the strawberries, and arrange them on top. Remove the ring and cut into 12 pieces.

Gooseberry Galette

Carbohydrates ●●◖		50 min.
Fat ●●●		(+ 30 min. resting)
		(+ 45 min. baking)

Per serving: approx. 256 calories
8 g protein · 12 g fat · 29 g carbohydrates

FOR 12 SERVINGS:
FOR THE CRUST:
1⅔ cups (400 mL/200 g) coarsely ground whole wheat flour
2 tbsp (30 mL/30 g) butter
1 egg
3 tbsp (45 mL) sugar
Pinch salt
½ tsp (2 mL) grated lemon zest
¼ cup (50 mL) milk
FOR THE FILLING:
⅓ cup (75 mL/30 g) ground almonds
½ tsp (2 mL) ground cinnamon
4 cups (1 L/600 g) gooseberries
½ cup (125 mL/125 g) low-fat quark or puréed cottage cheese
2 eggs
Seeds of ½ vanilla bean
A few drops bitter almond flavoring
Sweetener
1 tbsp (15 mL) slivered almonds

1 Knead together the flour, butter, egg, sugar, salt, lemon zest and milk. Wrap in plastic wrap and refrigerate for 30 minutes. Preheat the oven to 350°F (180°C). Grease a 10-inch (25 cm) springform pan. Roll out the dough slightly larger than the pan and line the bottom and partway up the sides. Pierce in several place with a fork and place parchment paper and pie weights on top. Bake for 15 minutes. Leave to cool, then remove weights and paper.

2 Combine the ground almonds and cinnamon and sprinkle over the crust, then distribute the gooseberries. Mix the eggs, quark, vanilla, bitter almond and sweetener. Pour over the gooseberries and spread smooth. Sprinkle with the slivered almonds. Bake for 30 minutes. Leave to cool. Cut into 12 pieces and serve.

Nectarine–Strawberry Yogurt Flan, top
Gooseberry Galette, bottom

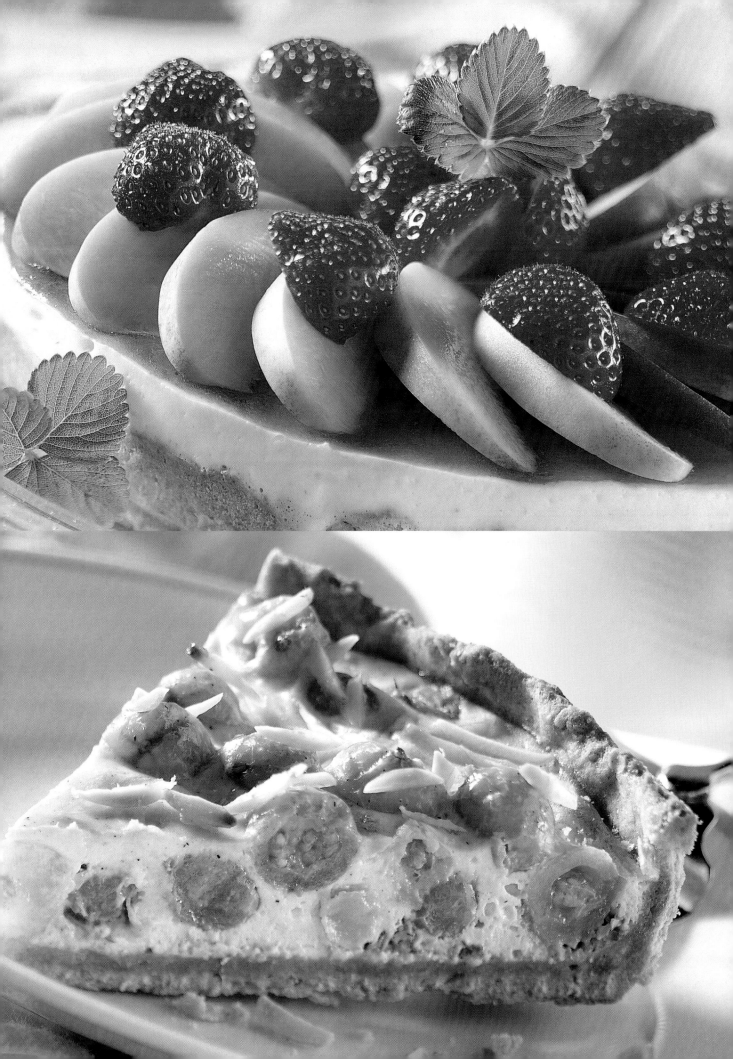

Orange Loaf Cake

Carbohydrates ●◖	20 min.
Fat +	(+ 1 hr. 10 min. baking)

Per serving: approx. 211 calories
2 g protein · 15 g fat · 18 g carbohydrates

FOR 10 SLICES:
Bread crumbs
⅔ cup (150 mL/150 g) butter
½ cup (125 mL/100 g) sugar
2 eggs
2 vanilla beans
2 tbsp (30 mL) baking powder
Grated zest and juice of 1 orange
¾ cup (175 mL/80 g) flour

1 Preheat the oven to 325°F (160°C). Grease a 9- x 5-inch (23 x 13 cm) loaf pan and sprinkle with bread crumbs. Beat the butter and sugar until creamy and smooth. Beat in eggs one at a time. Split the vanilla beans lengthwise and scrape out the seeds. Stir baking powder and vanilla seeds into the flour. Stir into the butter mixture along with the orange zest and orange juice. Combine thoroughly.

2 Pour the batter into the prepared pan and spread smooth. Bake on a rack in the second position from the bottom of the oven for 1 hour and 10 minutes, until golden. Let cool for 5 minutes, then remove from the pan and leave to cool completely on a wire rack. Cut into 10 slices and serve.

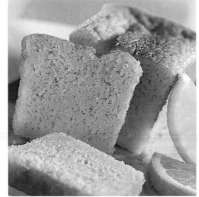

Apple–Rice Tart

Carbohydrates ●●◖	1 hr.
Fat ●●●	(+ 30 min. resting)
	(+ 55 to 60 min. baking)

Per serving: approx. 231 calories
6 g protein · 9 g fat · 29 g carbohydrates

FOR 12 SERVINGS:
FOR THE PASTRY:
1¼ cup (300 mL/150 g) all-purpose flour
2 tbsp (30 mL) sugar
Pinch salt
1 egg
¼ cup (50 mL/50 g) butter
FOR THE FILLING:
1 vanilla bean
2 cups (500 mL) milk
Pinch salt
1 tbsp (15 ml) sugar
¾ cup (175 mL/150 g) brown rice
1 piece lemon zest
3 eggs, separated
4 tart apples
2 whole cloves; 1 cinnamon stick
¼ cup (50 mL) each dry white wine and water
Sweetener
3 tbsp (45 mL) slivered almonds

1 Knead together the flour, sugar, egg and butter until smooth. Wrap and refrigerate for 30 minutes. Preheat the oven to 350°F (180°C). Grease a 10-inch (25 cm) springform pan. Roll out the dough and line the bottom and sides. Pierce in several places with a fork. Place parchment paper and pie weights on top and bake for 15 minutes. Leave to cool.

2 Split and scrape the vanilla bean. Combine milk, salt, sugar, rice, lemon zest and vanilla seeds and pod. Bring to a boil, stirring constantly. Simmer, covered, on low heat until rice is cooked. Leave to cool, then remove the vanilla pod and lemon zest. Whisk 2 egg yolks and stir in. Beat the egg whites until stiff and fold in.

3 Peel and cut the apples in wedges and cook with the cloves, cinnamon, wine, water and sweetener until almost tender. Drain and leave to cool, then remove cloves and cinnamon.

4 Spread ½ the rice mixture over the partly baked crust. Distribute the apples and cover with the remaining rice. Whisk the remaining egg yolk and brush over the top. Sprinkle with almonds. Bake for 40 to 45 minutes. Leave to cool. Cut into 12 pieces and serve.

Apple–Rice Flan, right

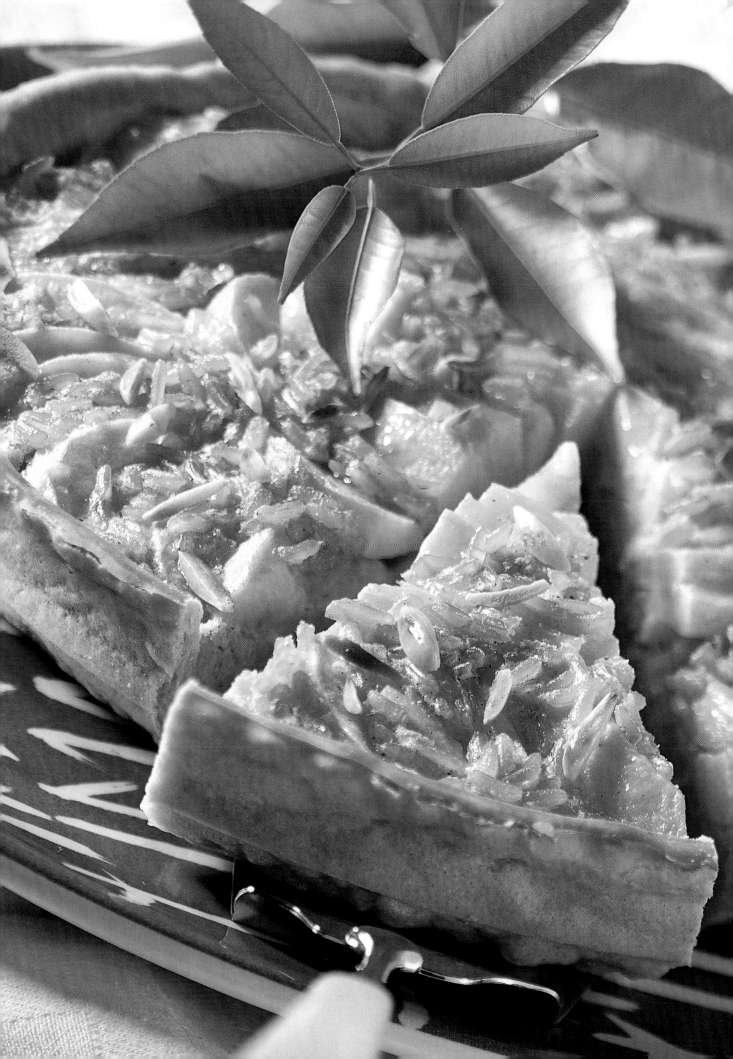

Pear–Nut Pie

Carbohydrates ●●	1 hr.
++	(+ 30 minutes resting)
Fat	(+ 45 min. baking)

Per serving: approx. 314 calories
25 g protein · 21 g fat · 24 g carbohydrates

FOR 12 SERVINGS:
FOR THE PASTRY:
1 cup (250 mL/125 g) pastry flour
1⅓ cups (325 mL/125 g) ground hazelnuts
1 tsp (5 mL) baking powder
3 tbsp (45 mL) sugar
Pinch salt
1 tsp (5 mL) grated orange zest
⅓ cup (75 mL/80 g) butter
1 egg
FOR THE FILLING:
5 medium pears (about 2 lb/900 g)
¾ cup (175 mL) dry white wine
1 tbsp (15 mL) sugar
1 small piece lemon zest
¾ cup (175 mL/100 g) chopped walnuts
¼ cup (50 mL/50 g) crème fraîche or sour cream
1 egg

1 Combine flour, ground hazelnuts, baking powder, sugar, salt, orange zest, butter and egg.
Knead until smooth. Wrap in plastic wrap and
refrigerate for 30 minutes. Preheat the oven to
350°F (180°C). Grease a 10-inch (25 cm) springform pan. Roll out the dough ⅔ larger than the
pan. Line the bottom and press into the sides.
Cover with parchment paper and pie weights, and
bake for 20 minutes. Cool, then remove paper and
weights.

2 Peel and slice the pears and cook with the wine,
lemon zest and sugar for 5 minutes. Drain and
leave to cool.

3 Sprinkle walnuts over the partially baked crust,
then arrange the pear slices. Whisk together the
crème fraîche and egg and spread over the pears.

4 Roll out the remaining dough to fit the pan and
place over the filling. Press down to form an
edge and pierce several holes in the top. Bake for 25
minutes. Leave to cool. Cut into 12 pieces and
serve.

Whole-Grain Fruit Bread

| Carbohydrates ●● | 30 min. |
| Fat ●●● | (+ 1 hr. baking) |

Per serving: approx. 211 calories
6 g protein · 12 g fat · 20 g carbohydrates

FOR 12 SLICES:
1½ cups (375 mL/200 g) mixed dried fruit (unsulphured
    preferred)
¾ cup (175 mL/100 g) blanched skinned hazelnuts
¼ cup (50 mL/50 g) soft butter
2 eggs, separated
1 tsp (5 mL) grated lemon zest
1 tsp (5 mL) grated orange zest
½ tsp (2 mL) ground coriander seeds
½ tsp (2 mL) ground cinnamon
Pinch ground allspice
¾ cup (175 mL/100 g) coarsely ground whole wheat flour
1¼ cups (300 mL/100 g) quick-cooking rolled oats
2 tsp (10 mL) baking powder
Salt
3 tbsp (45 mL/300 g) blanched almond halves

1 Soak the dried fruit and hazelnuts in warm
water for 1 hour; drain, reserving the liquid. Cut
the fruit into pieces.

2 Beat the butter and egg yolks until creamy. Add
lemon and orange zest, ground coriander, cinnamon and allspice. Stir in the flour, rolled oats and
baking powder. Add as much of the soaking water
as needed to make a smooth dough.

3 Preheat the oven to 325°F (160°C). Grease a
10- x 6-inch (25 x 15 cm) loaf pan. Beat the egg
whites with a pinch of salt until stiff. Fold into the
batter with the fruit and hazelnuts. Pour into the
pan, spread smooth, and garnish with almond
halves. Bake for 1 hour. Cool slightly, then turn out
of the pan and leave to cool completely on a wire
rack. Wrap in aluminum foil and allow to rest for
at least 1 day in the refrigerator to bring out the
flavors. Cut into 12 slices and serve.

Pear–Nut Pie, top
Whole-Grain Fruit Bread, bottom

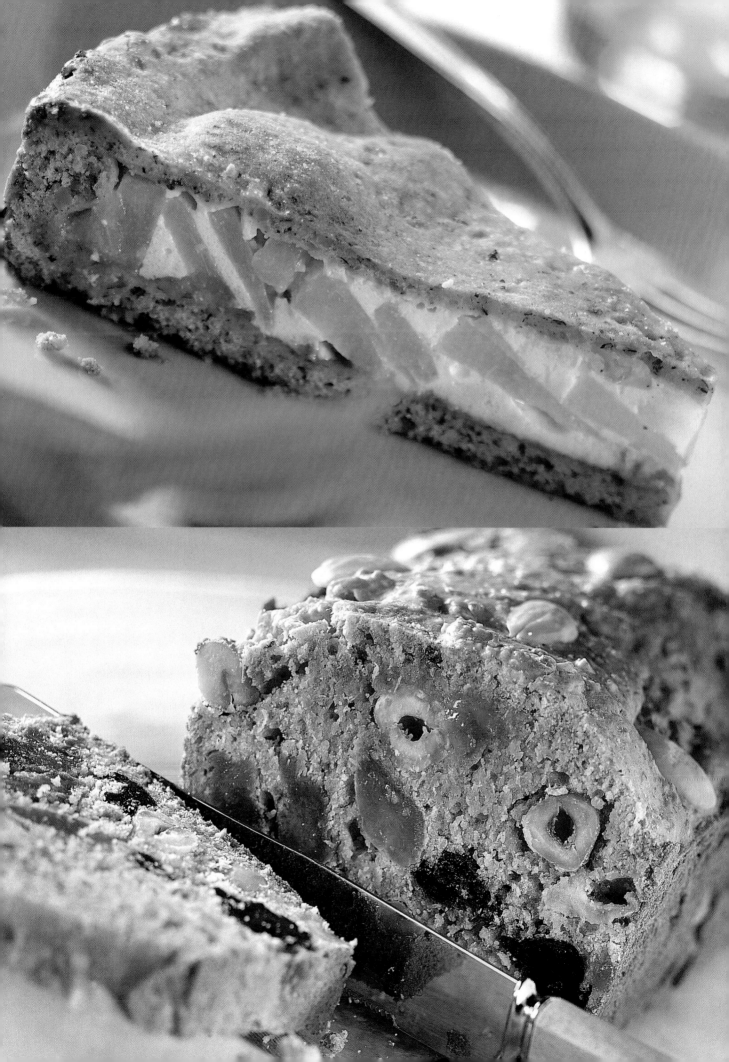

Index

Adult-onset diabetes (type 2), 7–8
Alcoholic beverages and diabetes, 15
Almonds: Spiced Almond Bars, 200
Apples
    Apple-Blueberry Pancakes, 160
    Apple-Celery Root Salad, 54
    Apple-Pear Tart, 204
    Apple-Quark Yogurt, 172
    Apple-Raisin Turnovers, 192
    Apple-Raspberry Jell, 168
    Apple-Rice Tart, 224
    Crunchy Apple Slices, 202
    Crunchy Muesli with Apples and Bananas, 25
    Honey-Apple Crêpes, 162
    Matjes Herring and Apple-Bean Salad, 96
    Quark-Apple Turnovers, 192
Apricots
    Apricot Cheesecake, 216
    Apricot Creams, 212
    Apricot Galette, 204
    Millet Pudding with Apricots and Dried Cranberries, 172
    Whole-Grain Muesli with Apricots and Yogurt, 24
Artichokes: Risotto with Artichokes, 144
Arugula Salad with Melon, 57
Asparagus
    Asparagus, Strawberry and Avocado Salad, 58
    White Asparagus with New Potatoes and Chervil Sauce, 74
Aubergine. See Eggplant
Avocados: Asparagus, Strawberry and Avocado Salad, 58

Baked goods. See Bars and Squares; Bread sticks; Breads; Brioches; Cheesecakes; Galettes; Muffins; Rolls and buns; Scones; Tarts; Torte; Turnovers

Baked Salmon with Cucumber Salad, 100
Baking and diabetes, 20
Bananas: Crunchy Muesli with Apples and Bananas, 25
Barley Soup with Parmesan Cheese, 68
Barley with Beets, 152
Bars and squares
    Crunchy Apple Slices, 202
    Granola Bars, 201
    Hazelnut Squares, 202
    Spiced Almond Bars, 200
Beans, dried. See Chickpeas; Lentils
Beans, green
    Lamb with Beans and Red Peppers, 120
    Matjes Herring and Apple-Bean Salad, 96
Beef
    Beef à la Ficelle, 122
    Beef Patties with Herbs and Red Pepper, 114
    Beef Stew with Tomatoes and Olives, 122
    Rosemary Beef Stew, 122
    Spicy Chili Con Carne, 156
Beets
    Barley with Beets, 152
    Creamed Beet Juice Soup, 65
Belgian Endive-Sprout Salad, 54
Berries. See also names of specific berries
    Berry-Buttermilk Tarts, 188
    Berry Cake with Vanilla Whipped Cream, 214
    Melon-Berry Salad, 34
Beverages
    alcoholic, and diabetes, 15
    Cherry-Whey Cocktail, 33
    non-alcoholic, and diabetes, 14
    Pear-Buttermilk Flip, 32
    Red Fitness Drink, 32
    Sea Buckthorn-Buttermilk Shake, 33

Black Olive and Sun-Dried Tomato Loaves, 180
Blood sugar (blood glucose), 6
Blueberries
    Apple-Blueberry Pancakes, 160
    Blueberry Muffins, 190
    Blueberry-Semolina Cake, 218
    Clafoutis, 196
Body Mass Index (BMI), chart, 17
Bouillabaisse Provençale, 104
Braised Chicken Legs with Roasted Potatoes and Cabbage Salad, 124
Bread sticks: Caraway Bread Sticks, 182
Breads
    Black Olive and Sun-Dried Tomato Loaves, 180
    Ciabatta with Thyme, 178
    Spelt-Walnut Bread, 178
    Whole-Grain Fruit Bread, 226
Breakfasts
    Coconut Muesli with Papaya, 24
    Crunchy Muesli with Apples and Bananas, 25
    Whole-Grain Muesli with Apricots and Yogurt, 24
Brioches: Spelt Brioches, 184
Broccoli-Red Pepper Vegetable Mix, 90
Broccoli Soup with Thyme Cream, 66
Brown Rice Jambalaya, 146
Brown Rice with Carrots, 146
Brussels Sprout, Pear and Prosciutto Salad, 62
Buckwheat Torte with Red Currants, 210
Bulgur
    Bulgur with Tomatoes and Peppers, 150
    Stuffed Eggplant (Aubergine) with Bulgur, 84

Buttermilk
Berry-Buttermilk Tarts,
188
Buttermilk-Lime Ice Cream,
164
Pear-Buttermilk Flip, 32
Sea Buckthorn-Buttermilk
Shake, 33

Cabbage
Braised Chicken Legs with
Roasted Potatoes and
Cabbage Salad, 124
Green-Cabbage Salad with
Shiitakes, 60
Pasta with Cabbage, 142
Rolls with Smoked Salmon,
Chinese Cabbage and
Green-Pepper Cream, 44
Savoy Cabbage Rolls with
Semolina-Carrot Stuffing,
88
Cakes
Berry Cake with Vanilla
Whipped Cream, 214
Blueberry-Semolina Cake,
218
Carrot-Potato Cake, 206
Dark Pound Cake, 208
English Teacake, 206
Orange Loaf Cake, 224
Walnut-Ginger Cakes, 201
[no ginger in recipe]
Yogurt Cake with Fresh Figs,
208
Capers: Rice with Cucumbers and
Capers, 146
Caraway Bread Sticks, 182
Carbohydrates and diabetes, 11
Carpaccio: Cucumber
Carpaccio with Tomato
Dressing, 56
Carrots
Brown Rice with Carrots, 146
Carrot-Nut Muffins, 190
Carrot-Potato Cake, 206
Carrot-Raisin Salad, 36

Cream of Carrot Soup with
Pistachios, 66
Quinoa with Carrots and
Leeks, 150
Savoy Cabbage Rolls with
Semolina-Carrot Stuffing,
88
Sweet Creamed Carrots, 50
Cashews: Fruit Salad with Cashew
Sauce, 25
Catfish with Tomatoes, 108
Cauliflower: East Indian Potato-
Cauliflower Curry, 88
Celery-Pear Salad, 36
Celery root
Apple-Celery Root Salad, 54
Lentils and Celery Root, 60
Champagne: Chilled Raspberry-
Champagne Cocktail, 168
Cheese
Barley Soup with Parmesan
Cheese, 68
Cream Cheese and Fruit
Sandwich, 26
Pumpkin Rolls with Blue
Cheese, 28
Ricotta Cream with Kiwi-
Gooseberry Purée, 162
Rolls with Ricotta Cream, 26
Spelt Gnocchi with Cheese
Sauce, 152
Spinach-Feta Tarts, 186
Strawberry-Cream Cheese
Waffles, 194
Supertoast with Cream
Cheese, 28
Veal Rouladen with Ham and
Cheese, 118
Zucchini-Olive Crostini with
Feta, 38
Cheesecakes
Apricot Cheesecake, 216
Grape Cheesecake, 220
Mandarin Cheesecake, 220
Cherries
Cherry Pudding with
Almonds, 162

Cherry-Quark Strudel, 216
Cherry-Whey Cocktail, 33
Soft-Frozen Cherry Yogurt,
165
Chervil: White Asparagus with
New Potatoes and Chervil
Sauce, 74
Chicken
Braised Chicken Legs with
Roasted Potatoes and
Cabbage Salad, 124
Chicken and Curry Cream
Sandwich, 46
Chicken Breasts in Curry
Sauce with Basmati Rice,
126
Chicken Breasts with Rice
and Peas, 124
Chicken Skewers with Lentil
Sauce, 128
Chicken Stir-Fry, 132
Chicken Tonnato with
Vegetables, 126
Chinese Fondue, 132
Exotic Fruit Salad with
Chicken Breast, 62
Chickpeas
Chickpea Pâté on Rye, 40
Eggplant (Aubergine) with
Chickpeas, 154
Chili Con Carne, Spicy, 156
Chilled Raspberry-Champagne
Cocktail, 168
Chinese Fondue, 132
Chives: Tuna and Chive Cream
Baguettes, 44
Choux Ring with Tropical Fruit,
212
Chutney, Vegetable Skewers with
Red-Pepper Chutney, 154
Ciabatta with Thyme, 178
Clafoutis, 196
Coconut Muesli with Papaya, 24
Cod with Summer Vegetables,
98
Courgette. See Zucchini
Couscous with Rabbit, 134

Cranberries
    Millet Pudding with Apricots and Dried Cranberries, 172
    Saddle of Venison with Cranberry Sauce and Lamb's Lettuce, 136
Cream Cheese and Fruit Sandwich, 26
Cream of Carrot Soup with Pistachios, 66
Cream puffs, Raspberry Cream Puffs, 192
Creamed Beet Juice Soup, 65
Creamed Ham Rolls, 30
Crêpes
    Crêpes Stuffed with Sauerkraut, 92
    Honey-Apple Crêpes, 162
    Whole Wheat Crêpes with Plum Compote, 160
Crispbread Pizzas, 186
Crostini
    Crostini with Tomato Ragout, 40
    Zucchini-Olive Crostini with Feta, 38
Crunchy Apple Slices, 202
Crunchy Muesli with Apples and Bananas, 25
Cucumbers
    Baked Salmon with Cucumber Salad, 100
    Cucumber Carpaccio with Tomato Dressing, 56
    Rice with Cucumbers and Capers, 146
    Turkey-Cucumber Clay Pot Casserole, 130
Currants, red: Buckwheat Torte with Red Currants, 210
Curried dishes
    Chicken and Curry Cream Sandwich, 46
    Chicken Breasts in Curry Sauce with Basmati Rice, 126

Curried Lentil Casserole, 84
East Indian Potato-Cauliflower Curry, 88
Lamb Curry with Tomatoes and Zucchini (Courgette), 120
Lentil Curry with Rice, 156
Shrimp Curry with Rice, 110

Dark Pound Cake, 208
Desserts. *See also* chapter on baked goods, pages 174–226
    Apple-Blueberry Pancakes, 160
    Apple-Quark Yogurt, 172
    Apple-Raspberry Jell, 168
    Buttermilk-Lime Ice Cream, 164
    Cherry Pudding with Almonds, 162
    Chilled Raspberry-Champagne Cocktail, 168
    Exotic Rice Pudding, 172
    Frozen Raspberry Yogurt, 165
    Fruit Salad in Melon Boats, 169
    Ginger-Pear Granita, 166
    Green Fruit Jell with Vanilla Sauce, 169
    Honey-Apple Crêpes, 162
    Mango Sorbet on Marinated Oranges, 164
    Millet Pudding with Apricots and Dried Cranberries, 172
    Red Fruit Jell with Yogurt Sauce, 170
    Ricotta Cream with Kiwi-Gooseberry Purée, 162
    Soft-Frozen Cherry Yogurt, 165
    Walnut Ice Cream, 166
    Whole Wheat Crêpes with Plum Compote, 160
    Yogurt Mousse with Marinated Figs, 170

Diabetes
    and blood glucose, 6
    and hypoglycemia, 8, 19, 21
    and physical activity, 18–19
    and weight control, 16–17
    dealing with, 6–7
    diet and nutrition, 8, 9–15, 20–21
    metabolic syndrome, 8
    special products, 21
    type 1 (juvenile-onset), 7
    type 2 (adult-onset), 2, 6, 7–8
Dill: Shrimp and Dill Cream Baguettes, 42
Dried-Fruit Purée, 51
Duck: Sweet and Sour Duck, 134

East Indian Potato-Cauliflower Curry, 88
Egg dishes
    Hard-Cooked Eggs with Potatoes and Herb Sauce, 90
    Olive Omelet, 80
    Pan-Fried Vegetables with Eggs, 78
    Spanish Omelet with Vegetables, 78
    Spanish Potato-Fennel Omelet, 90
    Vegetable Ragout with Poached Eggs, 82
Eggplant (aubergine)
    Eggplant with Chickpeas, 154
    Eggplant with Tomatoes and Mint Yogurt, 76
    Stuffed Eggplant with Bulgur, 84
Endive: Belgian Endive-Sprout Salad, 54
English Teacake, 206
Exercise and diabetes, 18–19
Exotic Fruit Salad with Chicken Breast, 62
Exotic Rice Pudding, 172
Exotic Stir-Fry, 102

Fats and diabetes, 13, 20
Fennel
    Millet Risotto with Fennel,
        148
    Spanish Potato-Fennel
        Omelet, 90
Fiber and diabetes, 11, 20
Figs
    Yogurt Cake with Fresh
        Figs, 208
    Yogurt Mousse with
        Marinated Figs, 170
Fish and seafood
    Baked Salmon with
        Cucumber Salad, 100
    Bouillabaisse Provençale, 104
    Catfish with Tomatoes, 108
    Chicken Tonnato with
        Vegetables, 126
    Cod with Summer Vegetables,
        98
    Exotic Stir-Fry, 102
    Fish Fillets with Zucchini
        (Courgette) and Tomatoes,
        108
    Grilled Red Bream or Red
        Snapper with Tarragon, 100
    Grouper with Orange, 108
    Matjes Herring and Apple-
        Bean Salad, 96
    Oven-Baked Fillets with
        Vegetables, 104
    Plaice Pouches, 106
    Plaice with Tomato Polenta,
        98
    Rice with Squid and
        Vegetables, 144
    Salmon with Fettuccine, 98
    Shrimp and Dill Cream
        Baguettes, 42
    Shrimp Curry with Rice, 110
    Smoked Trout Fillets with
        Warm Potato Salad, 96
    Steamed Trout, 102
    Stir-Fried Shrimp, 110
    Swordfish-Zucchini
        (Courgette) Kebabs, 106

Flans
    Lime-Almond Flan, 214
    Nectarine-Strawberry Yogurt
        Flan, 222
    Orange-Rice Flan, 218
    Rhubarb Flan, 210
Fondue: Chinese Fondue, 132
Frozen Raspberry Yogurt, 165
Fruit. See also Berries; names of
    specific fruits
    Choux Ring with Tropical
        Fruit, 212
    Cream Cheese and Fruit
        Sandwich, 26
    Dried-Fruit Purée, 51
    Exotic Fruit Salad with
        Chicken Breast, 62
    Fruit Salad in Melon Boats,
        169
    Fruit Salad with Cashew
        Sauce, 25
    Fruit Tarts, 188
    Fruity Rice Salad, 34
    Green Fruit Jell with Vanilla
        Sauce, 169
    Phyllo Fruit Baskets, 194
    Red Fruit Jell with Yogurt
        Sauce, 170
    Whole-Grain Fruit Bread,
        226

Galettes
    Apricot Galette, 204
    Gooseberry Galette, 222
    Savory Galette, 182
Ginger-Pear Granita, 166
Glucose, 6
    blood, regulating, 6
Glycemic index (GI), 11; chart, 12
Gnocchi
    Spelt Gnocchi with Cheese
        Sauce, 152
    Vegetable Ragout with
        Saffron Gnocchi, 74
Gooseberries
    Gooseberry Galette, 222
    Gooseberry Jam, 50

Ricotta Cream with Kiwi-
        Gooseberry Purée, 162
Granola Bars, 201
Granola Buns, 176
Grape Cheesecake, 220
Grapefruit: Stuffed Grapefruit, 34
Green-Cabbage Salad with
    Shiitakes, 60
Green Fruit Jell with Vanilla
    Sauce, 169
Grilled Red Bream or Red
    Snapper with Tarragon, 100
Grouper with Orange, 108

Ham
    Creamed Ham Rolls, 30
Ham Crescents, 180
    Veal Rouladen with Ham and
        Cheese, 118
    Vegetable-Ham Wraps, 42
Hard-Cooked Eggs with Potatoes
    and Herb Sauce, 90
Hazelnut Squares, 202
Herring, Matjes Herring and
    Apple-Bean Salad, 96
Honey-Apple Crêpes, 162
Hypoglycemia, 8
    symptoms, 19
    ways of preventing, 21

Ice cream
    Buttermilk-Lime Ice Cream,
        164
    Walnut Ice Cream, 166

Jambalaya: Brown Rice Jambalaya,
    146
Jams
    about, 49
    Gooseberry Jam, 50
    Pumpkin-Orange Jam, 48
    Strawberry-Pineapple Jam, 48
Jellies, about, 49
Juvenile-onset diabetes (type 1), 7

Kebabs: Swordfish-Zucchini
    (Courgette) Kebabs, 106

Kiwi: Ricotta Cream with Kiwi-Gooseberry Purée, 162
Kohlrabi with Grainy Mustard Dressing, 56

Lamb Curry with Tomatoes and Zucchini (Courgette), 120
Lamb with Beans and Red Peppers, 120
Lamb's Lettuce: Saddle of Venison with Cranberry Sauce and Lamb's Lettuce, 136
Lasagna
    Tomato Lasagna, 140
    Vegetarian Lasagna, 140
Lean Pea Soup, 70
Leeks
    Leek Turnovers, 184
    Mushroom-Leek Soup, 65
    Orange-Leek Salad, 55
    Quinoa with Carrots and Leeks, 150
Lentils
    Chicken Skewers with Lentil Sauce, 128
    Curried Lentil Casserole, 84
    Lentil Curry with Rice, 156
    Lentils and Celery Root, 60
    Pork with Lentils, 116
    Turkey Cutlet with Lentils, 128
Lettuce Salad with Croutons, 55
Light Potato Salad with Snow (Mange-Tout) Peas, 57
Lime
    Buttermilk-Lime Ice Cream, 164
    Lime-Almond Flan, 214
Lovage: Open-Face Tomato Sandwich with Lovage, 38

Macaroons, Oatmeal, 200
Mandarin Cheesecake, 220
Mango Sorbet on Marinated Oranges, 164
Marmalades, about, 49

Matjes Herring and Apple-Bean Salad, 96
Meats. See also specific kinds of meat
    Beef à la Ficelle, 122
    Beef Patties with Herbs and Red Pepper, 114
    Beef Stew with Tomatoes and Olives, 122
    Couscous with Rabbit, 134
    Lamb Curry with Tomatoes and Zucchini (Courgette), 120
    Lamb with Beans and Red Peppers, 120
    Pork and Peppers, 114
    Pork Cutlets with Vegetables, 114
    Pork with a Savory Topping, 116
    Pork with Lentils, 116
    Rosemary Beef Stew, 122
    Saddle of Venison with Cranberry Sauce and Lamb's Lettuce, 136
    Spicy Chili Con Carne, 156
    Veal Rouladen with Ham and Cheese, 118
    Veal with Swiss Chard and Potatoes, 118
    Venison Medallions with Chanterelles, Onions and Pears, 136
Melon
    Arugula Salad with Melon, 57
    Fruit Salad in Melon Boats, 169
    Melon-Berry Salad, 34
Metabolic syndrome, 8
Millet Pudding with Apricots and Dried Cranberries, 172
Millet Risotto with Fennel, 148
Millet Soufflé with Peas, 148
Minerals and diabetes, 14
Mini-Panettones, 196

Mousse: Yogurt Mousse with Marinated Figs, 170
Muesli
    Coconut Muesli with Papaya, 24
    Crunchy Muesli with Apples and Bananas, 25
    Whole-Grain Muesli with Apricots and Yogurt, 24
Muffins
    Blueberry Muffins, 190
    Carrot-Nut Muffins, 190
Mushrooms
    Green-Cabbage Salad with Shiitakes, 60
    Mushroom-Leek Soup, 65
    Tuna-Mushroom Salad, 58
    Venison Medallions with Chanterelles, Onions and Pears, 136
Mustard: Kohlrabi with Grainy Mustard Dressing, 56

Nectarine-Strawberry Yogurt Flan, 222
Nut Crescents, 198
Nutrition, 8, 9–15, 20–21
    combining foods, 9
    pyramid (chart), 10

Oatmeal Macaroons, 200
Olives
    Beef Stew with Tomatoes and Olives, 122
    Black Olive and Sun-Dried Tomato Loaves, 180
    Olive Omelet, 80
    Zucchini-Olive Crostini with Feta, 38
Omelets
    Olive Omelet, 80
    Spanish Omelet with Vegetables, 78
    Spanish Potato-Fennel Omelet, 90
Onions
    Onion Soup, 64

Venison Medallions with Chanterelles, Onions and Pears, 136

Open-Face Tomato Sandwich with Lovage, 38

Open-Face Turkey Breast and Remoulade Sandwich, 30

Oranges
Grouper with Orange, 108
Mandarin Cheesecake, 220
Mango Sorbet on Marinated Oranges, 164
Orange-Leek Salad, 55
Orange Loaf Cake, 224
Orange-Pear Relish, 51
Orange-Rice Flan, 218
Pumpkin-Orange Jam, 48

Oven-Baked Fillets with Vegetables, 104

Pan-Fried Vegetables with Eggs, 78

Pancakes
Apple-Blueberry Pancakes, 160
Potato Pancake with Sour Cream, 92

Panettones, Mini, 196

Papaya: Coconut Muesli with Papaya, 24

Pasta dishes
Pasta with Cabbage, 142
Pesto Spaetzle, 142
Salmon with Fettuccine, 98
Spelt Gnocchi with Cheese Sauce, 152
Spelt Spaetzle, 142
Tomato Lasagna, 140
Vegetable Casserole with Pasta and Pesto, 82
Vegetable Ragout with Saffron Gnocchi, 74
Vegetarian Lasagna, 140

Pastries
Apricot Creams, 212
Choux Ring with Tropical Fruit, 212

Spiced Plum-Nut Danishes, 198

Pâté: Chickpea Pâté on Rye, 40

Pears
Apple-Pear Tart, 204
Brussels Sprout, Pear and Prosciutto Salad, 62
Celery-Pear Salad, 36
Ginger-Pear Granita, 166
Orange-Pear Relish, 51
Pear-Buttermilk Flip, 32
Pear-Nut Pie, 226
Pear Tarte Tatin, 204
Quark with Pear on Pumpernickel, 26
Venison Medallions with Chanterelles, Onions and Pears, 136

Peas
Chicken Breasts with Rice and Peas, 124
Lean Pea Soup, 70
Millet Soufflé with Peas, 148

Peas, snow (mange-tout): Light Potato Salad with Snow Peas, 57

Peppers, sweet
Beef Patties with Herbs and Red Pepper, 114
Broccoli-Red Pepper Vegetable Mix, 90
Bulgur with Tomatoes and Peppers, 150
Lamb with Beans and Red Peppers, 120
Pork and Peppers, 114
Red-Pepper Quark on Pumpernickel, 40
Red Peppers with Polenta Stuffing, 86
Rolls with Smoked Salmon, Chinese Cabbage and Green-Pepper Cream, 44
Vegetable Skewers with Red-Pepper Chutney, 154

Pesto
Pesto and Sprouts on Rye Rolls, 30
Pesto Spaetzle, 142
Vegetable Casserole with Pasta and Pesto, 82

Phyllo Fruit Baskets, 194

Pie: Pear-Nut Pie, 226

Pineapple: Strawberry-Pineapple Jam, 48

Pistachio nuts: Cream of Carrot Soup with Pistachios, 66

Pizza: Crispbread Pizzas, 186

Plaice Pouches, 106

Plaice with Tomato Polenta, 98

Plums
Spiced Plum-Nut Danishes, 198
Whole Wheat Crêpes with Plum Compote, 160

Polenta
Plaice with Tomato Polenta, 98
Red Peppers with Polenta Stuffing, 86

Pork
Pork and Peppers, 114
Pork Cutlets with Vegetables, 114
Pork with a Savory Topping, 116
Pork with Lentils, 116

Potatoes
Braised Chicken Legs with Roasted Potatoes and Cabbage Salad, 124
East Indian Potato-Cauliflower Curry, 88
Hard-Cooked Eggs with Potatoes and Herb Sauce, 90
Light Potato Salad with Snow (Mange-Tout) Peas, 57
Potato Pancake with Sour Cream, 92

Potato Soup with Smoked
Salmon, 68
Pumpernickel with Herbed
Potato Cream, 38
Smoked Trout Fillets with
Warm Potato Salad, 96
Spanish Potato-Fennel
Omelet, 90
Twice-Cooked Potatoes with
Quark and Tomato Salad,
76
Veal with Swiss Chard and
Potatoes, 118
White Asparagus with New
Potatoes and Chervil Sauce,
74
Poultry. *See* Chicken; Duck;
Turkey
Preserves
about, 49
Dried-Fruit Purée, 51
Gooseberry Jam, 50
Pumpkin-Orange Jam, 48
Strawberry-Pineapple Jam,
48
Prosciutto: Brussels Sprout, Pear
and Prosciutto Salad, 62
Protein and diabetes, 12
Puddings
Cherry Pudding with
Almonds, 162
Clafoutis, 196
Exotic Rice Pudding, 172
Millet Pudding with Apricots
and Dried Cranberries, 172
Pumpernickel
Pumpernickel with Herbed
Potato Cream, 38
Quark with Pear on
Pumpernickel, 26
Red-Pepper Quark on
Pumpernickel, 40
Pumpkin
Pumpkin Rolls with Blue
Cheese, 28
Pumpkin-Orange Jam, 48
Pumpkin-Seed Rings, 178

Quark
Apple-Quark Yogurt, 172
Quark-Apple Turnovers, 192
Quark with Pear on
Pumpernickel, 26
Quick Quark Rolls, 176
Red-Pepper Quark on
Pumpernickel, 40
Twice-Cooked Potatoes with
Quark and Tomato Salad,
76
Quick and Easy Tomato Soup, 70
Quick Quark Rolls, 176
Quinoa with Carrots and Leeks,
150

Rabbit: Couscous with Rabbit,
134
Raisins
Apple-Raisin Turnovers, 192
Carrot-Raisin Salad, 36
Raisin Scones, 190
Raspberries
Apple-Raspberry Jell, 168
Chilled Raspberry-
Champagne Cocktail, 168
Frozen Raspberry Yogurt, 165
Raspberry Cream Puffs, 192
Red bream: Grilled Red Bream or
Red Snapper with Tarragon,
100
Red Fitness Drink, 32
Red Fruit Jell with Yogurt Sauce,
170
Red-Pepper Quark on
Pumpernickel, 40
Red Peppers with Polenta
Stuffing, 86
Red snapper: Grilled Red Bream
or Red Snapper with Tarragon,
100
Relish: Orange-Pear Relish, 51
Rhubarb Flan, 210
Rice
Apple-Rice Tart, 224
Brown Rice Jambalaya, 146
Brown Rice with Carrots, 146

Chicken Breasts in Curry
Sauce with Basmati Rice,
126
Chicken Breasts with Rice
and Peas, 124
Exotic Rice Pudding, 172
Exotic Stir-Fry, 102
Fruity Rice Salad, 34
Lentil Curry with Rice, 156
Rice with Cucumbers and
Capers, 146
Rice with Squid and
Vegetables, 144
Risotto with Artichokes, 144
Shrimp Curry with Rice, 110
Spring Soup with Rice, 64
Turkey with Brown Rice
Risotto, 130
Zucchini (Courgette) Boats
with Rice Stuffing, 86
Ricotta Cream with Kiwi-
Gooseberry Purée, 162
Risottos
Millet Risotto with Fennel,
148
Risotto with Artichokes, 144
Turkey with Brown Rice
Risotto, 130
Rolls and buns
Granola Buns, 176
Ham Crescents, 180
Nut Crescents, 198
Pumpkin Rolls with Blue
Cheese, 28
Pumpkin-Seed Rings, 178
Quick Quark Rolls, 176
Rolls with Ricotta Cream,
26
Rolls with Smoked Salmon,
Chinese Cabbage and
Green-Pepper Cream, 44
Rolls with Ricotta Cream, 26
Rosemary Beef Stew, 122
Rye bread
Chickpea Pâté on Rye, 40
Pesto and Sprouts on Rye
Rolls, 30

Saddle of Venison with Cranberry Sauce and Lamb's Lettuce, 136

Saffron: Vegetable Ragout with Saffron Gnocchi, 74

Salads
  Apple-Celery Root Salad, 54
  Arugula Salad with Melon, 57
  Asparagus, Strawberry and Avocado Salad, 58
  Baked Salmon with Cucumber Salad, 100
  Belgian Endive-Sprout Salad, 54
  Braised Chicken Legs with Roasted Potatoes and Cabbage Salad, 124
  Brussels Sprout, Pear and Prosciutto Salad, 62
  Carrot-Raisin Salad, 36
  Celery-Pear Salad, 36
  Cucumber Carpaccio with Tomato Dressing, 56
  Exotic Fruit Salad with Chicken Breast, 62
  Fruit Salad in Melon Boats, 169
  Fruit Salad with Cashew Sauce, 25
  Fruity Rice Salad, 34
  Green-Cabbage Salad with Shiitakes, 60
  Kohlrabi with Grainy Mustard Dressing, 56
  Lentils and Celery Root, 60
  Lettuce Salad with Croutons, 55
  Light Potato Salad with Snow (Mange-Tout) Peas, 57
  Matjes Herring and Apple-Bean Salad, 96
  Melon-Berry Salad, 34
  Orange-Leek Salad, 55
  Smoked Trout Fillets with Warm Potato Salad, 96
  Salads, Stuffed Grapefruit, 34
  Tuna-Mushroom Salad, 58

Twice-Cooked Potatoes with Quark and Tomato Salad, 76

Salmon
  Baked Salmon with Cucumber Salad, 100
  Potato Soup with Smoked Salmon, 68
  Rolls with Smoked Salmon, Chinese Cabbage and Green-Pepper Cream, 44
  Salmon with Fettuccine, 98

Sandwiches and snacks
  Chicken and Curry Cream Sandwich, 46
  Chickpea Pâté on Rye, 40
  Cream Cheese and Fruit Sandwich, 26
  Creamed Ham Rolls, 30
  Crostini with Tomato Ragout, 40
  Open-Face Tomato Sandwich with Lovage, 38
  Open-Face Turkey Breast and Remoulade Sandwich, 30
  Pesto and Sprouts on Rye Rolls, 30
  Pumpernickel with Herbed Potato Cream, 38
  Pumpkin Rolls with Blue Cheese, 28
  Quark with Pear on Pumpernickel, 26
  Red-Pepper Quark on Pumpernickel, 40
  Rolls with Ricotta Cream, 26
  Rolls with Smoked Salmon, Chinese Cabbage and Green-Pepper Cream, 44
  Shrimp and Dill Cream Baguettes, 42
  Supertoast with Cream Cheese, 28
  Tuna and Chive Cream Baguettes, 44
  Turkey Snacks with Dip, 36
  Vegetable-Ham Wraps, 42

Vegetable Salad Sandwich, 46
Zucchini-Olive Crostini with Feta, 38

Sauerkraut: Crêpes Stuffed with Sauerkraut, 92

Savory Galette, 182

Savoy Cabbage Rolls with Semolina-Carrot Stuffing, 88

Scones: Raisin Scones, 190

Sea Buckthorn-Buttermilk Shake, 33

Seafood. See Fish and seafood; names of specific kinds of fish and seafood

Shrimp
  Shrimp and Dill Cream Baguettes, 42
  Shrimp Curry with Rice, 110
  Stir-Fried Shrimp, 110

Smoked Trout Fillets with Warm Potato Salad, 96

Snacks. See Sandwiches and snacks

Soft-Frozen Cherry Yogurt, 165

Sorbet: Mango Sorbet on Marinated Oranges, 164

Soufflé: Millet Soufflé with Peas, 148

Soups
  Barley Soup with Parmesan Cheese, 68
  Broccoli Soup with Thyme Cream, 66
  Cream of Carrot Soup with Pistachios, 66
  Creamed Beet Juice Soup, 65
  Lean Pea Soup, 70
  Mushroom-Leek Soup, 65
  Onion Soup, 64
  Potato Soup with Smoked Salmon, 68
  Quick and Easy Tomato Soup, 70
  Spring Soup with Rice, 64

Spaetzle
  Pesto Spaetzle, 142
  Spelt Spaetzle, 142

Spanish Omelet with Vegetables, 78

Spanish Potato-Fennel Omelet, 90

Spelt Brioches, 184

Spelt Gnocchi with Cheese Sauce, 152

Spelt Spaetzle, 142

Spelt-Walnut Bread, 178

Spiced Almond Bars, 200

Spiced Plum-Nut Danishes, 198

Spicy Chili Con Carne, 156

Spinach-Feta Tarts, 186

Spinach Gratin, 80

Spring Soup with Rice, 64

Sprouts
    Belgian Endive-Sprout Salad, 54
    Pesto and Sprouts on Rye Rolls, 30

Squares. *See* Bars and Squares

Squid: Rice with Squid and Vegetables, 144

Steamed Trout, 102

Stews
    Beef Stew with Tomatoes and Olives, 122
    Rosemary Beef Stew, 122

Stir-Fries
    Chicken Stir-Fry, 132
    Exotic Stir-Fry, 102
    Stir-Fried Shrimp, 110

Strawberries
    Asparagus, Strawberry and Avocado Salad, 58
    Nectarine-Strawberry Yogurt Flan, 222
    Red Fitness Drink, 32
    Strawberry-Cream Cheese Waffles, 194
    Strawberry-Pineapple Jam, 48

Strudel: Cherry-Quark Strudel, 216

Stuffed Eggplant (Aubergine) with Bulgur, 84

Stuffed Grapefruit, 34

Sugar and diabetes, 20

Supertoast with Cream Cheese, 28

Supplements and diabetes, 21

Sweet and Sour Duck, 134

Sweet Creamed Carrots, 50

Sweeteners, 11-12

Swiss chard: Veal with Swiss Chard and Potatoes, 118

Swordfish-Zucchini (Courgette) Kebabs, 106

Tarts
    Apple-Pear Tart, 204
    Apple-Rice Tart, 224
    Berry-Buttermilk Tarts, 188
    Fruit Tarts, 188
    Pear Tarte Tatin, 204
    Spinach-Feta Tarts, 186

Thai Vegetables, 84

Tomatoes
    Beef Stew with Tomatoes and Olives, 122
    Black Olive and Sun-Dried Tomato Loaves, 180
    Bulgur with Tomatoes and Peppers, 150
    Catfish with Tomatoes, 108
    Crostini with Tomato Ragout, 40
    Cucumber Carpaccio with Tomato Dressing, 56
    Eggplant (Aubergine) with Tomatoes and Mint Yogurt, 76
    Fish Fillets with Zucchini (Courgette) and Tomatoes, 108
    Lamb Curry with Tomatoes and Zucchini (Courgette), 120
    Open-Face Tomato Sandwich with Lovage, 38
    Plaice with Tomato Polenta, 98
    Quick and Easy Tomato Soup, 70
    Tomato Lasagna, 140

Twice-Cooked Potatoes with Quark and Tomato Salad, 76

Torte: Buckwheat Torte with Red Currants, 210

Trout
    Smoked Trout Fillets with Warm Potato Salad, 96
    Steamed Trout, 102

Tuna
    Chicken Tonnato with Vegetables, 126
    Tuna and Chive Cream Baguettes, 44
    Tuna-Mushroom Salad, 58

Turkey
    Open-Face Turkey Breast and Remoulade Sandwich, 30
    Turkey-Cucumber Clay Pot Casserole, 130
    Turkey Cutlet with Lentils, 128
    Turkey Snacks with Dip, 36
    Turkey with Brown Rice Risotto, 130

Turnovers
    Apple-Raisin Turnovers, 192
    Leek Turnovers, 184
    Quark-Apple Turnovers, 192

Twice-Cooked Potatoes with Quark and Tomato Salad, 76

Type 1 diabetes (juvenile-onset), 7

Type 2 diabetes (adult-onset), 7–8

Veal Rouladen with Ham and Cheese, 118

Veal with Swiss Chard and Potatoes, 118

Vegetables. *See also* names of specific vegetables
    Broccoli-Red Pepper Vegetable Mix, 90
    Cod with Summer Vegetables, 98

Crêpes Stuffed with Sauerkraut, 92
Curried Lentil Casserole, 84
East Indian Potato-Cauliflower Curry, 88
Eggplant (Aubergine) with Tomatoes and Mint Yogurt, 76
Hard-Cooked Eggs with Potatoes and Herb Sauce, 90
Olive Omelet, 80
Oven-Baked Fillets with Vegetables, 104
Pan-Fried Vegetables with Eggs, 78
Potato Pancake with Sour Cream, 92
Red Peppers with Polenta Stuffing, 86
Rice with Squid and Vegetables, 144
Savoy Cabbage Rolls with Semolina-Carrot Stuffing, 88
Spanish Omelet with Vegetables, 78
Spanish Potato-Fennel Omelet, 90
Spinach Gratin, 80
Stuffed Eggplant (Aubergine) with Bulgur, 84
Thai Vegetables, 84
Twice-Cooked Potatoes with Quark and Tomato Salad, 76

Vegetable Casserole with Pasta and Pesto, 82
Vegetable-Ham Wraps, 42
Vegetable Ragout with Poached Eggs, 82
Vegetable Ragout with Saffron Gnocchi, 74
Vegetable Salad Sandwich, 46
Vegetable Skewers with Red-Pepper Chutney, 154
White Asparagus with New Potatoes and Chervil Sauce, 74
Zucchini (Courgette) Boats with Rice Stuffing, 86
Vegetarian Lasagna, 140
Venison
Saddle of Venison with Cranberry Sauce and Lamb's Lettuce, 136
Venison Medallions with Chanterelles, Onions and Pears, 136
Vitamins and diabetes, 14

Waffles: Strawberry-Cream Cheese Waffles, 194
Walnut-Ginger Cakes, 201 [no ginger in recipe]
Walnut Ice Cream, 166
Watermelon: Red Fitness Drink, 32
Weight control and diabetes, 16–17
Whey: Cherry-Whey Cocktail, 33
White Asparagus with New Potatoes and Chervil Sauce, 74

Whole-Grain Fruit Bread, 226
Whole-Grain Muesli with Apricots and Yogurt, 24
Whole Wheat Crêpes with Plum Compote, 160

Yogurt
Apple-Quark Yogurt, 172
Eggplant (Aubergine) with Tomatoes and Mint Yogurt, 76
Frozen Raspberry Yogurt, 165
Nectarine-Strawberry Yogurt Flan, 222
Red Fruit Jell with Yogurt Sauce, 170
Soft-Frozen Cherry Yogurt, 165
Whole-Grain Muesli with Apricots and Yogurt, 24
Yogurt Cake with Fresh Figs, 208
Yogurt Mousse with Marinated Figs, 170

Zucchini (courgette)
Fish Fillets with Zucchini and Tomatoes, 108
Lamb Curry with Tomatoes and Zucchini, 120
Swordfish-Zucchini Kebabs, 106
Zucchini Boats with Rice Stuffing, 86
Zucchini-Olive Crostini with Feta, 38